SKIN DISEASE
IN CHILDHOOD AND
ADOLESCENCE

Skin Disease in Childhood and Adolescence

Elisabeth Higgins

MA, MRCP
Senior Lecturer
and Consultant Dermatologist
King's College Hospital

Anthony du Vivier

MD, FRCP
Consultant Dermatologist
King's College Hospital

Blackwell
Science

© 1996 by
Blackwell Science Ltd
Editorial Offices:
Osney Mead, Oxford OX2 OEL
25 John Street, London WC1N 2BL
23 Ainslie Place, Edinburgh EH3 6AJ
238 Main Street, Cambridge
   Massachusetts 02142, USA
54 University Street, Carlton
   Victoria 3053, Australia

Other Editorial Offices:
Arnette Blackwell SA
   1, rue de Lille, 75007 Paris
   France

Blackwell Wissenschafts-Verlag GmbH
   Kurfürstendamm 57
   10707 Berlin, Germany

   Feldgasse 13, A-1238 Wien
   Austria

First published 1996

Set by Excel Typesetters, Hong Kong
Printed and bound in Italy by
Vincenzo Bona srl, Turin

A catalogue record for this title
is available from the British Library

ISBN 0-86542-835-2

Library of Congress
Cataloging-in-Publication Data

Higgins, Elisabeth.
   Skin disease in childhood and adolescence
/ Elisabeth Higgins, Anthony du Vivier.
      p.   cm.
   Includes bibliographical references and
index.
   ISBN 0-86542-835-2
   1. Pediatric dermatology.   I. du
Vivier, Anthony.   II. Title.
   [DNLM: 1. Skin Diseases — in infancy &
   childhood.   2. Skin Diseases — in
   adolescence. WS 260 H636s 1996]
   RJ511.H54   1996
   618.92′5 — dc20
   DNLM/DLC   95-6273
   for Library of Congress
                                     CIP

DISTRIBUTORS

Marston Book Services Ltd
PO Box 87
Oxford OX2 0DT
(Orders: Tel: 01865 791155
         Fax: 01865 791927
         Telex: 837515)

North America
Blackwell Science, Inc.
238 Main Street
Cambridge, MA 02142
(Orders: Tel: 800 215-1000
              617 876-7000
         Fax: 617 492-5263)

Australia
Blackwell Science Pty Ltd
54 University Street
Carlton, Victoria 3053
(Orders: Tel: 03 9347-0300
         Fax: 03 9349 3016)

Contents

Preface

This book is an illustrated guide to skin diseases seen in the early part of life. Although the emphasis is on childhood disorders, there is no universally agreed definition as to when paediatric care ends and adult medicine begins. Therefore this volume considers those skin disorders which may arise in childhood and adolescence. While this text is by no means exhaustive, it is hoped that it will provide the reader with a broad introduction to the subject. Emphasis has been given to the more common cutaneous problems, but rarer congenital syndromes have been included if they are important. Nearly all the conditions discussed are illustrated in colour, with emphasis on the clinical features, key physical signs and possible differential diagnoses. Space does not permit a detailed review of aetiology in every instance, but advice is given on the management of each disorder, and guidelines on the use of topical steroids appear at the end. It is hoped that this format will provide a valuable practical aid to the understanding and diagnosis of skin diseases in this age group. This book is primarily aimed at general practitioners, undergraduates and residents in training who require an introduction to dermatology in the young. We hope that we may inspire their enthusiasm for the subject and allow them to make the more common diagnoses with confidence.

Elisabeth Higgins
Anthony du Vivier
London

Acknowledgements

We would like to express our gratitude to all the clinicians who so kindly allowed us to use examples from their own cases in this book, and who are acknowledged individually throughout the text. In particular, we are indebted to our colleague Dr Andrew Pembroke, who was in charge of the Paediatric Skin Clinic at King's College Hospital for many years and responsible for the care of many of the children illustrated in this book.

We owe special thanks to Mr Barry Pike and all the staff of the Medical Photography Department at King's College Hospital for their skill, technical help and the unerring quality of their clinical photographs, which play such a vital part in demonstrating the features of the different skin diseases.

Finally, we are grateful to Edward Wates and Rebecca Huxley at Blackwell Science for their enthusiasm and support, but most of all we would like to thank our families for their encouragement and patience during the completion of this project.

Chapter 1
Introduction to the Skin

Introduction

The skin is the largest organ in the body. Rather than being a simple inert covering, it is an active regenerative structure, with a vital role in physiological homeostasis. The functions of the skin are wide-ranging (Table 1.1), but it is most important in providing a protective barrier, both against physical trauma and infection and in regulating heat and fluid loss.

Any disease process which disrupts the integrity of the skin results in a breakdown of this barrier function. If the disease is extensive, the effects can be especially far-reaching. Neonates in particular have a large surface area to volume ratio and are especially vulnerable to heat and fluid loss in severe inflammatory conditions, such as erythroderma.

Mature skin is composed of epidermis, dermis and an underlying layer of subcutaneous fat (Fig. 1.1). The epidermis is the stratified layer of cells capable of regeneration. Beneath the epidermis lies the connective tissue of the dermis, containing the appendages. The junction between the epidermis and dermis is a complex, multilayered structure (Fig. 1.2).

Mature epidermis is a dynamic structure. The cells of the basal layer constantly proliferate and the keratinocytes so formed mature and move up through the layers of the epidermis, eventually losing their nuclei, to form the horny outer layer of the skin (the stratum corneum), before being shed. This epidermal cycle takes 30 days in healthy skin, but may be considerably accelerated in certain disease states, e.g. psoriasis.

Development of the skin

The skin is derived from ectoderm (epidermis) and mesoderm (the dermis). By 4 weeks after conception the embryonic skin is composed of a rudimentary structure, the periderm overlying a basal cell layer. The periderm has multiple projectory villi on its surface; which are believed to play a role in secretion and absorption of nutrients in the fetus. The periderm persists until about the 24th week of gestation.

Between the eighth and 11th weeks of development, an intermediate cell layer forms and begins to stratify, so that the number of cell layers gradually

Table 1.1 Functions of the skin

Physiological	Prevention of fluid loss
	Thermoregulation
	sweating
	piloerection
	vasodilatation/constriction
Barrier properties	Protection against
	infection
	ultraviolet radiation
	physical trauma
	chemical trauma
Metabolic	Vitamin D metabolism
Neurological	Sensory function
	tactile
	pain

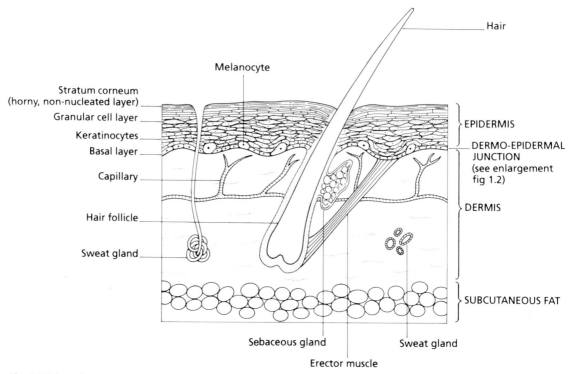

Fig. 1.1 Schematic representation of the structure of mature human skin.

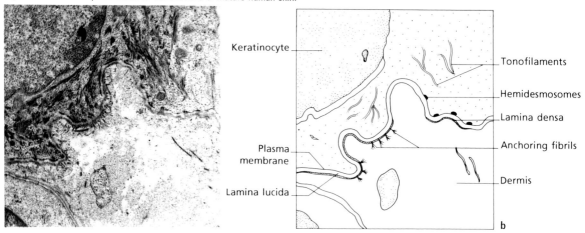

Fig. 1.2 (a) Electron photomicrograph of the dermo-epidermal junction depicted in (b) (courtesy of Dr P McKee). (b) Schematic diagram of the dermo-epidermal junction.

increases, up to the 26th week of gestation. During the period between 14 and 24 weeks of fetal life, the basal layer develops buds which eventually invaginate into the dermis to form the appendages (hair follicles, sebaceous and sweat glands) (Fig.

1.3). Certain keratins are specific to fetal skin, but those keratins associated with mature skin are initially expressed in the hair follicles, and by 24 weeks of gestation are present throughout the epidermis.

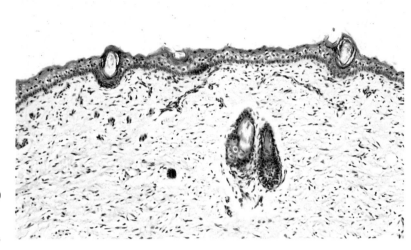

Fig. 1.3 Section of the fetal skin at 20 weeks' gestation, showing the rudimentary development of hair follicles (courtesy of Professor R. Eady).

Three additional groups of cells develop in the skin, and their presence may help in determining the age of fetal skin. Langerhans cells, which have immunoregulatory functions in later life, are present from the age of 6 weeks. The melanocytes, derived from the neural crest, migrate to the dermo-epidermal junction by 12 weeks' gestation, although pigmentation cannot be identified before the age of 4–6 months. Finally, Merkel cells, the function of which is unknown, but which may represent primitive nerve cells, can be identifed in fetal skin by 18 weeks.

The skin is mature by 30 weeks' gestation (Fig. 1.4), but very premature babies born before this time have extremely fragile, easily traumatized skin, with poor barrier properties, which is vulnerable to infection and can severely complicate their care (Fig. 1.5).

Dermatological examination

Assessing a patient with a cutaneous problem is essentially the same as in any other branch of medicine, in that the process involves taking a history, examining the skin and then performing appropriate special investigations as indicated. However, there are some specific aspects of taking a dermatological history and examining the skin which merit particular attention.

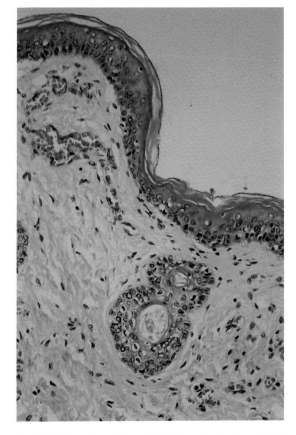

Fig. 1.4 Section of normal neonatal skin demonstrating the presence of a fully stratified epidermis and mature appendages (courtesy of Dr M. Newbold).

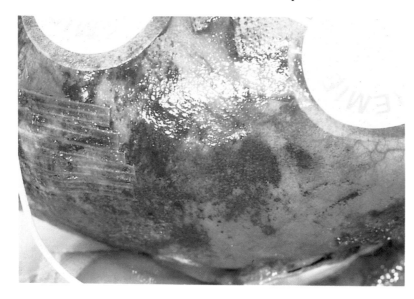

Fig. 1.5 Severe cutaneous pseudomonas infection in a premature baby of 24 weeks' gestation.

The history

The following questions should be asked in trying to establish the nature of the cutaneous problem, e.g. the presence of a rash. It is particularly important to take a detailed drug history, including establishing if any over-the-counter preparations have been taken or applied, as these may well modify (or even be responsible for) the clinical signs, yet are often not considered relevant or worthy of mention by the patient or the family.

- How long has the eruption been present?
- Is it static, spreading or intermittent?
- Has the child had a similar episode in the past?
- Where did the rash start?
- How has it progressed/spread?
- Is it itchy/symptomatic?
- Are any close contacts similarly affected?
- Are there any aggravating or relieving factors?
- What treatment has been given and have any medications been taken (including any proprietary preparations)?
- Is there any past history of relevance?
- Is there any family history of skin disease (e.g. atopy) or any other disorder?
- Has there been recent travel abroad?
- Have there been any changes recently in home circumstances (e.g. move house/school, parental marital problems, etc.)?
- Are there any pets?

Examining the skin

The principle in examining the skin is to establish the overall pattern of the eruption. It is therefore imperative to examine the whole skin in most instances, other than for simple matters such as straightforward viral warts.

The following points should be taken into account when examining the skin.

- Is it a localized or generalized phenomenon?
- Is the eruption primarily symmetrical (and therefore likely to be endogenous in origin) or asymmetrical (and therefore likely to be exogenous in origin)?
- Does it primarily affect the flexures (e.g. atopic eczema) or extensor surfaces (e.g. psoriasis) of the body, or is it non-specific?
- Is the eruption palpable?
- Are the individual lesions macular, papular, vesicular, pustular, plaques, nodules or wheals (see 'Glossary of dermatological terms', below)?
- Is there any secondary infection?
- Are the mucous membranes, hair or nails involved?

• Is there any associated systemic upset (e.g. fever, lymphadenopathy, organomegaly)?

Special investigations

Investigations which may be specifically indicated in dermatology include the following.
• *Skin swabs* for microbiology.
• *Skin smears of blister fluid* for virology (electron microscopy) and *skin swabs* in viral transport medium for viral culture.
• *Skin scrapings/plucked hairs* for mycology (potassium hydroxide preparation for direct microscopy and dry scrapings for culture).
• *Wood's light examination* for fluorescence (e.g. some fungal eruptions) and to highlight pigmentary irregularities.
• *Skin biopsy* for routine histology, direct immuno-fluorescence or occasional electron microscopy.

Glossary of dermatological terms

Atrophy Loss of substance of the epidermis, dermis or both. There is thinning, wrinkling and transparency of the skin.

Bulla A large, tense blister filled with clear fluid.

Crust A dried exudate that previously was serous, purulent or haemorrhagic.

Erosion Superficial loss of part of the epidermis.

Excoriation A shallow excavation of the skin secondary to scratching, resulting in bleeding.

Lichenification Thickening of the skin with exaggeration of the skin creases.

Macule A non-palpable (flat) lesion less than 1 cm in diameter.

Necrosis Death of the skin.

Nodule A firm, raised lesion greater than 0.5 cm in diameter.

Papule A small, domed, raised lesion less than 0.5 cm in diameter.

Patch A flat lesion greater than 1 cm in diameter.

Plaque A well-circumscribed, palpable thickening of the skin, greater than 1 cm in diameter.

Pustule A small, tense accumulation of purulent fluid within the epidermis.

Sclerosis An induration or hardening of the skin.

Telangiectasia Dilatation of capillaries.

Ulcer Full-thickness loss of the epidermis.

Vesicle A small, fluid-filled blister.

Wheal Localized dermal oedema and erythema.

Chapter 2
Neonatal Disorders

Introduction

The neonatal period is defined as the first 4 weeks of life. The most frequent problems and those specific to the newborn are discussed in this chapter, but other conditions that may be seen during this period are also included in Chapters 3 (Developmental Disorders and Genodermatoses), 10 (Naevi) and 20 (The Skin in Systemic Disease).

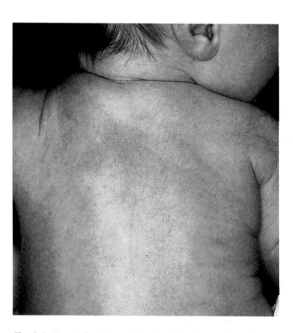

Fig. 2.1 *Neonatal erythema.* There is a blotchy macular erythema which is most prominent on the trunk (courtesy of Mr C. Chandler).

Physiological disorders

Neonatal erythema

DEFINITION

A normal response in which prominent hyperaemia develops in the first few hours after birth.

CLINICAL FEATURES

A generalized erythema (Fig. 2.1) is apparent. But it fades within 48 hours of birth.

Cutis marmorata

DEFINITION

Mottling of the skin which develops as a physiological response to lower temperatures.

CLINICAL FEATURES

A purplish-blue reticulate pattern (livedo) can be seen, most prominently on the limbs (Fig. 2.2). The condition usually fades on warming, but may be faintly apparent at room temperature in some neonates.

DIFFERENTIAL DIAGNOSES

1 Cutis marmorata telangiectatica congenita (see p. 125): a rare developmental anomaly in which there is a

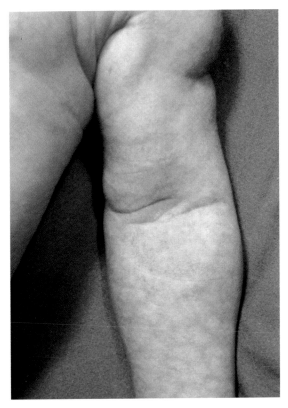

Fig. 2.2 *Cutis marmorata*. A purplish reticulate patterning occurs during infancy, particularly on the limbs and in response to cold. It is a temporary, physiological phenomenon.

a florid and persistent livedo, which may be associated with other congenital malformations.

2 In older children a persistent livedo may be a sign of a connective tissue disorder or hypothyroidism.

MANAGEMENT

The mottling gradually disappears after infancy.

Sebaceous gland hyperplasia

DEFINITION

Common, transient papules seen especially over the nose in the newborn, secondary to the effect of maternal androgens.

CLINICAL FEATURES

Profuse, small, yellowish-white papules develop at the orifices of the pilosebaceous unit. They may occur anywhere on the body, but tend to be most pronounced on the face, especially over the nose (Fig. 2.3) and forehead. They may appear in conjunction with milia (see below).

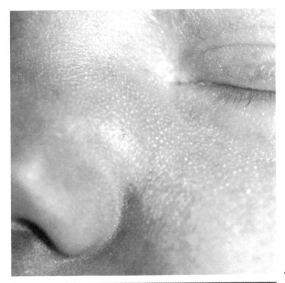

a

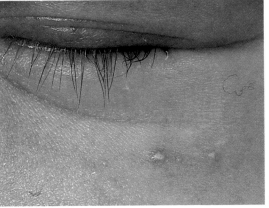

b

Fig. 2.3 (a) *Sebaceous gland hyperplasia*. Multiple, uniform, minute, yellow papules occur, especially on the nose, cheeks and forehead. They represent the effect of maternal androgens on the sebaceous glands (courtesy of C. Lawrence, 1993). *Colour Atlas and Text of Physical Signs of Dermatology*. Lawrence C. and Cox N.H. (eds), Mosby Year Books, Europe Ltd. **(b)** Larger lesions may resemble acne.

DIFFERENTIAL DIAGNOSES

1 Milia: these are white rather than yellow.
2 Infantile acne: the papules tend to be larger, more inflamed and more persistent.

MANAGEMENT

The papules resolve without treatment within a few weeks, as the influence of maternal androgens diminishes.

Milia

DEFINITION

Small keratin retention cysts within the upper dermis.

CLINICAL FEATURES

Superficial, 1–2 mm, whitish papules (Fig. 2.4) may occur anywhere on the body, but particularly over the face. When they occur on the alveolar margin and palate they are called Epstein's pearls or Bohn's nodules.

MANAGEMENT

Spontaneous rupture of the cysts usually occurs within 6 weeks of birth.

Pathological disorders

Miliaria

DEFINITION

A vesicular eruption due to the retention of eccrine sweat.

AETIOLOGY

Although the eccrine sweat glands are fully developed by 36 weeks' gestation, they are often functionally immature at birth. They can easily become obstructed, producing a condition known as miliaria.

Miliaria crystallina occurs when the opening of the sweat duct becomes blocked so that sweat is retained within the stratum corneum, and miliaria rubra occurs ('prickly heat') when the duct is blocked at a deeper level so that sweat is retained in the dermis.

CLINICAL FEATURES

Miliaria may develop at any age, but is particularly common during the neonatal period.

Miliaria crystallina

Widespread, tiny (1–2 mm), clear vesicles arise from normal skin. The lesions are very superficial, and rupture within a few hours.

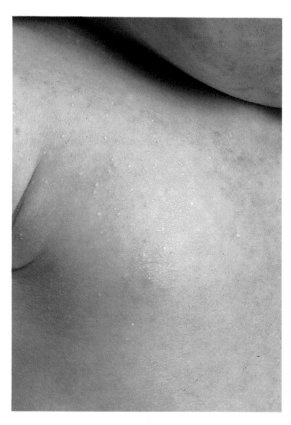

Fig. 2.4 *Milia*. Small, white papules may occur, anywhere on the body, but are most common on the face. They are keratin retention cysts which spontaneously rupture and disappear after a few weeks (courtesy of the Institute of Dermatology).

Miliaria rubra

Larger (1–4 mm) vesicles develop on an erythematous base, which may become quite urticated (Fig. 2.5). Although the vesicles are sterile, they often appear pustular, due to trapped cellular debris. True infection by staphylococci may also occur as a secondary event. The lesions are most numerous at flexural sites (e.g. the neck and groin), and any conditions which produce occlusion, such as plastic pants, will exacerbate the condition. Situations which promote overheating, such as phototherapy and the use of incubators, are particularly likely to induce miliaria. If the lesions are numerous, the baby may become quite restless and uncomfortable. The rash fades after 2–3 days, but recurrences are common.

MANAGEMENT

Avoidance of those factors (e.g. occlusion and excessive heat) which predispose to the condition, as far as practical.

Erythema toxicum neonatorum

DEFINITION

A transient condition most commonly seen in full-term infants, in which erythematous macules develop on the trunk.

AETIOLOGY

The cause of the condition is unknown; despite the name, it is not thought to be due to a toxin. It is more common in full-term than in preterm babies.

CLINICAL FEATURES

This condition is common, affecting as many as half of all full-term babies. Large (2–3 cm in diameter) asymptomatic erythematous patches develop which may have a central sterile vesicle which is rich in eosinophils (Fig. 2.6). There may be a peripheral eosinophilia if the cutaneous lesions are extensive. The eruption is most prominent on the trunk.

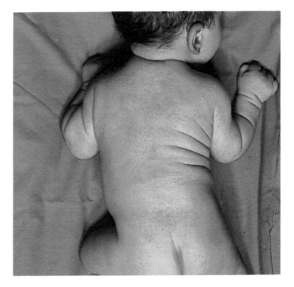

Fig. 2.5 *Miliaria rubra.* Widespread, small vesicles containing clear fluid occur within the first couple of weeks, due to obstruction of functionally immature sweat glands.

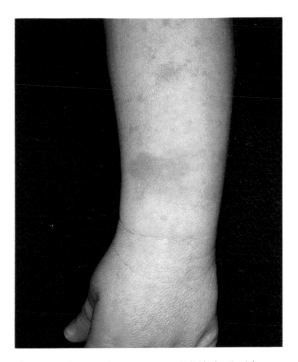

Fig. 2.6 *Erythema toxicum neonatorum.* Individual urticarial areas occur, often with a central blister. The lesions are short-lived and the infant is otherwise well (courtesy of Mr C. Chandler).

1 Transient neonatal pustulosis: the lesions contain neutrophils rather than eosinophils.
2 Viral infections: the virus can rapidly be identified on a vesicular smear, by electron microscopy.

MANAGEMENT

Reassurance is all that is required, as the lesions fade spontaneously within 2–3 days.

Transient neonatal pustulosis
(transient neonatal pustular melanosis)

DEFINITION

A sterile, neutrophilic pustular eruption associated with macular pigmentation, which is most prevalent in healthy black children.

AETIOLOGY

Its cause is unknown, but this condition has been considered to be a variant of erythema toxicum neonatorum.

CLINICAL FEATURES

The disorder affects up to 5% of black babies and is ten times more common in black children compared with those of other races. Small, flaccid, superficial pustules (Fig. 2.7) are present at birth. They may occur anywhere on the skin, but particularly on the face and trunk. The pustules are fragile and rupture quickly, and when they dry they form a superficial brown crust with a collarette of scale. As this resolves in black children it may leave a pigmented macule which persists for several months. The macule is usually indiscernible in babies of other races.

DIFFERENTIAL DIAGNOSES

1 Infantile acropustulosis: the distribution helps distinguish the condition.
2 Erythema toxicum neonatorum: the lesions are surrounded by erythema and the pustules contain eosinophils, not neutrophils.
3 Impetigo: a Gram's stain can rapidly identify the presence of staphylococci.
4 Scabies: the presence of burrows is diagnostic.
5 Herpes simplex infection: the virus can be identified by electron microscopy or culture.

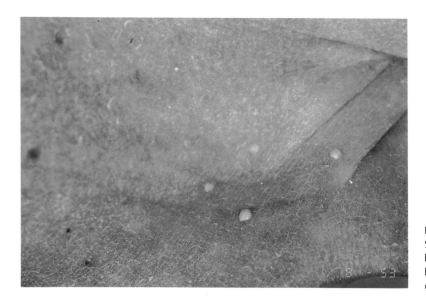

Fig. 2.7 *Transient neonatal pustulosis.* Small, sterile pustules are present at birth which rupture quickly, leaving behind a pigmented macule (courtesy of Dr M. Clement).

MANAGEMENT

There is no specific treatment for the eruption.

Infantile acropustulosis

DEFINITION

A recurrent, pruritic, vesiculopustular eruption of the hands and feet, often seen in black infants.

AETIOLOGY

The cause is unknown. It is more prevalent in boys. Although it can affect all races, in the USA it has been shown to be more common in black children.

CLINICAL FEATURES

The eruption usually begins within the first 3 months as small red papules, which evolve over the course of 24 hours into intra-epidermal vesicles and finally subcorneal pustules. It affects the palms, soles and lateral borders of the feet (Fig. 2.8), but can occur on the dorsal aspect of the hands and toes, and other sites of the body. The pustules recur in crops about every 4 weeks, each episode lasting 1–2 weeks. The lesions are usually intensely pruritic. Attacks diminish in severity and frequency with time, and resolve completely by the age of 2 years.

DIFFERENTIAL DIAGNOSES

1 Scabies: this can be difficult to distinguish from acropustulosis because of the similar sites, and many children are given acaricides in error. Burrows should be searched for.
2 Transient neonatal pustulosis: the distribution of infantile acropustulosis on the extremities helps to distinguish the two conditions.

MANAGEMENT

1 Reassurance that this is a benign, non-infectious and ultimately self-limiting condition.
2 Antihistamines may help the pruritus.
3 Topical steroids given early, when new lesions develop, can sometimes prevent an incipient attack developing further.
4 Dapsone has been reported to be effective, but its use is rarely justified.

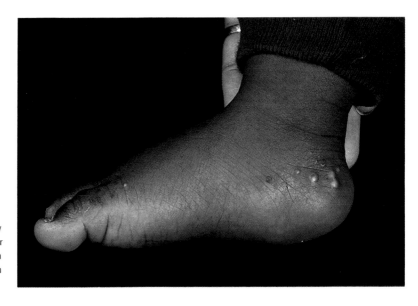

Fig. 2.8 *Infantile acropustulosis.* Itchy sterile vesicles lasting a few days occur on the palms and soles, particularly in Afro-Caribbean children. The condition may persist for up 1 year.

Subcutaneous fat necrosis of the newborn

DEFINITION

A rare disorder of babies during the neonatal period in which there is granulomatous necrosis of the subcutaneous fat.

AETIOLOGY

Several factors have been implicated in the development of this disorder.

1 The subcutaneous fat of the neonate is more highly saturated than that of adults, and appears to be more vulnerable to cold-induced injury. Similar lesions may occur in infants rendered hypothermic during cardiac surgery.

2 Tissue hypoxia secondary to obstetric complications (e.g. traumatic delivery, maternal pre-eclampsia) has been put forward as a possible cause of fat necrosis.

3 Subcutaneous fat necrosis may be associated with hypercalcaemia.

CLINICAL FEATURES

Thickened plaques can be felt within the subcutaneous tissues of the buttocks, thighs, back (Fig. 2.9) and cheeks. They vary in size from small nodules to large plaques several centimetres across (Fig. 2.10). The lesions are more common in full- or post-term babies. They are usually present at birth, but may develop in babies up to the age of 6 weeks. Features of hypercalcaemia such as vomiting and failure to thrive may occur.

DIFFERENTIAL DIAGNOSES

1 Sclerema neonatorum: a diffuse, yellowish thickening of connective tissue seen in the first few days of life in severely ill babies and associated with a high mortality.

2 Neonatal cold injury: tight, shiny plaques of skin which feel cold to the touch develop over the trunk in small-for-dates babies who have become hypothermic. It used to be seen before central heating was commonplace, but is now rare in western countries.

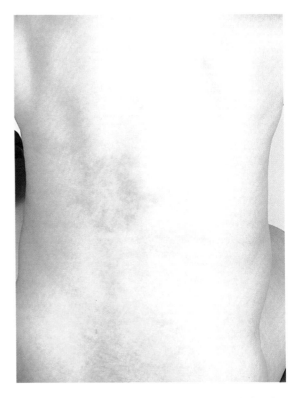

Fig. 2.9 *Subcutaneous fat necrosis of the newborn.* A thickened subcutaneous plaque was evident on the back, shortly after birth.

MANAGEMENT

The lesions slowly resolve over the course of several months, but may take longer in cases of hypercalcaemia. They may leave some residual atrophy.

Neonatal purpura fulminans

DEFINITION

A serious condition due to an inherited abnormality of clotting, characterized by large haemorrhagic plaques which rapidly become necrotic.

AETIOLOGY

In the newborn the condition is due to homozygous protein C deficiency. In older children a similar

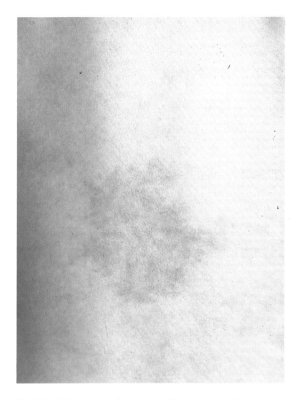

Fig. 2.10 *Subcutaneous fat necrosis of the newborn.* The subcutaneous tissue can be felt to be thickened and hard. There may be one or several lesions.

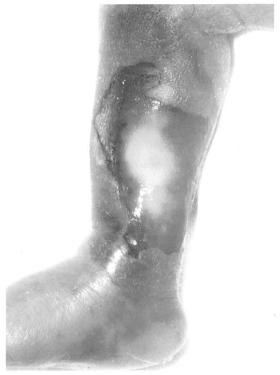

Fig. 2.11 *Neonatal purpura fulminans.* Large, firm haemorrhagic plaques which progress to necrosis in a child with homozygous protein C deficiency (courtesy of Professor H. Gamsu).

clinical picture may be seen in serious infections, when acquired protein C deficiency develops (e.g. meningococcal septicaemia).

CLINICAL FEATURES

Widespread dermal vein thrombosis results in tender ecchymoses surrounded by erythematous skin, which rapidly become haemorrhagic and necrotic (Fig. 2.11). Thromboses may develop in other organs and the condition is associated with a significant mortality.

MANAGEMENT

Prompt protein C replacement by means of fresh frozen plasma transfusions is required.

Cutaneous complications of prenatal diagnostic procedures

Amniocentesis pits

DEFINITION

Deep, punctate scars may appear in a small percentage of children as a direct complication of the procedure of amniocentesis performed during pregnancy.

AETIOLOGY

The scar arises from direct trauma to the skin by the amniocentesis needle. It is increasingly rare due to improved techniques.

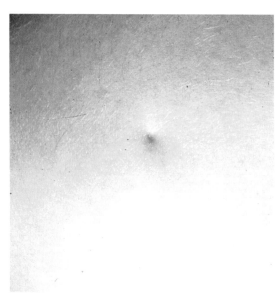

Fig. 2.12 *Amniocentesis pits.* Small punctate scars arise from trauma during amniocentesis (courtesy of Prof. Sharon Raimer).

CLINICAL FEATURE

A small dimple is seen at the site where the skin was punctured during the procedure (Fig. 2.12).

MANAGEMENT

No specific treatment is required.

Digital amputation

Loss of digits or phalanges has been observed following chorionic villous sampling for prenatal diagnosis. A similar clinical picture may also be seen due to the formation of amniotic constriction bands *in utero*.

Chapter 3
Developmental Disorders and Genodermatoses

Introduction

This chapter reviews those skin conditions which arise as isolated developmental anomalies or as more general familial syndromes, in which the cutaneous features are only a part. Most of them are quite rare.

Developmental disorders

Aplasia cutis

DEFINITION

A congenital absence of skin over part of the scalp.

AETIOLOGY

The condition may occur as an isolated finding or familial trait. There is localized failure of development of either the epidermis, dermis, subcutis or all three layers. Occasionally, it may occur in association with other developmental defects (e.g. congenital heart disease).

CLINICAL FEATURES

The incidence of the condition is 1:3000 births. Well-demarcated hairless areas are present on the scalp (Fig. 3.1) from birth, most frequently over the vertex. They may be depressed and if the epidermis is involved they are ulcerated. The affected area may vary in size from a few millimetres to several centimetres across. Small lesions heal spontaneously

to leave atrophic scars. The defect is almost always confined to the skin, but deeper structures such as the dura and bone may occasionally be involved.

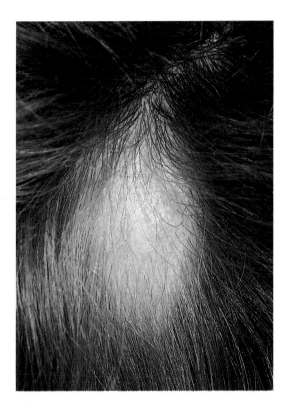

Fig. 3.1 *Aplasia cutis.* A well-demarcated area of hair loss is present on the scalp at birth, with accompanying loss of tissue, depending on how much epidermis, dermis or subcutis is missing (courtesy of Dr M. Clement).

COMPLICATIONS

1 Secondary infection of the ulcer is common.
2 Meningitis may complicate deeper lesions.

DIFFERENTIAL DIAGNOSES

1 Abrasions from fetal scalp electrodes: these can initially resemble aplasia cutis.
2 Secondary infection (e.g. herpes simplex) introduced from the maternal genital tract by instrumentation at delivery may produce a large ulcer mimicking aplasia cutis, but this can be excluded by virology.
3 Pressure ulcers: neonates who become hypoxic or hypovolaemic may develop pressure ulcers on the scalp. These ulcers heal to leave areas of scarring alopecia.
4 Sebaceous naevus (see p. 130): although initially flat in infants and associated with a patch of alopecia, the lesion becomes raised and has a distinctive orange-yellow colour. The surface of the naevus becomes progressively papilliferous with time.

MANAGEMENT

1 It is important to assess the extent of the defect, and to seek neurosurgical advice if subcutaneous structures are involved.
2 Small areas of aplasia cutis heal spontaneously by secondary intention, but the residual scarring alopecia is permanent.
3 Larger defects require plastic surgery and skin grafting for closure.

Dermoid cysts

DEFINITION

A developmental cyst containing the remnants of various epidermal appendages.

AETIOLOGY

Dermoid cysts are developmental inclusion cysts which form by the entrapment of epithelium along lines of embryonic fusion.

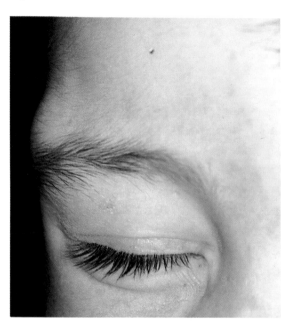

Fig. 3.2 *Dermoid cysts.* Dermoid cysts occur anywhere along planes of embryonic fusion, especially on the face. They are flesh-coloured, subcutaneous nodules.

CLINICAL FEATURES

Dermoid cysts are relatively rare. They are usually noted soon after birth and affect both sexes equally. They may occur anywhere along planes of embryonic fusion, but are most frequent on the face, especially on the nose, scalp or at the lateral aspect of the eyebrow. The lesions are flesh-coloured, smooth, mobile subcutaneous nodules (Fig. 3.2), which slowly enlarge with age. The cyst is lined by epidermis and contains a white cheesy material composed of a variety of cutaneous structures including hair and adnexal glands. They may become secondarily infected and inflamed. Deep lesions may be associated with a sinus tract, for example midline dermoids of the nose (Fig. 3.3) may be associated with a fistula from which a tuft of hair emanates.

DIFFERENTIAL DIAGNOSIS

Rarely, an extranasal glioma at the root of the nose may be confused with a dermoid cyst. If there is any

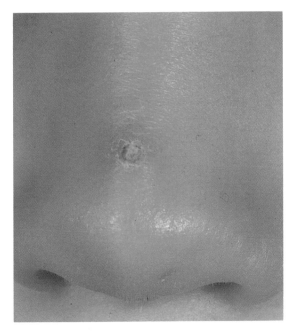

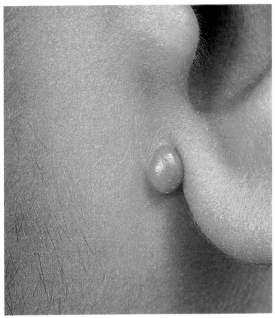

Fig. 3.3 *Median nasal fistula.* This sinus, through which a tuft of hairs may arise, is associated with a deep midline dermoid.

Fig. 3.4 *Accessory auricles.* Single or multiple flesh-coloured pedunculated nodules occur anywhere along the line from the ear to the angle of the mouth.

doubt, a CAT scan should be arranged prior to excision, as gliomas communicate with the sub-arachnoid space.

MANAGEMENT

Surgical excision is the treatment of choice.

Accessory auricles

DEFINITION

Small, additional rudimentary tragi which form during embryogenesis.

AETIOLOGY

The tragus of the ear is formed from the first bran-chial arch. Accessory auricles may be found any-where along these embryonic lines of development. They are usually isolated developmental anomalies, but in rare instances they may occur with other congenital facial abnormalities as part of a more generalized syndrome (e.g. the Treacher–Collins syndrome).

CLINICAL FEATURES

They are most common in the immediate pre-auricular area, but may be found anywhere in a line from the ear to the angle of the mouth, or in the cervical region along the sternocleidomastoid muscle. They are small, flesh-coloured pedunculated nodules, which may be soft or cartilaginous. They may be single (Fig. 3.4) or multiple and are occasionally bilateral.

MANAGEMENT

If the patient requests treatment, surgical excision is the management of choice. It can be performed under local anaesthetic.

The ichthyoses

This term is used to describe a heterogenous group of congenital disorders in which there is an abnormality of keratinization, resulting in generalized scaly skin.

Ichthyosis vulgaris

DEFINITION

A common, mild, familial form of ichthyosis in which coarse scaling is most prominent on the extensor surfaces.

AETIOLOGY

The condition is inherited as an autosomal-dominant trait, although different family members may be affected to quite variable degrees. Histopathologically, the granular layer of the epidermis is absent. The condition was said to be associated with atopy, but this is now disputed.

CLINICAL FEATURES

The incidence of ichthyosis vulgaris is 1 : 300 births. From early childhood, the skin is coarse with widespread areas of fine white scaling that produces a crazed appearance. The skin feels rough and dry, and is often worse in winter. The palms and soles may be affected, but the flexures are usually spared (Fig. 3.5). Keratosis pilaris may be prominent. The condition is quite variable in its severity and is often mild, but there may be extensive desquamation in more severely affected individuals. The hair, teeth and nails develop normally, but the cutaneous changes usually persist although there may be some improvement in adult life.

DIFFERENTIAL DIAGNOSES

1 Xeroderma: dry skin is a feature of many conditions, especially eczema, but it should be distinguished from the coarser, persistent scaling of ichthyosis. Xeroderma tends to be more exaggerated in the flexures, which are often spared in ichthyosis.

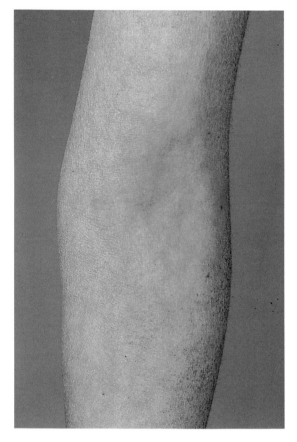

Fig. 3.5 *Ichthyosis vulgaris.* The skin is roughened with dry white scaling and notable sparing of the flexures.

2 Acquired ichthyosis: the acquisition of dry skin (Fig. 3.6) is unusual and may be associated with lymphoma.
3 Refsum's disease: this is a rare autosomal-recessive metabolic disorder caused by the accumulation of phytanic acid in the tissues. The ichthyosis of Refsum's disease becomes apparent during the second decade of life and is associated with retinitis pigmentosa and deafness. The diagnosis is confirmed by finding raised levels of phytanic acid in the serum.

MANAGEMENT

1 Mild cases may require no specific treatment.
2 Emollients, especially those containing urea, are

Fig. 3.6 *Acquired ichthyosis.* Ichthyosis is normally present at birth. An acquired dry skin may be associated with lymphoma. This teenager has Hodgkin's disease.

the mainstay of treatment and should be applied regularly and liberally.

3 Systemic retinoids are effective but not curative, and they are therefore rarely justified in this milder form of ichthyosis.

Collodion baby

DEFINITION

A temporary, tough, taut, shiny membrane covering the entire body surface at birth, which later peels to reveal one of the more severe variants of ichthyosis underneath.

AETIOLOGY

The condition is usually associated with lamellar ichthyosis or ichthyosiform erythroderma (see p. 21). Rarely, the collodion membrane may peel off to reveal normal skin.

CLINICAL FEATURES

A thick, shiny, inflexible membrane (Fig. 3.7) composed of stratum corneum, said to resemble collodion, is present at birth. The rigidity of the membrane may interfere with sucking, respiration and thermoregulation.

DIFFERENTIAL DIAGNOSIS

Harlequin fetus: a rare but serious condition where the baby is born (often prematurely) with a hard membrane over the skin surface which cracks to produce a pattern of large diamond-like (harlequin) fissures. There are associated facial abnormalities with marked ectropion, conjunctival oedema and small ears, which produce a grotesque appearance. The prognosis for such infants is grave, but a few have shown a response to systemic retinoids.

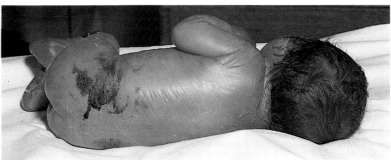

Fig. 3.7 *Collodion baby.* A temporary, taut, shiny membrane encases the fetus. It is shed within 2 weeks revealing either lamellar ichthyosis or ichthyosiform erythroderma.

MANAGEMENT

1 The treatment depends on the severity of the underlying skin disorder.

2 The thick collodion membrane impairs normal cutaneous function and affected babies may become dehydrated or hypothermic. Collodion babies should be nursed in humidified incubators to increase the pliability of the membrane and reduce respiratory difficulty.

Sex-linked recessive ichthyosis

DEFINITION

A rare form of ichthyosis characterized by large brownish scales.

AETIOLOGY

The condition is familial and inherited as a sex-linked, recessive trait. It is associated with steroid sulphatase deficiency which may be responsible for protracted, difficult labour in the mother.

CLINICAL FEATURES

The incidence is 1:6000 births. Large, dark scales (Fig. 3.8) produce a lizard-like skin (Fig. 3.9), which is most prominent at the sides of the neck. The palms and soles are spared, and slit-lamp examination may reveal associated corneal opacities. There may be associated hypogonadism.

DIFFERENTIAL DIAGNOSES

1 Lamellar ichthyosis: this is a much rarer (incidence, 1: 300,000), autosomal-recessive condition with prominent brownish-grey scales over most of the body surface from birth. The palms and soles are affected and scaling may be particularly verrucous over the large joints. Affected individuals have an increased susceptibility to infection.

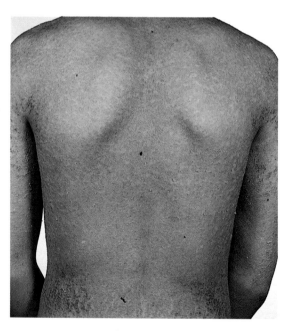

Fig. 3.8 *Sex-linked ichthyosis.* The coarse, large, dark scales make for a dirty appearance to the skin. The disorder is due to steroid sulphatase deficiency.

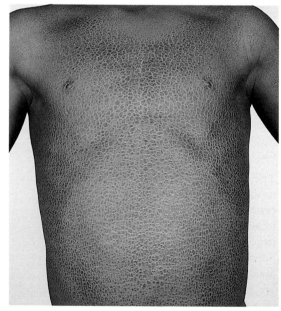

Fig. 3.9 *Sex-linked ichthyosis.* There are large, dark scales over most of the body surface from birth. The flexures are involved. There may be associated hypogonadism.

2 Sjögren–Larsson syndrome: this is a rare condition in which lamellar-like ichthyosis is present from the neonatal period. However, as the child develops, profound mental retardation, spastic paralysis and retinal degeneration become apparent.

MANAGEMENT

1 Emollients.
2 Weak salicylic acid preparations (2–6%) may remove the thick horny scale, but if they are overused they can produce irritation and even lead to excess absorption and salicylism.
3 In older patients who are severely affected, oral retinoids are effective but need to be taken on a long-term basis.

Epidermolytic hyperkeratosis (congenital bullous ichthyosiform erythroderma)

DEFINITION

A rare, inherited disorder, characterized by generalized erythema and blistering in the neonatal period, which is replaced by widespread hyperkeratosis as the individual ages.

AETIOLOGY

The condition is inherited as an autosomal-dominant trait, but many cases appear to be sporadic gene mutations.

CLINICAL FEATURES

The disease becomes evident during the immediate neonatal period. The baby's skin shows generalized erythema and scale with blistering, which may be localized or widespread. The bullae may result in large erosions which easily become secondarily infected. The erythema tends to become less prominent as the child grows, and the skin gradually becomes more verrucous (Fig. 3.10), particularly over the flexures. The blistering usually resolves by the age of 7–8 years, but may persist into adult life in about 20% of individuals. The nails may be dystrophic, but the hair is usually normal. In severely

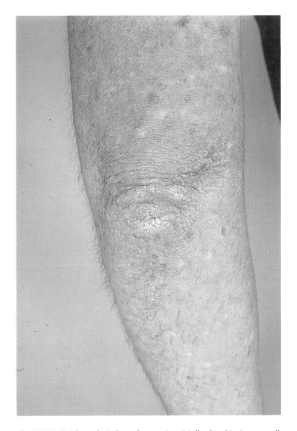

Fig. 3.10 *Epidermolytic hyperkeratosis.* Initially the skin is generally red, scaly and associated with blisters. It then becomes more verrucous, especially around the flexures (courtesy of St Mary's Hospital).

affected individuals, there may be ectropion and deformity of the ears. Histopathologically, the appearances of the skin are quite characteristic with giant keratohyaline granules and vacuolation of the granular layer.

DIFFERENTIAL DIAGNOSES

1 Epidermolysis bullosa: erythema is less prominent, but the ultimate diagnosis is based on the skin biopsy.
2 Non-bullous ichthyosiform erythroderma: erythema and generalized fine white scale (Fig. 3.11) develop in early childhood, but there is no history of blistering. The scalp hair may be sparse and in severe cases there is an associated ectropion.

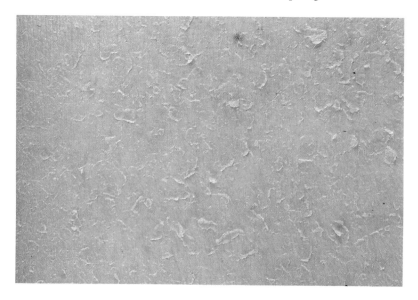

Fig. 3.11 *Non-bullous ichthyosiform erythroderma.* There is a generalized fine white scaling all over the skin, often sparse hair and ectropion.

MANAGEMENT

1 The diagnosis should be confirmed by the results of a skin biopsy.
2 Emollients should be applied to help reduce the scale.
3 Secondary sepsis should be treated appropriately.
4 Oral retinoids are the only definitive treatment and they need to be given for life. However, the age at which it is felt justified to commence such treatment is a specialist decision.

Other disorders of keratinization

Keratosis pilaris

DEFINITION

A common condition, prominent on the outer upper arms and thighs, in which the follicular orifice becomes plugged by hyperkeratotic scale with mild surrounding erythema.

AETIOLOGY

The disorder is inherited as an autosomal-dominant condition with variable penetrance. It may be seen associated with ichthyosis vulgaris and atopy.

CLINICAL FEATURES

The condition is most prevalent in childhood and adolescence. Small horny plugs (Fig. 3.12) obstruct the follicular orifice, which becomes dilated with a variable degree of perifollicular inflammation, and the skin feels rough. The disorder tends particularly to affect the outer aspects of the upper arms (Fig. 3.13) and thighs, but it may be more generalized and include the face (Fig. 3.14). It is asymptomatic, but may be of considerable cosmetic concern in severely affected individuals.

DIFFERENTIAL DIAGNOSIS

Lichen spinulosus: it is less common than keratosis pilaris and is characterized by the sudden appearance of localized plaques of spiny, follicular keratoses on the limbs. It may be precipitated by infection.

MANAGEMENT

1 Many mild cases require no treatment.
2 Emollients containing 20% urea are beneficial in reducing the scale.
3 Keratolytics (either 2% salicylic acid or weak preparations of Retin-A) may be helpful in more stubborn cases.

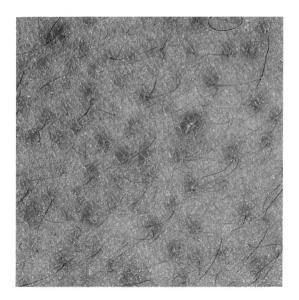

Fig. 3.12 *Keratosis pilaris.* Small horny plugs obstruct the follicular orifice. Pigmentation is prominent in dark-skinned races.

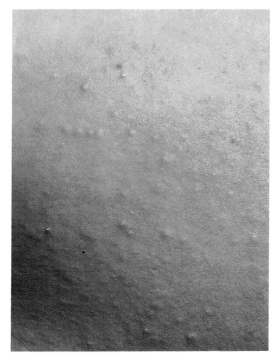

Fig. 3.14 *Keratosis pilaris.* The discrete, small, rough, grey papules may occur on the cheeks in more widespread cases.

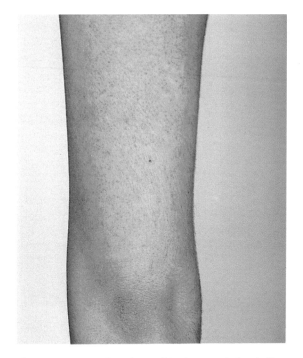

Fig. 3.13 *Keratosis pilaris.* The condition is symmetrical and affects the outer aspects of the upper arms and thighs. It is very common in adolescence, but may also be familial.

Ulerythema ophryogenes

DEFINITION

An unusual variant of keratosis pilaris affecting the face, especially the eyebrows, and associated with prominent erythema and some degree of atrophy.

AETIOLOGY

Some cases appear to be familial but many are sporadic. Boys tend to be more severely affected than girls.

CLINICAL FEATURES

From early childhood, scaly plugs are prominent in the lateral part of the eyebrows (Fig. 3.15). As the changes extend medially they may be accompanied by follicular destruction. The cheeks may also be affected.

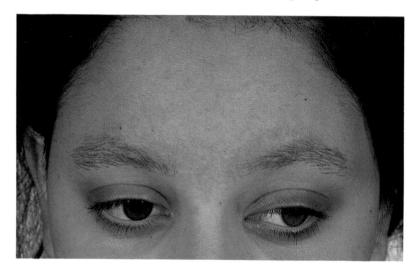

Fig. 3.15 *Ulerythema ophryogenes.* There is prominent erythema around the eyebrows with some atrophy.

MANAGEMENT

Emollients are the mainstay of treatment for this relatively persistent and recalcitrant condition, but topical retinoic acid may be of some benefit.

Erythrokeratoderma variabilis (Mendes da Costa syndrome)

DEFINITION

A genetically determined rare condition of circumscribed hyperkeratosis and erythema occurring in a persistent or variable manner.

AETIOLOGY

It is inherited probably as an autosomal dominant with variable expressivity. There is hyperkeratosis, acanthosis, dermal oedema and some cellular infiltration associated with a loss of keratinocytes.

CLINICAL FEATURES

There are erythematous hyperkeratotic plaques which are relatively fixed and figurate (Fig. 3.16) in appearance. They occur on the face, buttocks or limbs. In the variant known as Degos' syndrome (erythroderma en cocardes) there are round plaques of erythema with central scaling resembling rosettes

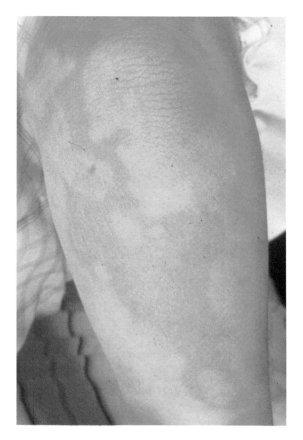

Fig. 3.16 *Erythrokeratoderma variabilis.* Fixed red hyperkeratotic plaques occur in a polycyclic, annular or comma-shaped fashion on the limbs or face (courtesy of Dr D. Atherton).

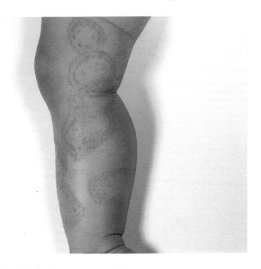

Fig. 3.17 *Erythrokeratoderma variabilis en cocardes.* There are circinate plaques of erytherma with inner scaling resembling rosettes (Fr. *cocardes*) which come and go on the limbs.

(Fig. 3.17) which arise and disappear at whim. They occur particularly on the limbs, and individual lesions may last several weeks.

MANAGEMENT

There is no specific treatment but topical steroids may reduce the inflammation.

The genodermatoses

Neurofibromatosis

DEFINITION

An inherited neurocutaneous disorder characterized by a distinctive triad of cutaneous lesions (café-au-lait spots, axillary freckling and multiple neurofibromas) and associated with multiple hamartoma formation and a high incidence of a variety of malignancies.

AETIOLOGY

The condition displays autosomal-dominant in-heritance with variable penetrance, but some cases arise as somatic mutations. Two distinct variants of neurofibromatosis have now been described: NF1 (Von Recklinghausen's disease) with involvement of the skin, skeleton, central nervous system and endo-crine system and NF2, a rarer but more localized form of the disease, characterized by bilateral acoustic neuromas but with minimal or no cutaneous changes. The gene for NF1 has now been localized to chromosome 17 and that of NF2 to chromosome 22. It is thought that the NF1 gene acts by inhibiting a tumour-supressor gene.

CLINICAL FEATURES

The incidence of NF1 is 30:100,000 births. The skin may appear normal at birth, but throughout childhood, multiple ovoid areas of pale macular pigmentation appear called café-au-lait spots (Fig. 3.18). Solitary café-au-lait spots may be found in normal individuals, but the presence of six or more

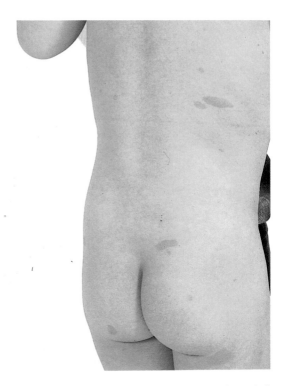

Fig. 3.18 *Neurofibromatosis.* The skin is normal at birth but multiple pigmented ovoid macules appear early in life as in this 2-year-old child.

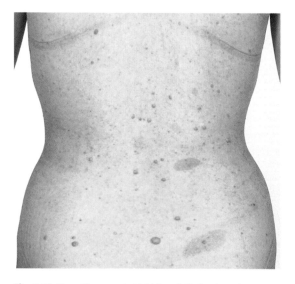

Fig. 3.19 *Neurofibromatosis.* Multiple soft flesh-coloured neurofibromas develop from adolescence onwards.

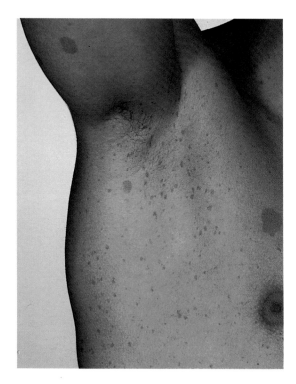

Fig. 3.20 *Neurofibromatosis.* Axillary freckling is pathognomonic of the condition.

lesions greater than 5 mm in diameter in a child under the age of 6 years (or greater than 15 mm in diameter in an adolescent) would strongly suggest a diagnosis of NF1. With time, multiple soft, flesh-coloured nodules (Fig. 3.19) appear on the skin and freckling develops in the axillary vault (Fig. 3.20), but may not be prominent until the late teens. The neurofibromas, which can be indented easily, may be small or large. Subcutaneous lesions, which are connective tissue hamartomas, may grow to an enormous size (plexiform neurofibromas) and be very disfiguring. Associated findings are listed in Table 3.1.

Hamartomas of the iris (Lisch nodules), which are visible as greyish-white lesions on slit-lamp examination, develop early in the disease and are a useful screening investigation for children from affected families, as they are often evident before the cutaneous signs.

DIFFERENTIAL DIAGNOSES

1 LEOPARD syndrome: multiple lentigines occur in association with sensineural deafness but no neurofibromas.
2 McCune–Albright syndrome: giant segmental pigmented macules occur in association with skeletal cysts and precocious puberty.

MANAGEMENT

1 The diagnosis is a clinical one based on the oculocutaneous signs and family history.
2 Affected children need careful assessment, including baseline electro-encephalography, audiometry and psychomotor testing. They should be under regular neurological follow-up to look for possible

Table 3.1 Extracutaneous features of neurofibromatosis 1

Meningiomas and other central nervous system tumours
Epilepsy
An increased incidence of learning difficulties
Bone cysts
Endocrine disease, especially phaeochromocytomas
A high incidence of malignant disease

complications including the development of asymptomatic optic gliomas.

3 Affected families should be referred for genetic counselling. Prenatal diagnosis is now possible in specialist centres.

Tuberous sclerosis (Bourneville's disease, epiloia)

DEFINITION

An inherited neurocutaneous syndrome, comprising epilepsy and mental retardation together with characteristic skin changes, namely adenoma sebaceum, ash-leaf macules, periungual fibromas and connective-tissue naevi.

AETIOLOGY

The disease is transmitted as an autosomal-dominant condition with high penetrance. Genetic linkage studies show that about half the affected families show linkage to chromosome 9 and half to chromosome 16. However, about 60% of cases appear to arise as spontaneous mutations.

CLINICAL FEATURES

The incidence of tuberous sclerosis is estimated at 1:10,000. The condition is not usually evident at birth, but becomes manifest during early childhood as seizures and developmental delay (hence the term *epiloia* – *epi*lepsy, *lo*w intelligence and *a*denoma sebaceum). The characteristic oval hypopigmented patches (ash-leaf macules) (Fig. 3.21) are present in over 80% of affected individuals from early childhood. They may be seen more clearly under Wood's light examination. Although the small, pink papules (Fig. 3.22) over the nose and cheeks are termed adenoma sebaceum, they are actually angiofibromas which do not develop until later in childhood, but become progressively more numerous thereafter. Other cutaneous features include connective-tissue naevi over the lumbosacral area (the shagreen patch) and periungual fibromas. Associated systemic findings include phacomas of the retina, cardiac rhabdomyosarcomas and hamartomas of the kidney.

Severely affected patients have a reduced life expectancy.

MANAGEMENT

1 The diagnosis is a clinical one based on the spectrum of neurocutaneous signs.
2 Affected individuals should be under the care of a neurologist for management of their epilepsy.

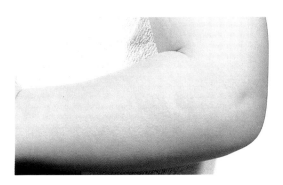

Fig. 3.21 *Tuberous sclerosis.* Oval hypopigmented macules, the shape of an ash leaf, are present early in life. They may be more obvious under Wood's light examination.

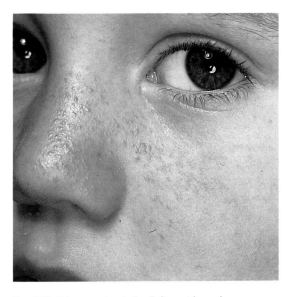

Fig. 3.22 *Tuberous sclerosis.* Small, firm, pink papules occur over the nose and cheeks: adenoma sebaceum.

3 Affected families should be referred for genetic counselling.

4 Dermabrasion, electrodessication and laser therapy have all been found to improve the cosmetic appearance of adenoma sebaceum, but the lesions will slowly recur.

Incontinentia pigmenti (Bloch–Sulzberger syndrome)

DEFINITION

An uncommon inherited neurocutaneous disorder in which the initial vesicular skin lesions become warty and pigmented with time. The syndrome is associated with a variety of problems of the central nervous system, especially epilepsy.

AETIOLOGY

The inheritance of the syndrome is sex-linked dominant and the condition is usually considered to be lethal in males.

CLINICAL FEATURES

The cutaneous features of the syndrome become evident during the first weeks of life, but evolve through different stages as the child grows. Initially, vesicles (Fig. 3.23) develop on a background of erythema in a linear distribution (Fig. 3.24). At this stage, eosinophilic spongiosis is a histological characteristic. Over the course of the next few weeks, the vesicles resolve and are replaced by hyperkeratotic papules (Fig. 3.25), most prominently seen on the limbs. These in turn are superseded by hyperpigmented macular lesions often arranged in a whorled configuration following Blaschko's developmental lines. These subsequently fade, to leave the final streaks of hypopigmentation and atrophy, which may be quite subtle. The nails may be abnormal. Other systems may be involved with dental anomalies, ocular defects, seizures and mental retardation.

DIFFERENTIAL DIAGNOSES

1 Epidermolysis bullosa in the neonate: this may be confused with incontinentia pigmenti, but the two conditions should be clearly distinguishable on skin biopsy.

2 Hypomelanosis of Ito: this may appear similar to the hypopigmented stage of incontinentia pigmenti, but the former has no history of initial vesicular or hyperpigmented lesions.

3 Goltz syndrome (focal dermal hypoplasia): this is

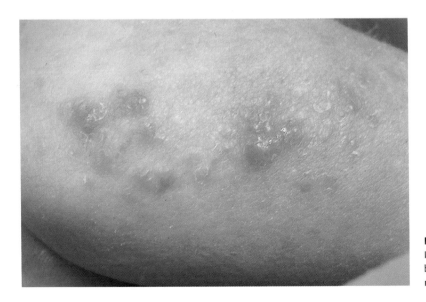

Fig. 3.23 *Incontinentia pigmenti.* Initially vesicles develop on a background of erythema within the first month of life.

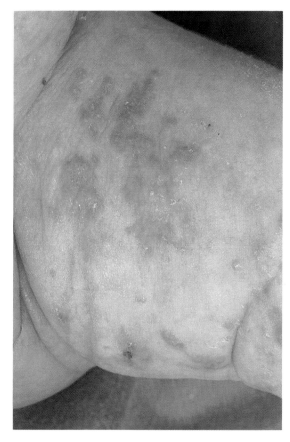

Fig. 3.24 *Incontinentia pigmenti.* The vesicles are distributed in a streaky or linear manner over a limb.

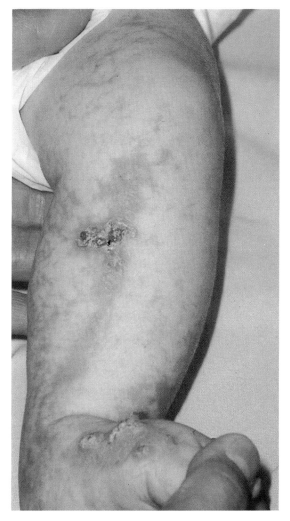

Fig. 3.25 *Incontinentia pigmenti.* As the lesions evolve, they become hyperkeratotic and whorled and finally hyperpigmented. It is lethal in males and associated with neurological, ocular and dental abnormalities.

also an X-linked dominant condition in which areas of atrophy follow a linear distribution. The key abnormality is that the dermis is absent in areas, with herniation of the subcutaneous fat. Although the condition may resemble the late stages of incontinentia pigmenti, its history and histology are distinct.

MANAGEMENT

1 The diagnosis is established on the basis of the constellation of clinical signs and the characteristic skin biopsy.

2 A detailed family history of cutaneous problems in childhood, seizures or previous miscarriages may help to establish the inheritance. Mothers of affected children should be examined for hypopigmented streaks on the limbs.

3 Once the diagnosis is confirmed, the child should have careful neurological and ophthalmic assessments to look for associated complications.

4 Affected families should receive appropriate genetic counselling, as a woman with incontinentia pigmenti has a 1 : 4 chance of future miscarriage and 1 : 2 of her daughters will be affected.

Anhidrotic ectodermal dysplasia

DEFINITION

A congenital syndrome in which there are an absence of sweat glands, sparse hair and dental anomalies.

AETIOLOGY

The condition is X-linked recessive and therefore the majority of cases occur in males. Female carriers may exhibit limited features of the full syndrome.

CLINICAL FEATURES

The incidence of the syndrome is 1:100,000 births. The first feature to cause concern is usually the sparse or absent hair, which is dry and brittle (Fig. 3.26). The eruption of the teeth is often delayed or absent. Conical incisors are characteristic. The nails may be brittle with linear ridging. Absence or reduction of sweating causes heat intolerance, which may present as unexplained fever in infancy. In some cases there may be a characteristic facies, with prominent forehead and large ears. One-third of affected individuals have some degree of mental retardation.

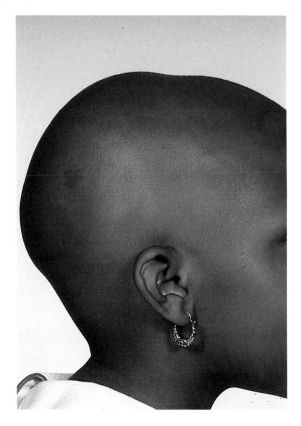

Fig. 3.27 *Hidrotic ectodermal dysplasia.* This young girl has never grown any hair.

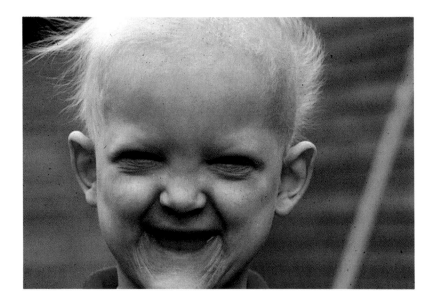

Fig. 3.26 *Anhidrotic ectodermal dysplasia.* This is a clinically and genetically heterogeneous group of disorders with absent or partial development of the hair, teeth, nails and sweat glands (courtesy of Dr A. Clark).

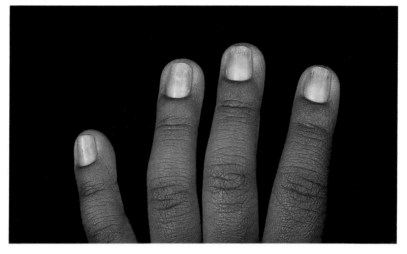

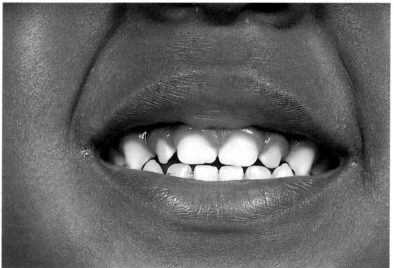

Fig. 3.28 *Hidrotic ectodermal dysplasia.* Although she has thickened nails (top); her teeth are normal (bottom).

DIFFERENTIAL DIAGNOSES

1 Hidrotic ectodermal dysplasia (Clouston's syndrome): although the scalp hair may be absent or sparse (Fig. 3.27), and the nails thickened, with an increased horizontal curvature, the dentition (Fig. 3.28) and sweating are normal.

2 Other ectodermal dysplasias: many variants of ectodermal dysplasia have now been described and classified according to the degree to which the hair, teeth, nails and sweat glands are affected. They are all rare, but detailed descriptions may be found in more specialized texts.

MANAGEMENT

1 The full syndrome is usually clinically obvious, but in more subtle cases examination of the rest of the family may establish the diagnosis.
2 Treatment is symptomatic with prevention of overheating and regular dental care.

Netherton's syndrome

DEFINITION

An inherited syndrome characterized by erythroderma, bamboo hair and a distinctive scaly eruption known as ichthyosis linearis circumflexa.

AETIOLOGY

The inheritance of the disorder is autosomal-recessive, but expression is variable and girls appear to be more frequently affected than boys.

CLINICAL FEATURES

Widespread erythema and scaling (Fig. 3.29) are usually present from the neonatal period. As the child grows, the erythematous component subsides, but may persist on the face. A dynamic scaling eruption produces a serpiginous pattern termed ichthyosis linearis circumflexa, in which plaques have a characteristic double collarette of scale. The hair is sparse and dry and appears spangled (Fig. 3.30). Light microscopy of the hair shaft reveals the abnormality trichorrhexis invaginata (see p. 196).

DIFFERENTIAL DIAGNOSES

1 Ichthyosiform erythroderma: this may be difficult to exclude in infancy.
2 Severe atopic eczema may resemble Netherton's syndrome, but the hair changes of the latter should point to the correct diagnosis.

COMPLICATIONS

Neonatal hypernatraemia has been reported.

MANAGEMENT

1 There is no specific treatment for the condition but liberal emollients will help the skin and topical steroids provide some temporary relief.

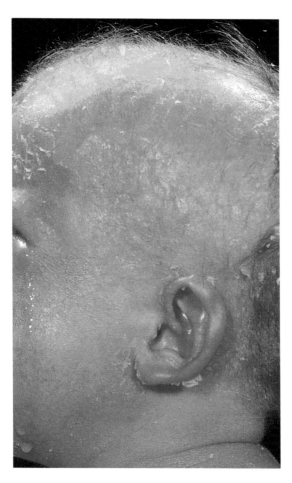

Fig. 3.29 *Netherton's syndrome.* There is widespread erythema and scaling initially especially on the face (courtesy of Dr D. Atherton).

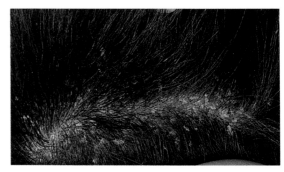

Fig. 3.30 *Netherton's syndrome.* The hair may be sparse and dry and characteristically is spangled in appearance due to bamboo-like nodes and fractures of the hair shaft.

2 The serum sodium should be monitored in young children because of the association with hypernatraemia.

3 Psoralens and ultraviolet A (PUVA) treatment has been found to be beneficial in some instances, and retinoids have been used in adults.

4 Any infection should be treated promptly as it can precipitate erythroderma.

Darier's disease

DEFINITION

An inherited disorder of keratinization, in which hyperkeratotic papules in a seborrhoeic distribution occur in association with a characteristic nail dystrophy.

AETIOLOGY

The condition is inherited as an autosomal-dominant trait with variable penetrance. Although the spectrum of clinical features is quite variable, the gene for all types of Darier's disease has been localized to chromosome 12. Histopathologically, there is dyskeratosis and suprabasal acantholysis in the epidermis with the formation of characteristic grains and corps ronds.

CLINICAL FEATURES

The majority of patients develop lesions during the second decade. Greasy, yellow-brown papules with a crusted surface (Fig. 3.31) develop on the skin, especially on the face and central trunk (Fig. 3.32). In flexural regions the lesions may coalesce to form large, hyperkeratotic plaques. Severely affected areas may weep and are prone to secondary infection by both bacteria and viruses (especially herpes simplex). The condition is often exacerbated by

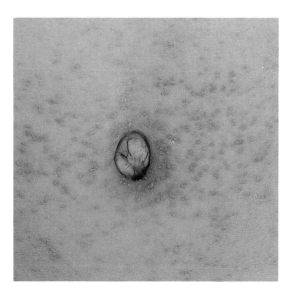

Fig. 3.31 *Darier's disease.* Greasy, pigmented papules are present. This is the 9-year-old brother of the 15-year-old child shown in Fig. 3.32.

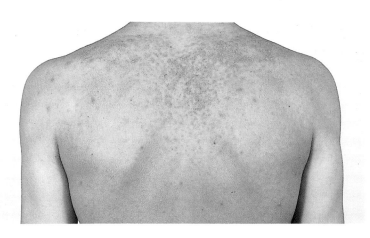

Fig. 3.32 *Darier's disease.* The upper back and front of the chest are commonly involved with symmetrical red-brown or pigmented papules.

sunlight. The nails may have linear white streaks and a characteristic V-shaped notch at the distal margin. Punctate pitting of the palms is a frequent feature of the disorder and flat, wart-like lesions may be seen on the backs of the hands.

DIFFERENTIAL DIAGNOSIS

Benign familial pemphigus (Hailey–Hailey disease) is histologically very similar, but it usually begins later in life than Darier's disease and tends to affect the axillae and groins, where it is often very erosive. Direct immunofluorescence can be helpful in distinguishing the two conditions.

MANAGEMENT

1 The diagnosis is made on the basis of the clinical appearance and skin biopsy.
2 Mild cases may require no treatment.
3 Patients should be advised to avoid excessive sun exposure.
4 Secondary infection should be treated appropriately and prophylactic antibiotics may sometimes be helpful.
5 More severe cases often respond to oral retinoids (Acetretin or Roaccutane), but treatment has to be continuous for control to be maintained.

Ehlers–Danlos syndrome

DEFINITION

A group of inherited disorders characterized by laxity and fragility of the skin and hyperextensibility of the joints.

AETIOLOGY

Ten different subtypes of the disorder have been described with different modes of inheritance. The primary defect is a disorder of collagen synthesis producing an overall deficiency of collagen.

CLINICAL FEATURES

The syndrome usually becomes apparent in childhood because of the excessive skin fragility and poor wound healing, with the formation of atrophic scars following injury (Fig. 3.33). The skin is lax over the joints and there is hypermobility of the joints (Fig. 3.34). There may be a history of easy bruising secondary to the increased fragility of the blood vessels (Fig. 3.35). In some variants of the disorder, scoliosis is prominent, and there may be collagen abnormalities in other tissues, e.g. the aorta, with associated risk of rupture.

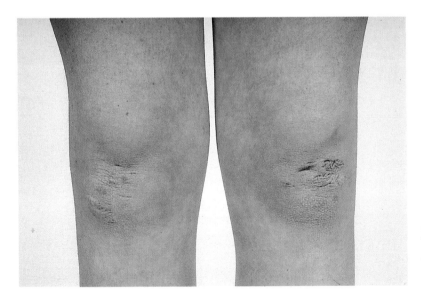

Fig. 3.33 *Ehlers–Danlos syndrome.* There is excessive skin fragility with poor wound healing and the formation of atrophic scars following injury (courtesy of Dr M. Clement).

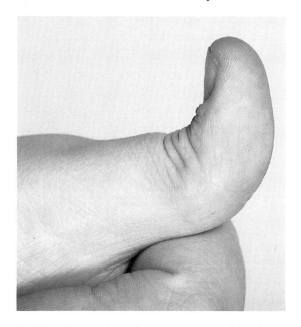

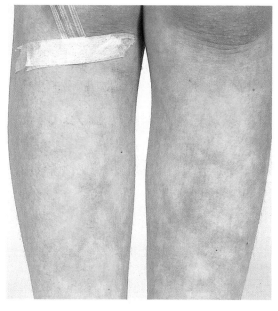

Fig. 3.34 *Ehlers–Danlos syndrome.* There is hypermobility of the joints and the skin is lax over them (courtesy of Dr M. Clement).

Fig. 3.35 *Ehlers–Danlos syndrome.* Frequent trauma is common, due to the increased fragility of the skin and poor wound healing.

DIFFERENTIAL DIAGNOSIS

Cutis laxa: In this condition, the skin hangs in loose folds and gives an appearance of premature ageing, but the joints are not hypermobile and there is no history of skin fragility.

MANAGEMENT

1 The diagnosis is clinical but confirmation of the subtype can be made by collagen analysis in reference laboratories.
2 Treatment is essentially supportive but it is important to avoid undue trauma.

Anderson–Fabry disease

DEFINITION

A rare in-born error of metabolism in which small cutaneous angiomas are associated with sudden attacks of pain, a risk of progressive renal disease and cerebrovascular haemorrhage.

AETIOLOGY

The syndrome is inherited as an X-linked recessive disorder. The primary defect is an abnormality in the metabolism of an α-galactosidase, ceramide-trihexosidase, with resultant accumulation of glycosphingolipid in endothelial cells throughout the skin and body.

CLINICAL FEATURES

Numerous small (pinpoint), bright red angiomas (Fig. 3.36) begin to develop around the umbilicus and groin from the early teens in affected individuals. The cutaneous lesions gradually increase in numbers, but other organ involvement may not be apparent until adulthood.

MANAGEMENT

1 The diagnosis is usually suggested by the clinical signs and a positive family history.
2 The features on skin biopsy may be suggestive,

Fig. 3.36 *Anderson–Fabry disease.*
Multiple, pinpoint, bright red angiomas
develop on the skin which are
associated with sudden periodic
excruciating attacks of pain in the limbs
with fever.

but confirmation of the enzyme abnormality requires fibroblast culture.
3 Individuals should be followed up for possible
renal and central nervous system complications.
4 Affected families should receive genetic
counselling.

Lipoid proteinosis

DEFINITION

A rare congenital syndrome in which the accumulation of an amorphous periodic acid–Schiff (PAS)-
positive material in the dermis produces multiple
papular lesions in the skin and mucous membranes.

AETIOLOGY

The disorder is thought to be inherited through
autosomal-recessive transmission and there is a high
incidence of parental consanguinity in affected
pedigrees.

CLINICAL FEATURES

Hoarseness is often apparent in early infancy due to
laryngeal deposits and respiratory obstruction may
result from extensive oropharyngeal deposits. The
cutaneous changes begin in early childhood as
multiple waxy-yellow papules on the face (especially
along the margins of the eyelids and lips; Fig. 3.37),
axillae and genitalia. In older individuals, diffuse
thickening of the skin may resemble solar elastosis.
If the scalp is affected, it may produce alopecia.

MANAGEMENT

There is no effective treatment.

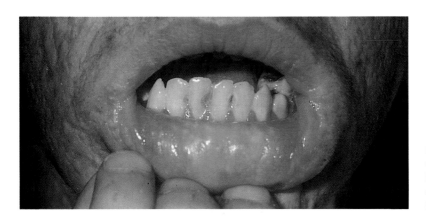

Fig. 3.37 *Lipoid proteinosis.* Firm,
waxy, white infiltrates develop on the
lips, tongue, pharynx, eyelids and
elsewhere. It presents in infancy with
hoarseness due to laryngeal deposits.

Chapter 4
Atopic Eczema

Introduction

Eczema is the most common skin problem seen in general practice, accounting for up to one third of all skin consultations. The terms *eczema* and *dermatitis* are synonymous and (although some reserve the term dermatitis for irritant or allergic – i.e. exogenous – causes) they are used interchangeably in this chapter.

Eczema is an inflammatory disorder of the skin. There are several forms, which are classified as depicted in Table 4.1. Atopic eczema is discussed here and other forms of eczema in Chapter 5. However, the salient pathological features are the same for all types of eczema. The characteristic histological hallmark is that of intra-epidermal oedema (spongiosis), which may be sufficiently marked in acute disease to cause rupture of the intercellular bridges, with the formation of vesicles. In subacute forms there is a variable degree of acanthosis, and in chronic lichenified forms, hyperkeratosis. Secondary changes from rubbing and infection may be superimposed, and there is dilatation of the blood vessels and a prominent lymphohistiocytic infiltrate in the dermis.

Atopic eczema

DEFINITION

The term atopy refers to a group of inherited disorders (asthma, urticaria, eczema and hay fever) in which type 1 hypersensitivity reactions are mediated via IgE. Atopic eczema describes a relapsing and remitting condition, common in childhood and associated with the atopic state.

AETIOLOGY

The precise aetiology of atopic eczema is still unknown, although it is accepted that there is an inherited tendency and that the disease is immunologically mediated.

Immunology

Levels of IgE are elevated in 80% of patients with atopic eczema, and a sensitivity to house-dust mite is usually demonstrated. There is evidence of decreased cell-mediated immunity, which accounts for the increased susceptibility of patients to viral infections.

Table 4.1 Classification of paediatric eczema

Endogenous	Atopic eczema
	Seborrhoeic dermatitis
	Pityriasis alba
	Lichen striatus
	Juvenile plantar dermatosis
	Pompholyx
	Eczema associated with systemic disease
Exogenous	Irritant dermatitis
	Allergic contact dermatitis
	Photoallergic dermatitis

Vascular

The vascular responses are abnormal, with a tendency to vasoconstriction. The skin is generally pale, and a linear blanching produced on stroking the skin is known as 'white dermographism'.

Food allergy

The role of food intolerance is controversial. A food allergy is often suspected by the parents of a child with atopic eczema, and many children are placed on *ad hoc* diets. However, true food sensitivity can only be demonstrated by carefully conducted exclusion diets, with the sequential reintroduction of possible culprit foods, as prick tests are unreliable in children. Such exclusion diets are laborious to conduct and require the strict supervision of a dietician, to ensure adequate nourishment is maintained.

There is some evidence emerging to suggest that restrictive diets during the first years of life (including the maternal diet during the period of breastfeeding) can reduce the risk of developing eczema in those children with a strong family history of atopy.

Environmental factors

1 The low relative humidity in winter and the presence of central heating, which produces a dry atmosphere, can exacerbate eczema.
2 There is also quite strong evidence that the modern urban lifestyle is implicated in the increasing prevalence of atopy. Atopic eczema is frequently seen in the children of immigrant populations living in the major cities. It is often rather more severe than in their native countries, where there may be no previous family history.

Psychological and emotional factors

Parental unrest, difficulties at school and other causes of unhappiness can have an adverse effect on the disease.

CLINICAL FEATURES

The clinical features of paediatric eczema are outlined in Table 4.2. The spectrum of disease is diverse, but severe atopic eczema (Fig. 4.1) is a miserable condition for both the child and parents, and can prove very frustrating because of its recurrent and chronic nature, and its sometimes disappointing response to treatment.

The diagnosis of atopic eczema is a clinical one. There is no diagnostic test for the disease, and prick tests, in particular, are unreliable in young children.

Prevalence

Precise assessment of the prevalence of atopy is difficult, but the incidence is increasing, and has doubled in recent years. Atopic eczema is now the most common problem seen in paediatric dermatology clinics. Nearly half the UK population shows evidence of atopy (by means of positive skin tests), and it is now estimated that at least 10% of children have atopic eczema.

Atopic eczema usually begins between the ages of 3 months and 2 years, but it can occur at any time. It is rare in very young infants.

Table 4.2 Physical signs of paediatric eczema

Acute	Weeping
	Erythema
	Pink papules
	Vesicles
	Secondary crust
	Excoriation
	Miserable child
Subacute	Erythema
	Oozing
	Crusting
	Thickened skin
Chronic	Dry skin (xerosis)
	Background erythema
	Lichenification
	Excoriation
	Postinflammatory pigmentary changes
	Dennie–Morgan fold (pronounced infraorbital fold)
	Pallor because of abnormal vasoconstriction responses

Eczema may be acute (vesicular; Fig. 4.2), subacute (with erythema oozing and crusting; Fig. 4.3) or chronic (and lichenified; Fig. 4.4). The individual with atopic eczema has an easily irritated skin, which is responsible for many of the physical signs. Itch is predominant. Excoriations are pronounced (Fig. 4.5), with multiple bleeding points which may become stuck to clothing, causing further discomfort. Secondary infection is common and can precipitate further attacks.

Sites

Any area may be affected, but the most prominent area of involvement changes with time. In infants, eczema tends to begin on the face (Fig. 4.6), especially the cheeks. With teething, thumb-sucking and other conditions that produce drooling, marked perioral eczema is seen, probably secondary to an irritant effect.

As the child begins to crawl, eczema is seen at sites of friction on the dorsal aspect of the ankles and extensor aspect of the knees. Once the child is walking, eczema most frequently localizes in the flexural creases (Fig. 4.7), although a 'reverse pattern' with extensor surface involvement is sometimes seen. This reverse pattern tends to reflect a poorer prognosis.

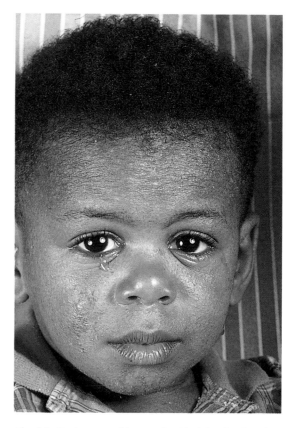

Fig. 4.1 *Atopic eczema.* It is uncomfortable, itchy, chronic and difficult for children and their parents to cope with.

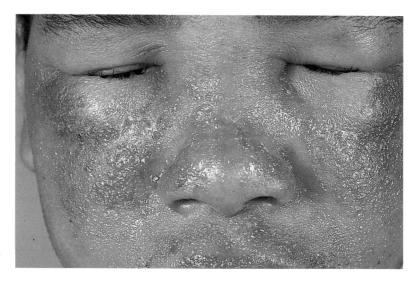

Fig. 4.2 *Eczema.* In acute eczema there are vesicles which weep and subsequently crust. Secondary sepsis is common.

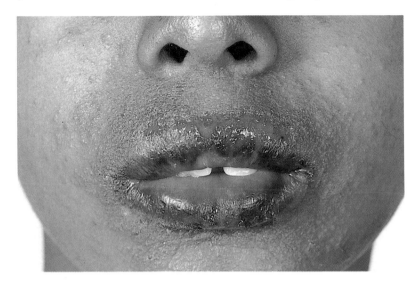

Fig. 4.3 *Atopic eczema.* There is oozing and crusting immediately around the lips with subacute papular erythema peripherally.

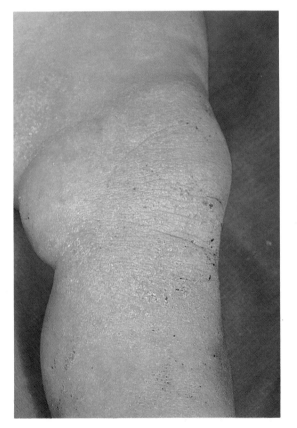

Fig. 4.4 *Atopic eczema.* In chronic eczema the skin is dry and scaly. The epidermis is thickened and skin markings exaggerated (lichenified) as a response to scratching.

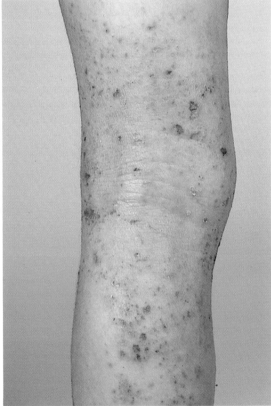

Fig. 4.5 *Atopic eczema.* Pruritus can be intense and the vigorous scratching produces numerous excoriations which bleed onto clothes and bedding.

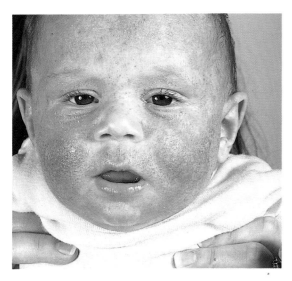

Fig. 4.6 *Atopic eczema.* In babies, eczema usually affects the face first, often beginning on the cheeks.

Ninety per cent of children with eczema will grow out of the disease by their teens, and the great majority will be free of symptoms much earlier. However, there is no predictive test to identify those individuals in whom the disease will persist into adult life, and there is no correlation between the severity of the disease in childhood and the likelihood that the condition will persist.

The skin of an individual with atopic eczema has a tendency to be very dry (xerosis), and ichthyosis and keratosis pilaris are common.

Specific patterns

1 Lichenification: this term means 'thickening of the skin with exaggeration of the skin markings, secondary to rubbing and scratching' (Fig. 4.8), and is a sign of chronicity. Lichenoid papules may be a particularly exaggerated feature in Afro-Caribbean children (Fig. 4.9).
2 Follicular eczema (Fig. 4.10): this condition is characterized by small follicular papules, which are often asymptomatic, occur especially on the trunk, and are particularly pronounced in children with pigmented skin.
3 Besnier's prurigo: this is a variant of eczema in

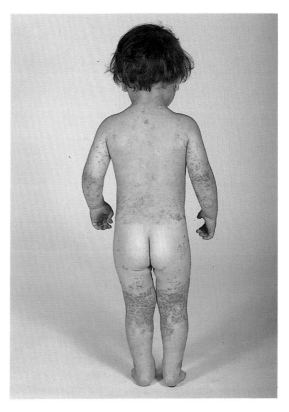

Fig. 4.7 *Atopic eczema.* As the child begins walking, the eczema tends to become more prominent on the limbs, especially around the flexures.

which excoriations predominate, with subsequent scarring and pigmentary changes.
4 Postinflammatory pigmentary changes: postinflammatory hypo- or hyperpigmentation (Fig. 4.11) is common in pigmented skin.
5 Atopic 'dirty neck': reticulate pigmentation can occur over the anterior neck in adolescents with atopic eczema, but is not common in young children.
6 Nail changes: the nails are not primarily affected in atopic eczema, unlike in psoriasis. However, if there is involvement of the digits around the nail fold, a secondary nail dystrophy may develop because of disruption of the growth of the nail matrix beneath the posterior nail fold, which produces horizontal ridging. The nails of a child with atopic eczema often appear buffed because they are constantly being rubbed against the skin.

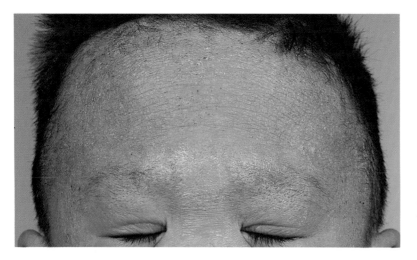

Fig. 4.8 *Atopic eczema.* Constant scratching induces epidermal thickening. The skin markings become more prominent. This lichenification may be localized or generalized.

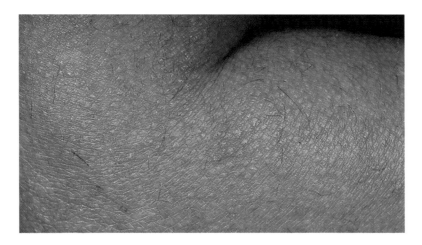

Fig. 4.9 *Atopic eczema.* A lichenoid pattern of flat-topped, itchy papules is often a marked feature on black skin.

Fig. 4.10 *Follicular eczema.* A so-called variant of eczema with small hyperkeratotic papules, not uncommon in black children. It is usually asymptomatic and unresponsive to treatment.

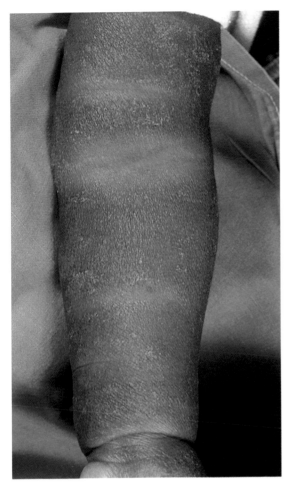

Fig. 4.11 *Atopic eczema.* Postinflammatory hyperpigmentation can dominate the dryness and scaliness of eczema in black skin.

DIFFERENTIAL DIAGNOSES

1 Wiskott–Aldrich syndrome: this X-linked recessive disease is characterized by thrombocytopenia, immunodeficiency and eczema. The skin is involved earlier than in atopic eczema, and is purpuric. The purpura and excessive bleeding from excoriations are clues to the diagnosis. These children are vulnerable to recurrent infection with bacteria (e.g. otitis media) and viruses (measles, etc.). They also have an increased risk of lymphoma and leukaemia, and rarely survive beyond the first decade. Eczema may also be associated with other forms of immuno-dysfunction, e.g. Job's syndrome.

2 Phenylketonuria: one quarter of children with phenylketonuria develop eczema, which responds to dietary restriction of phenylalanine.

MANAGEMENT

Although the disease eventually remits in 90% of children, the course is chronic, and most treatment is supportive rather than curative. Correct treatment (Table 4.3) is important, however, as undertreatment is common.

Over one third will also develop asthma or hay fever and, when the condition is severe, a combined approach to management with joint clinics between the paediatrician and dermatologist can be most helpful.

Caring for a child with severe atopic eczema is very demanding both in time and emotion. Many of the treatments are laborious and messy, and the remission they induce may only be short-lived. The role of a specialist nurse, both in demonstrating treatment and providing support to the parents, is invaluable. Patient information organizations such as the National Eczema Society are additional sources of information and support.

Emollients

Regular and liberal use of emollients (e.g. aqueous cream) and soap substitutes (e.g. emulsifying ointment) is the mainstay of treatment. In the acute phase of eczema, emollients are usefully applied as wet wraps (a fine-mesh gauze body suit soaked in aqueous cream, sometimes with the addition of

Table 4.3 First line treatment of atopic eczema

Treatment	Example
Emollients	Emulsifying ointment
Topical steroids	1% hydrocortisone
Bandaging	Calabands®
Treat secondary infection	Erythromycin
Sedative antihistamines	Chlorpheniramine
Reassurance/self-help groups	National Eczema Society

hydrocortisone). At other times, emollients may be applied directly to the skin, or used as a soap sub- stitute (dissolved in a jug of boiling water before adding to the bath).

Topical steroids

Active areas of eczema should be treated with topical steroids. There is prejudice against such medication, stemming from side effects which resulted from inappropriate use of these drugs in the past. Such fears need to be allayed, as undertreatment can be just as harmful and is common. A class IV steroid (1% hydrocortisone) is the most frequently used strength in children, and is the only preparation that should be used for the face. However, stronger preparations (class II) may occasionally be required at other sites for short periods, to gain control, before reducing to a class III or IV preparation. Combination steroid–antibiotic preparations are sometimes useful if recurrent infection is a problem.

Bandaging

Application of topical therapies beneath occlusive bandaging (e.g. Quinabands, Calabands) is soothing, improves penetration and reduces excoriation by protecting the skin. It is particularly helpful for lichenified and excoriated eczema but clioquinol (Quinabands) should be avoided in very young children.

Antihistamines

Non-sedative antihistamines are of no benefit in atopic eczema. Although sedative antihistamines have little effect on the pruritus of eczema, they may help a restless child to sleep, but care should be taken if the child also suffers from asthma, because of the possible risk of respiratory depression. Overuse of such sedative preparations may have a hangover effect and impair concentration at school during the day. Using chlorpheniramine maleate rather than trimeprazine tartrate can minimize this problem, because it has a shorter duration of action.

Tar and tar–steroid combinations

Tar preparations were commonly used in the past. Topical therapy with combination products (e.g. 5% liquor picis carbonis in 0.05% clobetasone butyrate) can be very beneficial in treating lichenification.

Exclusion diets

The role of dietary manipulation in the management of atopic eczema is controversial, but it should only be attempted under the supervision of a dietician, as there is a real danger of malnutrition (especially calcium deficiency) with unsupervised diets. High circulating levels of IgG antibody to β-lactoglobulin have now been shown to be useful in predicting which children are likely to benefit from dietary restriction.

Reduction of house-dust mites

Reducing dust levels in the home (e.g. by damp dusting, vacuuming and special mattress covers) will produce a degree of improvement in the skin.

Hospitalization

This not only facilitates time-consuming treatments, but is associated with an improvement *per se*, pro- bably due to low house-dust levels in the clinical environment. The advantages of in-patient treat- ment need to be balanced with the emotional effect of admission. Overall, there is now an increasing trend towards out-patient management for most cases.

Second-line therapy

1 Controlled trials have not shown oral supplements of evening primrose oil to be beneficial in treating atopic eczema. However, there is anecdotal evidence that they can be helpful in treating the lichenified eczema of Afro-Caribbean children.
2 Photochemotherapy (PUVA) has been successful in treating intractable eczema, but its use in children is reserved for extremely severe cases only, because of the risks of carcinogenesis.

3 Chinese herbal therapies are currently generating a lot of interest, but are still the subject of research to evaluate their true potential. The exact properties of the active ingredients are unknown, but they probably act through immunosuppression.

COMPLICATIONS

Secondary infections

Children with atopic eczema are vulnerable to infections, especially viral disease.

1 Bacterial infections: eczema frequently becomes secondarily infected, especially by staphylococci. Treatment is with courses of oral antibiotics guided by microbiological swabs and sensitivities. Resistance to common antibiotics can be a difficulty. If recurrent infections are a problem, it is worth excluding staphylococcal carriage (in the nose, axilla and perineum) in the child or the parents. Such staphylococcal carriage can be eradicated with topical mupirocin.

2 Viruses: it used to be thought that viral infections were more common in children with atopic eczema, but it has now been shown that these children have no increased susceptibility to common warts.

(a) Eczema herpeticum: superimposed herpes simplex infection spreads rapidly; in the days before effective antiviral therapy, it used to be associated with a significant mortality. Sheets of discrete vesicles (Fig. 4.12) that produce a studded appearance are the hallmark, particularly around the head and neck. The vesicles heal with crusting. While eczema herpeticum usually represents a primary infection, recurrences do occur. Vulnerable children should not be exposed to other family members with cold sores. Examination of vesicular fluid by electron microscopy provides rapid confirmation of the diagnosis, and treatment is with systemic acyclovir (200 mg orally (100 mg in children < 2 years) five times a day for 5 days).

(b) Mollusca contagiosum: children with atopic eczema are particularly susceptible to infection with mollusca.

Striae

Inappropriate use of potent topical steroids in the treatment of atopic eczema can result in cutaneous atrophy and striae, but such overtreatment is rare today. In contrast, the bad press of the past has resulted in a public backlash against the use of topical steroids, which can mean that children are denied optimum treatment.

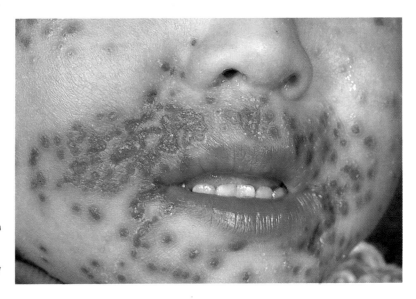

Fig. 4.12 *Eczema herpeticum.* The herpes simplex virus spreads rapidly on eczematous skin, forming crops of umbilicated vesicles. This young girl's eczema herpeticum was complicated by a dendritic corneal ulcer.

Chapter 5
Other Forms
of Eczema

Introduction

This chapter deals with variants of eczema distinct from atopic dermatitis, which is covered separately in Chapter 4. It includes other forms of endogenous eczema and those due to exogenous causes, such as irritant and allergic contact dermatitis (see Table 4.1).

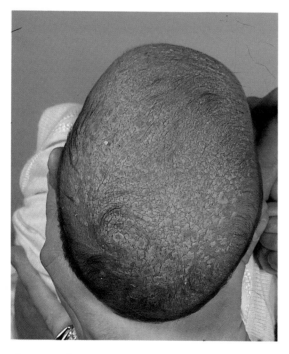

Fig. 5.1 *Cradle cap.* Thick, yellow, heaped-up scales, especially in the frontal area, are common in young babies.

Infantile seborrhoeic dermatitis

DEFINITION

A self-limiting eczematous eruption occurring during the first weeks of life, particularly on the face, scalp and flexures.

AETIOLOGY

The aetiology of this disorder is not fully established, but seborrhoeic dermatitis of infancy is distinct from the condition known as seborrhoeic dermatitis in adults, which is associated with the organism *Pityrosporum ovale*. Despite the name, there is no established link with sebum production.

CLINICAL FEATURES

In contrast to atopic eczema, which appears to be becoming more common, seborrhoeic dermatitis appears to be becoming less so. Onset is early, usually in the first 6 months of life, and often at the age of 2–6 weeks.

The key physical signs of the condition are outlined in Table 5.1. In its mildest form it constitutes simple cradle cap, in which large yellow scales become crusted on the scalp (Fig. 5.1). Most babies have a degree of this in the first few weeks of life. It may progress to involve other areas such as the napkin area (Fig. 5.2) and the face (Fig. 5.3), especially along the eyebrows and the retro-auricular folds. From these sites the dermatitis spreads (e.g.

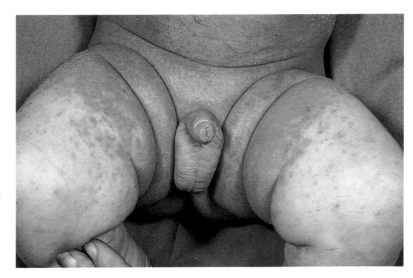

Fig. 5.2 *Seborrhoeic dermatitis.* Bright red erythema, which may be moist in the skin folds, is present with some scale. The napkin area is often most affected, but the baby is undisturbed by the condition.

down the sides of the face and to the skin flexures, particularly around the neck and axillae) and may rapidly become confluent. The skin is red, moist and glistening, with flaking at the edges of the involved areas. In contrast to irritant napkin dermatitis, the condition involves the skin creases, which may occasionally become eroded. Despite its extent, the infant is usually asymptomatic, and in stark contrast to a child with atopic dermatitis, appears content and unbothered by the eruption. The rash resolves over the course of 2–3 weeks and, with the exception of the napkin area, does not usually recur.

Seborrhoeic dermatitis may precede atopic eczema, and children who have seborrhoeic dermatitis appear to have a slightly increased risk of subsequently developing psoriasis.

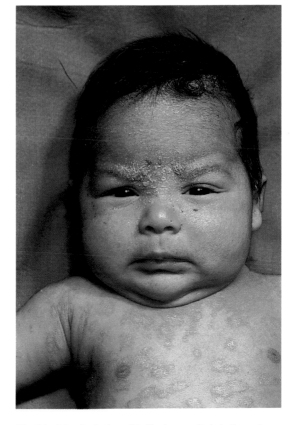

Fig. 5.3 *Seborrhoeic dermatitis.* The face, particularly the eyebrows, may be affected.

Table 5.1 Clinical features of seborrhoeic dermatitis

Scalp	Thick, greasy, yellow scales
Body	Erythema Fine, yellowish scale Affects face (eyebrows, cheeks, retro-auricular folds) and skin folds (often moist)

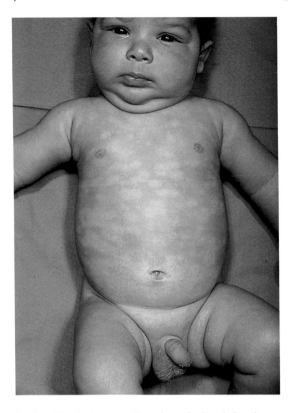

Fig. 5.4 *Seborrhoeic eczema.* The rash usually clears before the age of 3 months, but residual (temporary) postinflammatory hypopigmentation is common in black children's skins.

COMPLICATIONS

1 Infection: secondary infection may occur, e.g. with *Candida*.
2 Hypopigmentation: in Afro-Caribbean children secondary postinflammatory hypopigmentation may be prominent (Fig. 5.4) and a source of parental anxiety. Reassurance that these pigmentary changes are not permanent is all that is required.

DIFFERENTIAL DIAGNOSES

1 Atopic eczema (see Chapter 4): this is rare before the age of 3 months but is characterised by discomfort from pruritis. There is often a family history of atopy.
2 Napkin psoriasis (Fig. 5.5): the rash is composed of well-defined, dry, red, scaly plaques, extending up onto the trunk.
3 Leiner's disease (Fig. 5.6): this commences in the neonatal period and resembles severe seborrhoeic dermatitis culminating in erythroderma. It is accompanied by intractable diarrhoea and failure to thrive and is associated with immunodeficiency. Complement levels are reduced and there is impaired neutrophil chemotaxis, resulting in recurrent infections.

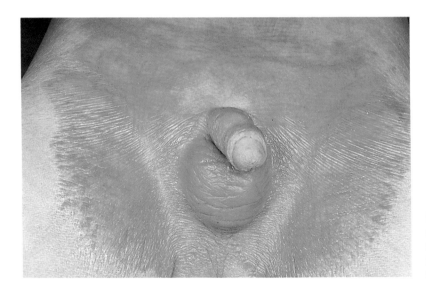

Fig. 5.5 *Napkin psoriasis.* When it occurs in the napkin area, it is well defined and the skin is dry and scaly rather than moist and glistening, as in eczema. It is rare in babies.

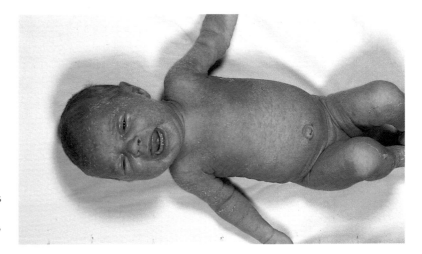

Fig. 5.6 *Leiner's disease.* The infant is erythrodermic and, unlike a child with seborrhoeic dermatitis, appears unwell, with diarrhoea and poor weight gain.

MANAGEMENT

Cradle cap

1 Mild: use arachis oil massaged into the scalp. Medicated shampoos and preparations containing salicylic acid are not recommended for use in the very young, because they are irritant and there is a risk of systemic absorption of salicylate through the scalp.
2 Severe: use 1% hydrocortisone lotion.

Seborrhoeic dermatitis

1 Daily bath with an emollient as soap substitute.
2 Weak topical steroids applied to the inflamed areas of the body are most useful if combined with an antifungal agent (e.g. hydrocortisone + either nystatin or an imidazole).
3 Topical preparations containing borage oil (rich in γ-linoleic acid) have recently been found to be highly effective in treating seborrhoeic dermatitis.

Irritant dermatitis

The newborn infant's skin is especially sensitive to irritants, the most common manifestation of which is napkin dermatitis. However, inappropriate use of topical antiseptics, impregnated baby wipes and some infant bath solutions may produce an irritant reaction in the very young. Even plastic hospital identity bracelets have been found to cause a transient dermatitis in some children.

Primary irritant napkin dermatitis (diaper dermatitis)

DEFINITION

An eczematous eruption occurring on the exposed areas of the perineum, secondary to the irritant effect of excreta.

AETIOLOGY

Prolonged contact with urine and faeces will produce irritation caused by the release of ammonia from bacterial degradation. A high urinary pH contributes and occlusion (e.g. by plastic pants) enhances the irritation by both disrupting the statum corneum and increasing penetration of the irritants. The resultant macerated and eroded skin frequently becomes colonized by *Candida albicans*, so perpetuating the dermatitis. The disorder may be found in children attending nurseries and crèches, where gastroenteritis is more common, but in general has become less frequent in recent years, due to the increased use of absorbant disposable nappies.

Some infants develop an unexplained transient but florid napkin dermatitis when they are teething.

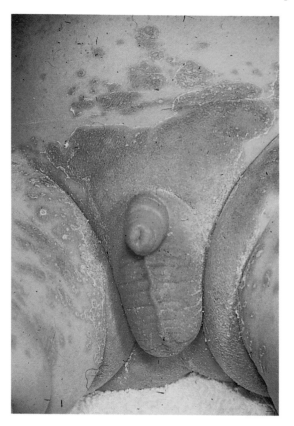

Fig. 5.7 *Napkin candidosis.* Individual satellite pustules are present away from the main body of the eruption.

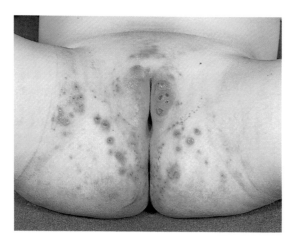

Fig. 5.8 *Jacquet's dermatitis.* This is a variant of irritant napkin dermatitis in which erosions predominate, usually as a result of poor parental care.

CLINICAL FEATURES

Clinical features of napkin dermatitis are outlined in Table 5.2. Napkin dermatitis is rare in the immediate neonatal period. It most frequently starts between the ages of 1 and 3 months, and reaches a peak incidence between 7 and 12 months. It is the most common cause of a rash in the napkin area, and it is estimated that at least 50% of all children are affected to some degree at some stage.

The key physical sign is of confluent erythema on the convex surfaces of the perineum (i.e. those areas in direct contact with the nappy) with sparing of the skin folds. The skin surface often appears glazed, and may become eroded in severe cases. The rash is usually quite well delineated, but can become disseminated.

Satellite pustules are seen if the skin becomes secondarily infected with *Candida* (from faecal contamination) (Fig. 5.7).

In severe examples, Jacquet's dermatitis erosions and vesicles may form (Fig. 5.8), which resembles eczema herpeticum (see p. 45), but no virus will be isolated.

DIFFERENTIAL DIAGNOSES

1 Seborrhoeic dermatitis: the deep skin creases are usually involved, and there is often evidence of the condition elsewhere (e.g. scalp or neck).
2 Napkin psoriasis: if scale is a very prominent feature, it may herald the development of psoriasis in later life.
3 Perianal dermatitis of the newborn: a form of irritant dermatitis, most common in formula-fed babies, in which a localized, annular area of erythema develops, 2–4 cm around the anal margin during the first weeks of life. Severe cases may become eroded.

Table 5.2 Clinical features of napkin dermatitis

Glazed erythema
Convex surface of perineum
Spares skin creases
May become eroded
Satellite pustules (represent secondary infection)

COMPLICATIONS

As in the case of seborrhoeic dermatitis, the affected area frequently becomes transiently hypopigmented in children with black skin.

MANAGEMENT

1 Attention to hygiene, with frequent napkin changes and, if possible, periods when the baby's skin is left exposed to air.
2 Clean soiled areas at each change, and dry thoroughly. Apply a barrier emollient at changing times (e.g. white soft paraffin or zinc and castor oil).
3 Mild topical steroids either alone or in combination with an anti-infective agent (e.g. nystatin, clioquinol or oxytetracycline).

Infantile gluteal granuloma

DEFINITION

Purplish-brown, ovoid nodules which develop as a complication of primary irritant napkin dermatitis.

AETIOLOGY

The condition appears to be a modern development, and has only been described in the last 20 years. It is thought that the occlusion produced by modern nappies may be responsible, but topical steroids used in the treatment of napkin dermatitis have also been implicated. The nodules may develop once the original napkin dermatitis has cleared.

CLINICAL FEATURES

Despite the name, the nodules are not confined to the gluteal region, but may occur anywhere within the perineum or thighs (Fig. 5.9). They tend to lie along the long axis of the skin creases.

MANAGEMENT

The nodules usually regress spontaneously over the course of several months, but topical steroids should be avoided. Reassurance and general advice about napkin care should be given.

Lip-licking dermatitis

DEFINITION

A well-circumscribed perioral dermatitis resulting from a habit tic.

AETIOLOGY

Repetitive licking of the skin produces an irritant, chaffing effect.

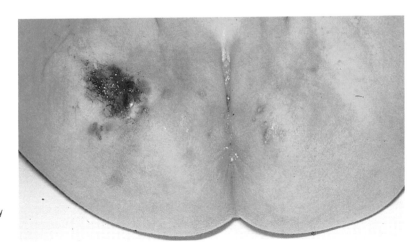

Fig. 5.9 *Infantile gluteal granuloma.* Purplish nodules occur in the napkin area. The lesions resolve spontaneously after some months (courtesy of Dr J. McLelland).

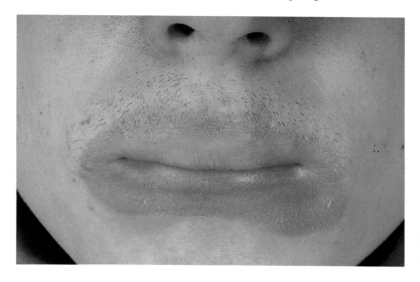

Fig. 5.10 *Lip-licking dermatitis.* This habit tic results in a well-circumscribed perioral irritant dermatitis.

CLINICAL FEATURES

The skin is dry with erythema and some scale. The condition occurs most prominently over the central part of the upper lip but may encircle the lips (Fig. 5.10).

DIFFERENTIAL DIAGNOSIS

Occasionally a similar appearance may occur with a food allergy or contact sensitivity to toothpaste.

MANAGEMENT

Treatment is to stop the lip-licking. Topical steroids should only be used in the short term. However, breaking the habit is hard and the behaviour may be denied by both parents and child. The use of emollients can be helpful because they provide a barrier and often have an unpleasant taste, so discouraging further licking.

Contact dermatitis

True allergic contact dermatitis (e.g. to nickel) is becoming more prevalent in children (Fig. 5.11), but remains relatively rare. However it is often underinvestigated. In the UK metals and topical steroids appear to be the most relevant allergens, but

in the USA it is plants of the *Rhus* species, which are normally responsible. Poison ivy (Fig. 5.12) and poison oak are such potent sensitizers that they merit special attention.

Rhus dermatitis

DEFINITION

An acute dermatitis resulting from exposure of a sensitive individual to the allergen occurring in members of the Anacardiaceae group of plants.

AETIOLOGY

All parts of the plant, but especially the root, are allergenic. *Rhus* dermatitis is extremely common in North America. Poison ivy occurs most frequently in the eastern part of the country, and poison oak in the western states.

CLINICAL FEATURES

Brushing against the plant produces a vesicobullous eruption in a haphazard, often linear pattern (Fig. 5.13). Indirect exposure (e.g. touching an animal which has been in contact with the plant) can cause an attack in a very sensitive subject, but produces a more diffuse dermatitis.

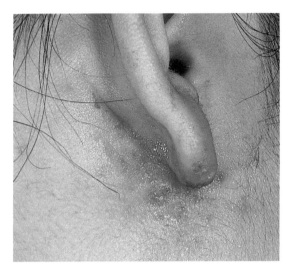

Fig. 5.11 *Contact dermatitis.* Itching, weeping, redness and scaling occur on the ear lobes and retro-auricular skin due to a delayed hypersensitivity to metal.

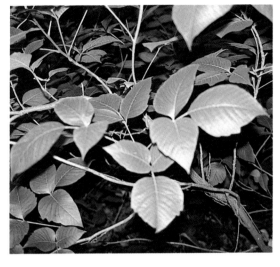

Fig. 5.12 *Poison ivy.* This weed is common in North America and is a potent contact sensitizer of the skin (courtesy of Dr C. Lovell).

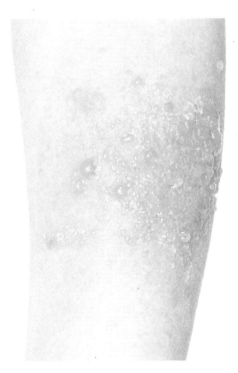

Fig. 5.13 *Poison ivy dermatitis.* An acute weeping, vesicular eruption occurs at the points of contact with the plant allergen (courtesy of Dr C. Lovell).

MANAGEMENT

1 Potent topical steroids are required.

2 In severe attacks a reducing course of oral steroids may be necessary.

3 Individuals who live or holiday in areas where the plants grow freely need to be taught to recognize and avoid the culprit vegetation.

Phytophotodermatitis

DEFINITION

An acute phototoxic eruption due to the interaction of sunlight and furocoumarins present in certain plants.

AETIOLOGY

The sap from certain species of plant (e.g. giant hogweed, cow parsley and rue) is phototoxic. Playing in overgrown gardens or meadows on a sunny day can result in the development of a striking dermatitis where the sap has come into contact with the skin.

CLINICAL FEATURES

The eruption consists of vesicular linear streaks of florid dermatitis, which frequently becomes bullous (Fig. 5.14). Lesions resolve to leave prominent post-inflammatory hyperpigmentation, which takes weeks to clear.

DIFFERENTIAL DIAGNOSIS

The eruption can be so severe, and the lesions produce such bizarre shapes, that the condition has been confused with non-accidental injury.

MANAGEMENT

Treatment is with a superpotent (grade I) topical steroid during the acute phase.

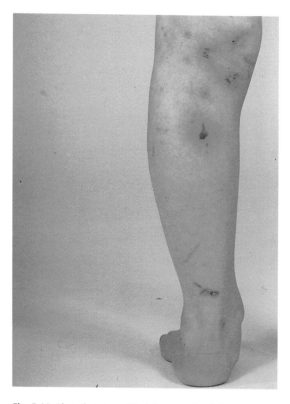

Fig. 5.14 *Phytophotodermatitis.* A linear, vesiculobullous eruption occurs as a result of a reaction between sunlight and furocoumarins which are photosensitizers in certain plants.

Pompholyx

DEFINITION

An endogenous eczema, characterized by a highly pruritic vesicular eruption of the palms and soles.

AETIOLOGY

Pompholyx may occur in atopic eczema, or as an isolated phenomenon. Irritants and allergens may occasionally produce this pattern of eczema, but often no cause can be found. Many patients have concomitant hyperhidrosis and the condition is sometimes known as dyshidrotic eczema.

CLINICAL FEATURES

The eruption occurs on the ventral aspect of the hands and feet. The palms and soles may be affected together or singly. Individual lesions are vesiculo-bulous, but can be seen to be multilocular in origin (Fig. 5.15). Erythema is often minimal. It is rare in very young children.

Resolution takes place with desquamation of the separated statum corneum over the course of 2–3 weeks.

MANAGEMENT

1 Rest.
2 Antiseptic soaks to dry up the vesicles (potassium permanganate 1:8000 solution or 10% aluminium acetate).
3 Potent topical steroids.

Juvenile plantar dermatosis

DEFINITION

A condition of dry erythema and fissuring confined to the plantar forefoot and unique to children.

AETIOLOGY

The eruption has only been described in the last 30 years. It is thought to be due to changes in modern

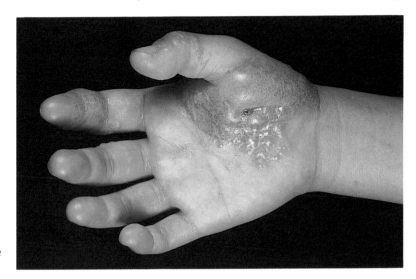

Fig. 5.15 *Pompholyx.* Florid, multiloculated vesicles coalesce to produce large bullae on the palms. The condition is intensely pruritic.

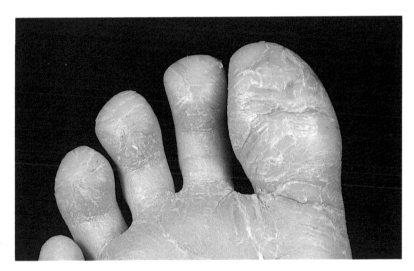

Fig. 5.16 *Juvenile plantar dermatosis.* There is chronic fissuring and a well-defined shiny erythema on the weight-bearing plantar skin. It is symmetrical.

hosiery and footwear, particularly the use of synthetic materials, and enclosed styles of shoes such as trainers, which promote occlusive conditions. The additional role of sweating and friction is unproven, and the relationship to atopy is controversial. Patch testing to the shoe battery is negative.

CLINICAL FEATURES

The disorder is most common between the ages of 8 and 14 years. The affected area becomes painful with a glazed red appearance (Fig. 5.16). The changes are most prominent around the ball of the foot and spare the toe creases. The problem tends to resolve during the teen years.

MANAGEMENT

Although cotton socks and open shoes are often recommended, many patients report that wearing these is of little benefit.

Topical steroids, on the whole, are ineffective, but urea containing emollients may be of value to affected children.

Lichen striatus

DEFINITION

A striking linear eruption composed of small pink papules, which follow Blaschko's lines, and occur most frequently on one of the limbs (Fig. 5.17).

AETIOLOGY

The aetiology of the condition is unknown, but the histology is eczematous, with varying degrees of spongiosis.

CLINICAL FEATURES

Lichen striatus may occur at any age but appears to be most prevalent in children aged between 5 and 15 years. The papules are hypopigmented in dark skins. It is asymptomatic, but the appearance may cause alarm. The disorder may affect the nails, which become ridged, if the eruption reaches the distal digits and involves the proximal nail folds.

DIFFERENTIAL DIAGNOSIS

The eruption needs to be distinguished from other linear rashes, especially epidermal naevi and linear lichen planus (Fig. 5.18).

MANAGEMENT

The condition is unresponsive to topical steroids. However, it is self-limiting, resolution taking between 3 and 18 months.

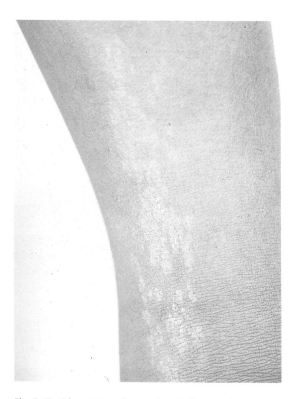

Fig. 5.17 *Lichen striatus.* Clusters of small, flat-topped, hypopigmented papules occur in a linear fashion along the long axis of a limb.

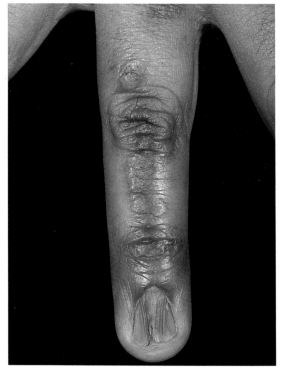

Fig. 5.18 *Linear lichean planus.* Purplish flat-topped papules occur in a linear manner and extend to involve the nail, with pterygium formation.

Pityriasis alba

DEFINITION

A non-specific process in which discrete areas of mild eczema resolve to leave hypopigmentation, especially on the face.

AETIOLOGY

The condition has been considered a variant of atopic eczema because it tends to occur in atopic patients, but it is not confined to this group. Exposure to the sun may highlight the condition in fair skin.

CLINICAL FEATURES

Lesions are small, up to a few centimetres in diameter, and may be composed of faint erythema, with fine surface scale. The face is the most usual site, but the upper trunk may also be affected. Often the patients only present with the final hypopigmentation (Fig. 5.19).

MANAGEMENT

The condition is self-limiting, but the pigmentary irregularities may take many months or years to fade. Simple bland emollients are all that are required to reduce the scale.

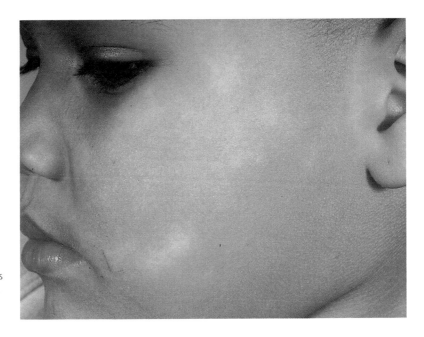

Fig. 5.19 *Pityriasis alba.* Multiple, asymptomatic, hypopigmented macules on the face. They are most prominent on pigmented skin and may be very persistent.

Introduction

Erythematous eruptions occurring as either plaques
or papules, in which the predominant feature is
scale, may be considered together as the papulo-
squamous disorders. They will often be considered
in the differential diagnosis of each other.

Psoriasis

There are several variants of psoriasis which may
affect children.

Chronic plaque psoriasis

DEFINITION

An inflammatory disease with an hereditary basis,
characterized by hyperproliferation of the epidermis.

AETIOLOGY

Psoriasis is a disorder characterized by hyperproliferation of the epidermis. Cellular kinetics are
increased tenfold, such that the epidermal turnover
time in psoriasis is reduced to 3 days. The hyperkeratotic changes in the epidermis are accompanied
by dilatation of the dermal capillaries and an inflammatory cell infiltrate. Lymphocytes are thought to
play a central role in the pathogenesis of psoriasis,
but neutrophils are also prominent histologically and
may form small collections (micro-abscesses) within
the epidermis.

The precise aetiology is not known, but there is a
strong family history in many cases. The disease is
inherited as an autosomal dominant with variable
penetrance, and there is linkage with certain histo-
compatability antigens (HLA), especially Cw6.

Psoriasis is often precipitated by infection and
over half the children presenting with psoriasis have
evidence of a recent streptococcal sore throat (e.g.
a positive throat swab or anti-streptolysin O titre).
Trauma is another important factor which can
initiate the disease (the Koebner phenomenon; Fig.
6.1). There is some evidence that cold weather and
emotional stress can also exacerbate the disease.

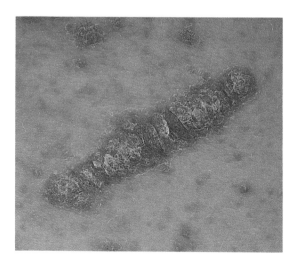

Fig. 6.1 *Koebner phenomenon.* Psoriasis may develop in sites of
trauma, for instance along scratch marks.

CLINICAL FEATURES

Thirty per cent of psoriatics develop their disease before 20, and 10% before 4 years. However, it is rare under the age of 2 years, but when it does occur in the very young it is usually in the napkin area (Fig. 6.2, see also Fig. 5.5). The mean age of onset in children is between 7 and 8 years. In adults, men and women are equally affected, but in children, girls are more frequently so. It is much more common in whites than blacks, but the disease is not uncommon in Asians.

Lesions consist of sharply demarcated erythematous plaques with coarse, adherent silvery scales (Fig. 6.3). The plaques may be itchy. The disease has a predilection for extensor surfaces (Fig. 6.4), but in children the face (especially around the eyes) and scalp are often the first areas to be affected (Fig. 6.5). The genitalia may be involved (Fig. 6.6). In contrast to adults, the palms, soles and nails are more frequently spared. If the nails are affected, it tends to be with pitting rather than onycholysis (Fig. 6.7). However, a solitary pustular acrodermatitis may be seen in association with psoriasis, called parakeratosis pustulosa (see p. 216). The disease follows a relapsing and remitting course.

DIFFERENTIAL DIAGNOSES

1 Tinea corporis: the lesions are usually asymmetrical or unilateral, in contrast to psoriasis, which is symmetrical.

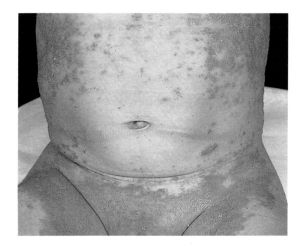

Fig. 6.2 *Napkin (diaper) psoriasis.* Psoriasis is rare before the age of 2 years, but occasionally may commence in the napkin area and spread elsewhere.

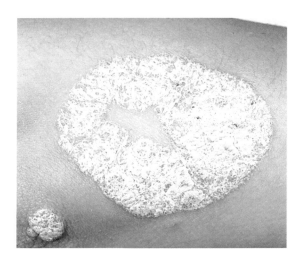

Fig. 6.3 *Psoriasis.* The plaques are very well defined, red in colour and have a thick white scale.

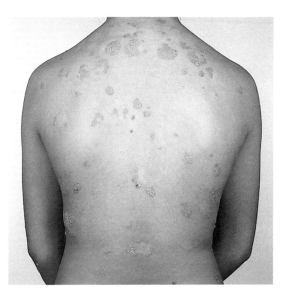

Fig. 6.4 *Psoriasis.* The lesions are relatively symmetrical and affect predominantly extensor surfaces.

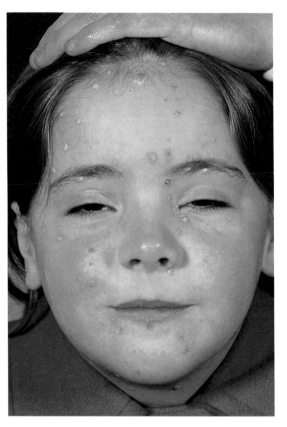

Fig. 6.5 *Psoriasis.* In children, the face and scalp may be the first sites to be affected.

2 Pityriasis rubra pilaris (see p. 69): follicular hyperkeratosis is characteristic.

COMPLICATIONS

Arthritis is less common in children than adults, but may precede the skin disease. It is seronegative and is usually a monoarthritis of a large joint such as the knee.

MANAGEMENT

Topical steroids

Mild topical steroids are ineffective in psoriasis. Potent and superpotent formulations are temporarily effective but need to be used judiciously, as the condition is chronic. However, they are easy to use and cosmetically acceptable and are therefore frequently prescribed as initial therapy. However, dermatologists usually prefer other treatment options.

Dithranol

Dithranol is an antimitotic agent. For in-patient management, it is usually applied according to the Ingram regime (gradually increasing strengths of

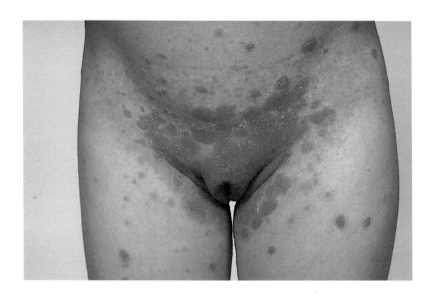

Fig. 6.6 *Psoriasis.* Lesions in the genital area may be very inflamed.

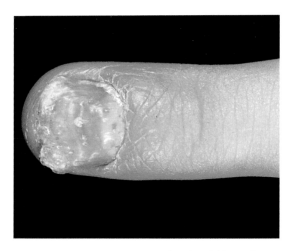

Fig. 6.7 *Psoriasis.* The nail may be affected in children with psoriasis, but this is less common than in adults.

dithranol in Lassar's paste applied daily under stockinette occlusion, in conjunction with tar baths and ultraviolet (UV) B therapy). Short-contact therapy, in which higher concentrations of dithranol (in a cream base) are left on the skin for half an hour and then washed off, may be more convenient at home. Care must be taken not to get the ointment onto the surrounding normal skin as it is an irritant and may cause burning and erythema. The preparation is effective, but sometimes unpopular because it is messy and stains the skin brown temporarily.

Tar

1 Tar shampoos are helpful for the scalp.
2 Tar preparations are used as a soap (20% liquor picis carbonis in emulsifying ointment) and as a photosensitizer in regimes involving UVB (e.g. Ingram, Goeckeman).
3 Tar may be combined with potent topical steroids in formulations such as 5% liquor picis carbonis in 0.05% clobetasone butyrate as a useful treatment for the hairline and flexures.

Ultraviolet B

Psoriasis often improves after a sunny holiday. Supervised courses of artificial UVB can be beneficial alone or as an adjunct to other treatments.

Systemic therapy

Systemic therapy is rarely justified in childhood, but in exceptional cases of erythrodermic psoriasis or severe recalcitrant disease, methotrexate or psoralens and ultraviolet A (PUVA) therapy may be employed under specialist supervision.

Acute guttate psoriasis

DEFINITION

A self-limiting variant of psoriasis, precipitated by infection and characterized by widely disseminated, small (droplet-sized) lesions.

AETIOLOGY

The eruption follows 2–3 weeks after an acute infection (Fig. 6.8). In most cases this is a throat infection due to *Streptococcus pyogenes*, but other infections, e.g. measles, may be implicated.

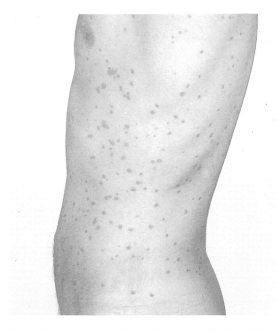

Fig. 6.8 *Guttate psoriasis.* A myriad of small drop-like (guttate) red papules with silver scale develop explosively a couple of weeks after an acute streptococcal throat infection.

CLINICAL FEATURES

Multiple, pale red plaques up to 1 cm in diameter are scattered all over the body, especially the trunk The eruption resolves over the course of 3 months.

DIFFERENTIAL DIAGNOSIS

In pityriasis rosea (see p. 63) the lesions have a collarette of scale and a herald patch is diagnostic.

MANAGEMENT

1 A course of UVB (often in conjunction with tar therapy) can lessen the intensity of the rash.
2 Emollients and a moderate topical steroid may provide symptomatic relief.

Pustular psoriasis

DEFINITION

A rare variant of psoriasis.

Fig. 6.9 *Generalized pustular psoriasis.* This is a rare, acute, widespread erythema studded over its surface with sterile pustules and associated with pyrexia and toxaemia.

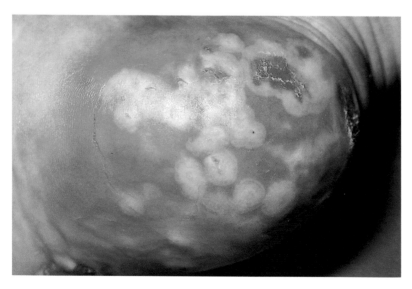

Fig. 6.10 *Localized pustular psoriasis.* Sterile pustules may develop on a background of erythema localized particularly to the palmar or plantar surfaces.

AETIOLOGY

The cause is unknown, but factors implicated in other forms of psoriasis are probably responsible.

CLINICAL FEATURES

Generalized pustular psoriasis is rare in children, but it may begin in infancy, and affects more boys than girls. There is often a prior history of an inflammatory eruption in the napkin area. Widespread pustules develop on erythematous skin (Fig. 6.9) with resolution by exfoliation. The acute episode may be accompanied by fever and malaise. Recurrences are common, but the disease usually follows a benign course. Some children may later develop chronic plaque psoriasis. A more localized variant has been described in older children (Fig. 6.10).

DIFFERENTIAL DIAGNOSES

1 Staphylococcal scalded skin syndrome: there is burning, erythema, desquamation and erosion but no pustules.
2 Pityriasis rubra pilaris type V (see p. 70): the islands of sparing, keratoderma and lack of pustules distinguish this condition from pustular psoriasis.

MANAGEMENT

1 Moderately potent topical steroids and emollients are effective in treating localized disease, but they can exacerbate the generalized form.
2 Systemic therapy, e.g. very small doses of methotrexate, may be required to control the disease. Oral retinoids have been used in children, but close monitoring is required to observe any bony abnormalities.
3 Dapsone or sulphapyridine are reported to be effective, if they can be tolerated.

Pityriasis rosea

DEFINITION

A common, self-limiting cutaneous eruption in young people with a characteristic evolution and distribution on the trunk.

AETIOLOGY

The cause is unknown; it is thought to be viral, but there is no objective evidence for this other than that the disease occasionally occurs in clusters, is reported in institutions and has a peak incidence in the spring and autumn. In the majority of cases no other family member is affected.

CLINICAL FEATURES

The disease is rare in the very young. There may be mild prodromal symptoms of an upper respiratory tract infection, but for the most part the rash begins with the appearance of a single, large, ovoid, erythematous lesion, known as the 'herald patch' (Fig. 6.11), most often on the shoulder. Smaller plaques

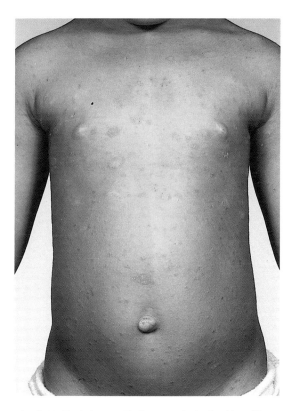

Fig. 6.11 *Pityriasis rosea.* The larger patch, the 'herald patch', over this 4-year-old girl's right chest was the first manifestation of the subsequent rash.

erupt over the trunk a few days later (Fig. 6.12). Lesions begin as small papules, which spread outwards (Fig. 6.13), producing a characteristic peripheral collarette of scale (Fig. 6.14). They tend to be distributed in parallel to the lines of the ribs. The rash spreads to the proximal limbs and may occasionally extend up onto the neck. The face is usually spared, but may be affected, especially in black children. The eruption is normally asymptomatic, but in severe cases may become quite urticated and itchy. It resolves over 3–6 weeks without scarring. A more chronic form of the eruption, an eczematide, may occur in Afro-Caribbean children (Fig. 6.15).

MANAGEMENT

No treatment is usually necessary. A moderately potent topical steroid may be used if the eruption is pruritic.

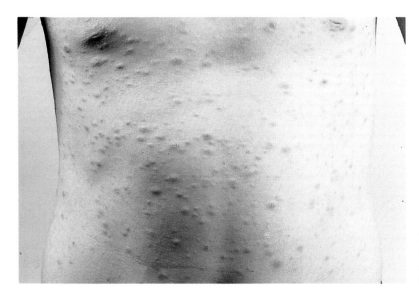

Fig. 6.12 *Pityriasis rosea.* The eruption commences several days after an initial solitary lesion. The torso is predominantly affected.

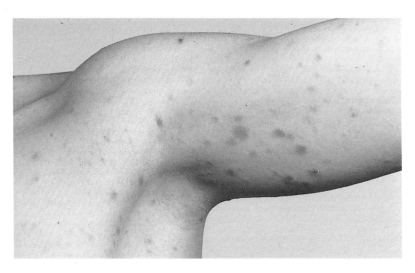

Fig. 6.13 *Pityriasis rosea.* The lesions may be papular at first, but expand into pink patches with an annular scale.

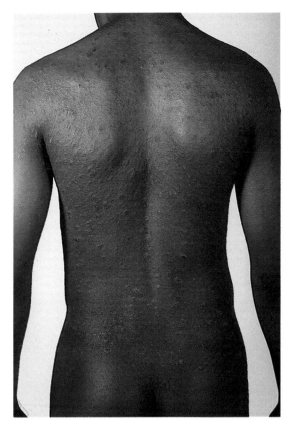

Fig. 6.14 *Pityriasis rosea.* The eruption affects the trunk, upper arms and thighs, but rarely the face, forearms or shins. The peripheral 'collarette' of scale is clearly seen.

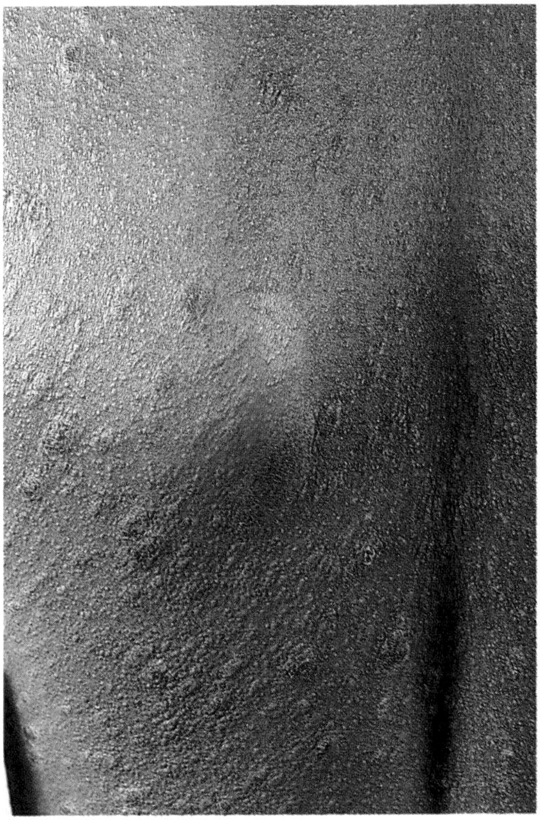

Fig. 6.15 *Pityriasis rosea.* In Afro-Caribbean children the initial erythema may be difficult to discern, but this close-up of Fig. 6.14 shows the pigmented patches with a peripheral collarette of scale.

Lichen planus

DEFINITION

An itchy, violaceous, mucocutaneous eruption, less common in children than adults, with a distinctive histology.

AETIOLOGY

The aetiology of this disorder is unknown. Histologically, there is band of thymus-derived lymphocytes immediately below the epidermis which results in liquefaction necrosis of the basal cells. The rete pegs are flattened outwards and have a saw-tooth-like appearance, and the melanin released from melanocytes is ingested by macrophages in the dermis. There is an increase in the granular cell layer. There are usually no precipitants but trauma (the Köebner response) and infection are reported and an association with hepatic disease is well recognized. It has been postulated that the thymus is protective, and that thymic function accounts for the rarity of lichen planus in childhood.

CLINICAL FEATURES

Lichen planus is uncommon in children. The largest series in childhood has been reported from India, where the disease is shown to be more common in boys. In children, the site and morphology of the disease do not follow the typical adult pattern.

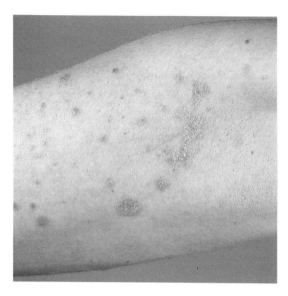

Fig. 6.16 *Lichen planus.* The papules or plaques are a distinctive violaceous or red-purple colour.

Intensely pruritic, violaceous (Fig. 6.16), hyperkeratotic papules and plaques occur most prominently over the wrists, ankles and trunk (Fig. 6.17). The fine white reticulum of scale over the surface of the lesions, the Wickham's striae, that is pathognomonic of classical lichen planus may not be obvious in children. Lesions often occur in sites of trauma, as a Koebner phenomenon. The lesions may be follicular, linear (see also Fig. 5.18) or occasionally bullous, but mucosal involvement is very rare in children (Fig. 6.18). The eruption lasts 12–18 weeks, and postinflammatory hyperpigmentation may be marked (Fig. 6.19). Nails are occasionally affected (Fig. 6.20; see also Fig. 5.18) in children as well as in adults.

DIFFERENTIAL DIAGNOSIS

In patients who have had a bone-marrow transplant, graft-versus-host disease may resemble lichen planus, but the clinical context and histology enable the correct diagnosis to be made.

MANAGEMENT

1 Superpotent topical steroids for short periods will relieve the pruritus.
2 In some rare cases (e.g. bullous disease) a reducing course of systemic steroids may be necessary.

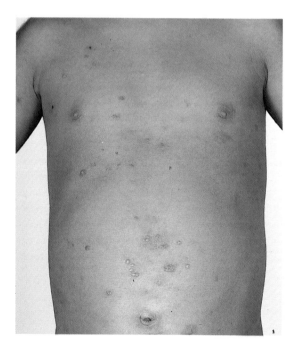

Fig. 6.17 *Lichen planus.* The lesions are flat-topped, purple papules and have a shiny surface; they are itchy, symmetrical and may be widespread on the trunk. This young patient developed lichen planus in association with cryptogenic cirrhosis.

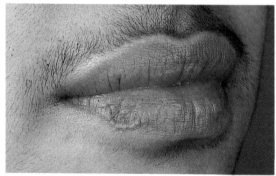

Fig. 6.18 *Lichen planus.* There is an annular white eruption on the lower lip.

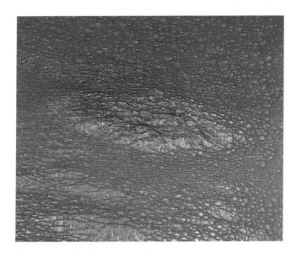

Fig. 6.19 *Lichen planus.* Postinflammatory hyperpigmentation occurs in all races but is marked in pigmented races.

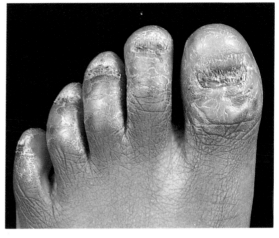

Fig. 6.20 *Lichen planus of the nail.* This is difficult to diagnose, for the condition is rare; in the absence of classical cutaneous lichen planus, biopsy may be necessary before the true nature of this destructive process is recognized.

Lichen nitidus

DEFINITION

A lichenoid eruption composed of clusters of pinpoint, flesh-coloured papules.

AETIOLOGY

The aetiology is unknown. The condition is histologically similar to classical lichen planus, but is immunologically distinct, which suggests that it is a different disorder.

CLINICAL FEATURES

The condition is uncommon, but typically occurs in children and adolescents. Myriads of small, monomorphic papules 1–2 mm in diameter (Fig. 6.21) erupt over the abdomen, arms or buttocks. Lesions have a flat-topped, shiny surface and are usually non-pruritic.

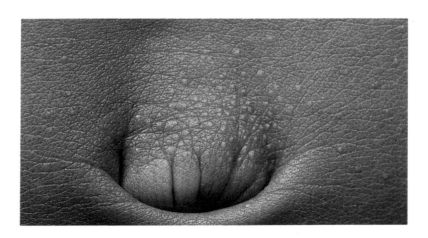

Fig. 6.21 *Lichen nitidus.* Small, monomorphic, flat-topped, flesh-coloured papules occur in the same sites as lichen planus.

The eruption may last a long time, but is eventually self-limiting. It is usually asymptomatic and rarely requires treatment.

Pityriasis lichenoides

DEFINITION

A reactive disorder with lymphocyte infiltration of the skin and a widespread polymorphic eruption of purpuric and necrotic papules.

AETIOLOGY

The cause of the condition is not known, but there is some evidence that it may be infective and mediated through immune complexes.

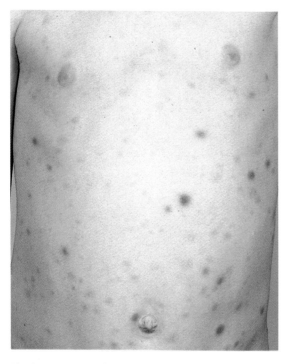

Fig. 6.22 *Pityriasis lichenoides varioliformis et acuta.* Crops of non-itchy pink or red papules which may be haemorrhagic, urticated or vesicular (and therefore mistaken for varicella) occur over a number of weeks on the trunk and limbs.

CLINICAL FEATURES

In children, the disorder most often occurs between the ages of 5 and 10 years. Two forms of the disease are recognized, an acute variant and a more chronic variant, but both types of lesion may be found simultaneously.

1 Pityriasis lichenoides varioliformis et acuta (Mucha–Habermann disease): crops of non-pruritic, pink, urticated papules appear on the trunk (Fig. 6.22) and along the inner aspect of the limbs. If they become vesicular, the condition may be mistaken for varicella. On rare occasions, the rash is accompanied by mild fever, but it is more often asymptomatic. The lesions are often purpuric. They may become necrotic centrally and heal to leave a small depressed scar. The papules appear in crops so that there are always lesions in different stages of evolution, hence the name varioliformis.

2 Pityriasis lichenoides chronica (guttate parapsoriasis): the eruption has a predilection for the inner aspect of the limbs (Fig. 6.23). Small, firm, reddish-brown papules (Fig. 6.24) with flecks of adherent (mica-like) scale develop which slowly flatten over the course of a month to leave a faint pigmented macule. As the rash clears, transient hypopigmentation may be seen, but there is no scarring.

DIFFERENTIAL DIAGNOSES

1 Chicken pox: if there is any clinical doubt, the two conditions can be distinguished by virology.

2 Secondary syphilis: palmoplantar lesions may occur in pityriasis lichenoides, but mucosal involvement is diagnostic of syphilis. Serology will confirm the diagnosis.

3 Guttate psoriasis (see p. 61): there is no purpura and the lesions are mostly truncal and do not become necrotic.

MANAGEMENT

1 A course of UVB is the most usual treatment, but the rash may recur on cessation of therapy.

2 Erythromycin has been found to be beneficial in some cases.

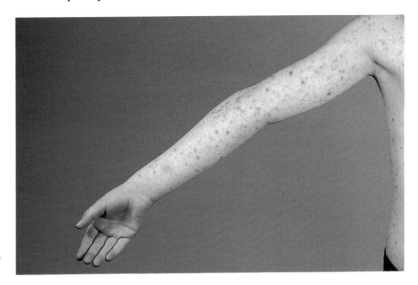

Fig. 6.23 *Pityriasis lichenoides chronica.* The eruption has a predilection for the inner aspect of the limbs and is symmetrical.

Fig. 6.24 *Pityriasis lichenoides chronica.* The papules may be a distinctive red-brown or pink colour with an adherent scale.

Pityriasis rubra pilaris (PRP)

DEFINITION

A rare disorder characterized by hyperproliferation of the epidermis, follicular keratosis, keratoderma and erythroderma.

AETIOLOGY

The aetiology is unknown, but genetic factors may be important.

CLINICAL FEATURES

Five variants of PRP have been described, but only types III–V affect children.

1 Type III (juvenile classical PRP): the disease begins in children between the ages of 5 and 10 years and may follow an acute infection. Orange-red plaques develop and the child may rapidly become erythrodermic (Fig. 6.25). A characteristic feature are small islands of normal skin within the erythematous plaques. Follicular plugging is usually prominent and there is a palmoplantar

keratoderma. The condition tends to clear within 1–2 years of its onset.

2 Type IV (juvenile onset – circumscribed): localized, sharply demarcated erythematous plaques develop on the knees (Fig. 6.26) and elbows. The lesions are reminiscent of psoriasis, but with prominent follicular keratoses ('nutmeg grater' skin). This variant follows a more chronic course than type III PRP, but may clear in the teens.

3 Type V (juvenile onset – atypical): the disease begins earlier, usually in infancy, with erythema and an accompanying keratoderma. The condition tends to persist.

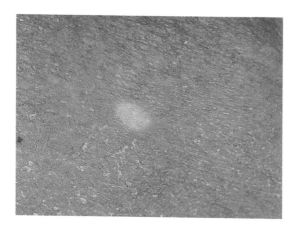

Fig. 6.25 *Juvenile classical pityriasis rubra pilaris.* The child is erythrodermic so virtually all the skin is involved, although some islands of normal skin are often visible.

DIFFERENTIAL DIAGNOSES

1 Psoriasis: follicular plugging distinguishes PRP from psoriasis (see p. 58). Histologically, there are no micro-abscesses in PRP.

2 Congenital ichthyosis: erythema and keratoderma may be prominent, but follicular plugging would suggest PRP.

MANAGEMENT

1 In the acute phase, rest and emollients are the mainstay of treatment.

2 In severe disease, oral retinoids may be used in adults but their use in children is more controversial.

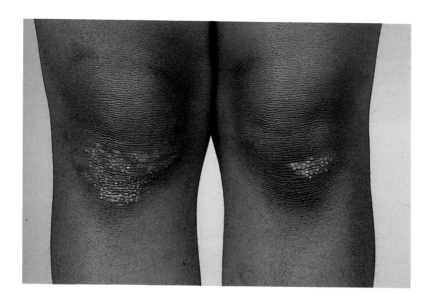

Fig. 6.26 *Juvenile onset circumscribed pityriasis rubra pilaris (type IV).* This is a more common variant, localized to the elbows and knees. Occurring particularly in childhood, it is often mistaken for psoriasis.

Introduction

Bacterial infections are common in childhood. The most prevalent tend to be relatively minor and readily treated with antibiotics. However, some of the rare and more serious infections are also discussed in this chapter.

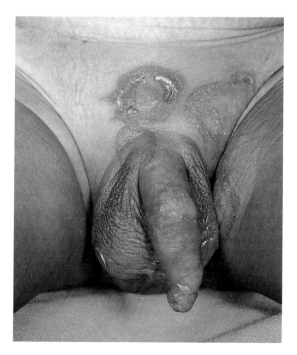

Fig. 7.1 *Impetigo.* The lesions are annular and contain pus. They may occur anywhere on the skin.

Impetigo

DEFINITION

A common, superficial, highly contagious bacterial infection of the skin.

AETIOLOGY

The condition is nearly always due to infection with *Staphylococcus aureus*, but occasionally streptococci may be responsible for non-bullous impetigo.

CLINICAL FEATURES

Annular erythematous lesions, 1–2 cm in diameter, with a honey-coloured crust on the surface may occur anywhere on the body (Fig. 7.1), but are most common on the face (Fig. 7.2). Multiple lesions are frequent, reflecting the infectious nature of the condition. Staphylococcal infections may become bullous (Fig. 7.3), especially in young children.

DIFFERENTIAL DIAGNOSIS

Blistering distal dactylitis is a condition where a solitary, superficial lake of pus may occur on the finger pulp. It is usually due to a streptococcus and responds rapidly to a course of penicillin.

COMPLICATIONS

Acute glomerulonephritis can complicate strepto-

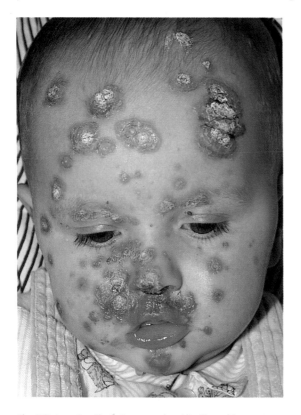

Fig. 7.2 *Impetigo.* The lesions spread rapidly. The golden crusts are apparent. *Staphylococcus aureus* is the most common cause.

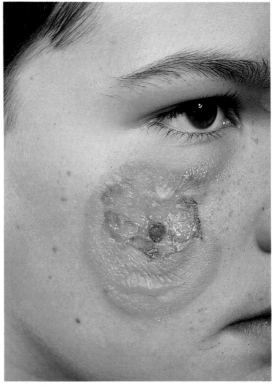

Fig. 7.3 *Impetigo.* The lesions start as blisters that contain a purulent fluid which subsequently becomes crusted. The face is a common site.

coccal impetigo, but is less common than it used to be in western countries.

MANAGEMENT

1 Prompt treatment is required to limit the spread of infection.

2 Topical antibiotics (chlortetracycline or fusidic acid) may be of value in minor cases, and are particularly helpful in softening and removing the crusts. Mupirocin is also effective, but its use is best restricted to cases of methicillin-resistant *S. aureus*, as indiscriminate community use encourages resistance.

3 A course of oral antibiotics is the treatment of choice. Flucloxacillin is most frequently used, or erythromycin if the child is allergic to penicillin.

4 The child is very contagious and should not go to school until the infection has resolved. At home, the child should have separate face-cloths and towels from the rest of the family, to help reduce cross-infection.

5 If repeated attacks occur, the child and other members of the family should be screened for carriage of *Staphylococcus* in the nose, axilla or groin. Staphylococcal carriers should be treated with chlorhexidene baths and applications of mupirocin cream.

Folliculitis

DEFINITION

A bacterial infection of hair follicles.

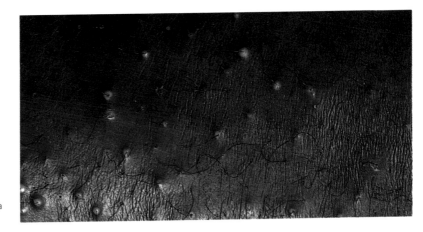

Fig. 7.4 *Folliculitis.* Small, discreet yellow pustules are centred around a follicular orifice.

AETIOLOGY

The infection is usually staphylococcal, but occasionally pseudomonas (acquired from jacuzzis and whirlpools) may be responsible. Occlusive conditions promote folliculitis and the infection may be precipitated by topical steroids.

CLINICAL FEATURES

Small yellow pustules (Fig. 7.4) are scattered over the affected area. Each lesion is centred around a follicular orifice and there may be surrounding erythema. Many eruptions are quite localized, but large, deep, painful abscesses (boils), termed furunculosis, may occur. Where several adjacent follicles become infected and discharge through multiple sinuses, the lesion is called a carbuncle.

MANAGEMENT

1 Swabs should be taken for microscopy and culture to identify the causal organism and determine its sensitivities.
2 Treatment is with appropriate oral antibiotics (usually flucloxacillin or erythromycin).
3 Large boils which are pointing should be incised to allow drainage of pus.
4 Diabetes should be excluded in cases of widespead infection.
5 If the infection becomes recurrent, the patient and immediate family should be screened for staphylococcal carriage (see above).

Ecthyma

DEFINITION

A deep necrotic infection of the skin.

AETIOLOGY

The infection is caused by *Staphylococcus aureus* and may arise from secondary infection of a penetrating injury or insect bite (Fig. 7.5).

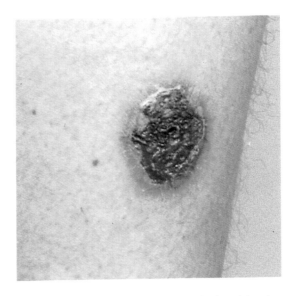

Fig. 7.5 *Ecthyma.* The infection occurs more deeply and there is a shallow ulcer under the crust.

A localized tender area of redness and induration develops around a necrotic ulcer covered by a thick black crust.

MANAGEMENT

The crust should be gently removed and the underlying slough cleaned with normal saline and covered with a non-adherent dressing. Oral antibiotics should be taken for 7–10 days, as for impetigo.

Staphylococcal scalded skin syndrome (Ritter's disease)

DEFINITION

A serious staphylococcal infection characterized by widespread, superficial epidermal necrolysis.

AETIOLOGY

The causative agent is a toxin-producing, coagulase-positive, group II *Staphylococcus*, usually phage type 71. The toxin is disseminated from the original focus of infection (e.g. the ear, umbilicus or circumcision scar) via the bloodstream to the skin. Occasionally, a sibling with impetigo may be the source of the infection.

CLINICAL FEATURES

The condition may affect people of any age, but it is most characteristic in young babies. The rash is preceded by tenderness and burning in the skin, and the infant is pyrexial, uncomfortable and restless. An initial faint erythema is rapidly followed by the development of oedema. The epidermis becomes puckered before separating to leave large glistening, denuded areas (Fig. 7.6). The head and flexures are initially affected but the condition rapidly becomes generalized. The epidermis is readily stripped off, the level of separation being subcorneal. A second, milder, 'peel' may occur 3–4 days after the initial episode.

DIFFERENTIAL DIAGNOSIS

Toxic epidermal necrolysis is a different disorder, often drug-induced and generally seen in adults rather than children. It is more severe. The epidermal split occurs at a deeper level (at the dermo–epidermal junction) and mucous membranes may be involoved.

MANAGEMENT

1 Prompt treatment is imperative, as without appropriate therapy the condition carries a 50% mortality.

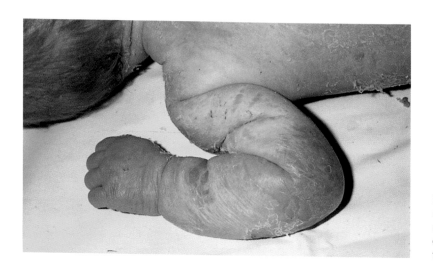

Fig. 7.6 *Staphylococcal scalded skin syndrome.* The child is pyrexial and restless. The skin is tender and the epidermis separates in sheets leaving the skin glistening and denuded.

2 Systemic antibiotics (e.g. flucloxacillin or a cephalosporin) are the key element of treatment.
3 Careful attention should be paid to fluid balance, body temperature and possible protein loss.

Dermatitis cruris pustulosa et atrophicans

DEFINITION

A superficial, pustular infection of the legs seen in Afro-Caribbean patients.

AETIOLOGY

The use of thick emollients produces occlusion of the follicular orifice, and promotes secondary infection by *Staphylococcus*.

CLINICAL FEATURES

Large (up to 1 cm in diameter), superficial lakes of pus are seen on the legs (Fig. 7.7). Each lesion is centred on a follicle (Fig. 7.8). The condition is commoner in women, but may occur in young girls if oily moisturizers are used to produce a glistening skin.

MANAGEMENT

1 Stop the use of emollients.
2 Short courses (5–7 days) of oral antibiotics (e.g. flucloxacillin).

Cellulitis

DEFINITION

A deep infection of the dermis and subcutaneous tissues.

AETIOLOGY

The condition is usually caused by a *Streptococcus*, but in children a unilateral facial cellulitis may complicate *Haemophilus influenzae* infection of the middle ear. Recurrent attacks of cellulitis may be secondary to lymphatic insufficiency or damage.

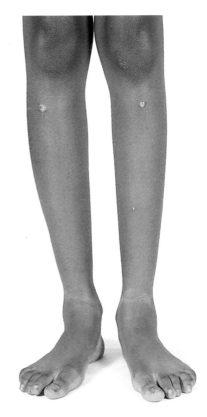

Fig. 7.7 *Dermatitis cruris pustulosa et atrophicans.* These pustular lesions usually occur on the limbs of black people and are secondary to follicular occlusion due to the application of oil to the skin with secondary sepsis.

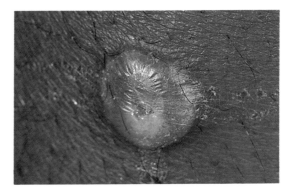

Fig. 7.8 *Dermatitis cruris pustulosa et atrophicans.* The pustular morphology of this form of folliculitis is apparent.

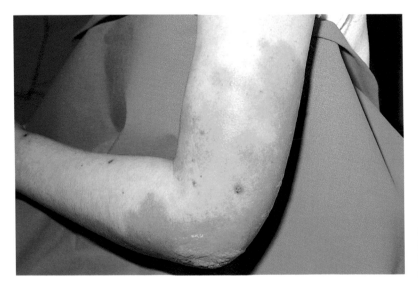

Fig. 7.9 *Cellulitis.* The skin is red, hot, tender and swollen and may even blister. The patient is pyrexial and unwell.

CLINICAL FEATURES

The patient is febrile and unwell. The affected area is often quite well localized. The skin is red, hot, tender and indurated (Fig. 7.9). Well-demarcated areas of cellulitis, especially when facial, are often termed erysipelas (Fig. 7.10). A limited, more superficial, cellulitis of the perineum occurs in children under the age of 10 years. Localized erythema and oedema develop in the vulval or perianal region.

Pain on defaecation may lead to secondary constipation. The condition responds rapidly to oral antibiotic therapy.

MANAGEMENT

1 Rest and, in the case of an involved limb, elevation.
2 Systemic antibiotics guided by microbiological sensitivities, e.g. penicillin for streptococcal infections and amoxycillin (or augmentin) for *Haemophilus*.

Scarlet fever (streptococcal toxic erythema)

DEFINITION

A systemic infection due to *Streptococcus pyogenes*, with a characteristic generalized erythematous rash. It has become much less common in western countries in recent years.

AETIOLOGY

Group A *Streptococcus* produces an erythrotoxin responsible for the high fever seen in the condition. The systemic infection usually spreads from a membranous tonsillitis.

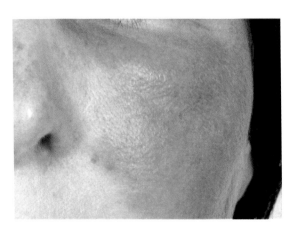

Fig. 7.10 *Erysipelas.* The infection involves the face and is typically unilateral.

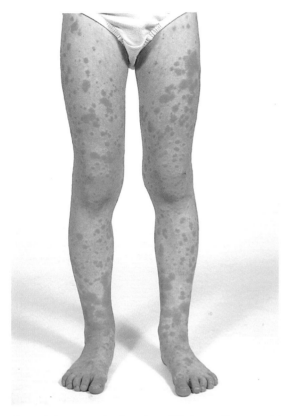

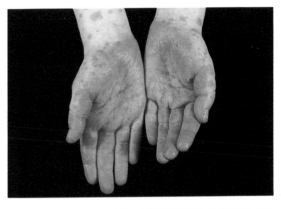

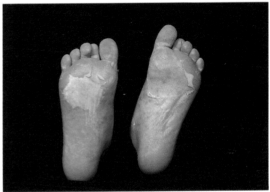

Fig. 7.11 *Streptococcal toxic erythema.* This 4-year-old was pyrexial and unwell. There is a blotchy erythema. The throat swab grew a group A *Streptococcus.* (The same patient as in Fig. 7.12.)

Fig. 7.12 *Streptococcal toxic erythema.* (a) There is a punctate erythema on the palms. (b) Subsequent to the erythema, there is desquamation, which is particularly noticeable on the palms and soles.

CLINICAL FEATURES

The incubation period of scarlet fever is 2–5 days. The cutaneous features begin with a punctate erythema, accompanied by fever and malaise. The skin involvement is most marked on the face (which is flushed, with perioral sparing), trunk and limbs (Fig. 7.11). The mucous membranes are bright red. The tongue is coated, with prominent papillae causing it to resemble a strawberry. The thick white coat peels off after a few days to reveal a bright red tongue, which resolves over the next 7 days. The erythematous lesions (Fig. 7.12a) resolve over the same period by desquamation, which is particularly obvious on the palms and soles (Fig. 7.12b).

COMPLICATIONS

The acute infection may be followed by:
1 glomerulonephritis;
2 rheumatic fever;
3 myocarditis.

MANAGEMENT

1 Early treatment with systemic penicillin is essential to minimize the occurrence of systemic complications.
2 If renal or cardiac complications ensue, specialist care is mandatory.

Meningococcal septicaemia

DEFINITION

A severe, life-threatening disseminated infection, in which haemorrhagic and necrotic cutaneous lesions develop in association with meningitis.

AETIOLOGY

The organism *Neiseria meningitidis* is spread via droplets. Once infection occurs, bacteraemia results in multiorgan involvement through immune-complex vasculitis.

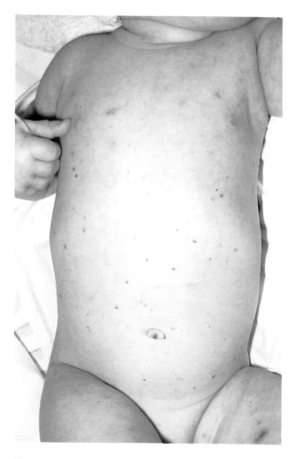

Fig. 7.13 *Meningococcal septicaemia.* There are widespread, small, purpuric papules secondary to direct invasion of cutaneous blood vessels by the *Neisseria* bacteria (courtesy of Dr C. Ball).

CLINICAL FEATURES

The incubation period is short. Small purpuric papules (Fig. 7.13) develop, characteristically on the lower legs, accompanied by fever and meningism. The lesions rapidly become disseminated and necrotic. The infection can affect any age group, but is most prevalent among children in the first decade of life.

COMPLICATIONS

1 The infection spreads through the bloodstream and therefore any organ may be affected, but meningitis is the most common presentation.
2 Disseminated intravascular coagulopathy may complicate the septicaemia.
3 Adrenal haemorrhage (Waterhouse–Friederickson syndrome) is a serious complication.

MANAGEMENT

1 High-dosage antibiotics (penicillin or chloramphenicol) should be given immediately the diagnosis is suspected. Delay of even a few hours can be fatal.
2 Rifampicin prophylaxis should be given to close contacts.

Cat-scratch disease

DEFINITION

An indolent disease characterized by granulomatous lymphadenitis.

AETIOLOGY

The disease is transmitted by cats. The exact organism is still uncertain, but there appears to be an overlap with the bacteria responsible for the condition bacillary angiomatosis seen in AIDS. It is a small bacillus, probably one of the proteobacteria, either *Alipia felis* or *Rochalimaea henselae*.

CLINICAL FEATURES

This is a rare disease, but the majority of cases occur

in children or teenagers. A small red papule develops at the site of inoculation (Fig. 7.14) (usually a scratch from a cat). It slowly expands, ulcerates and crusts over. The cutaneous signs may be quite minimal. There may be a low fever in about half the cases. Painful, regional lymphadenopathy develops within 2 weeks. The bacillus may be identified on skin or lymph node biopsy using the Warthin–Starry stain.

Complications

Encephalitis, osteomyelitis or septic shock may occur in immunocompromised patients.

MANAGEMENT

Most antibiotics are ineffective. The disease usually runs a benign course with full recovery in most cases. In severe infection, cephalosporins, amikacin or gentamicin may control the disease.

Lyme disease

DEFINITION

An arthropod-borne infection acquired in forested areas, which produces multiorgan involvement with a characteristic annular rash.

AETIOLOGY

The organism, a spirochaete, *Borrelia burgdorferi*, is transmitted by tick bites (the *Ixodes* tick). The infection is named after a town in Connecticut and is most prevalent in the eastern USA, but it has now been described throughout Australia and Europe, including the New Forest in the UK. Small mammals, especially rodents, are the main reservoir of infection, and deer, sheep and cattle are affected.

CLINICAL FEATURES

The peak incidence for infection is May and June. The disease may affect any age, including children. The characteristic eruption, erythema chronicum migrans, develops 1–2 weeks after the bite in 90% of cases, but onset may occasionally be delayed up to 5 weeks. The rash slowly expands outwards in an annular fashion from the original bite (Fig. 7.15).

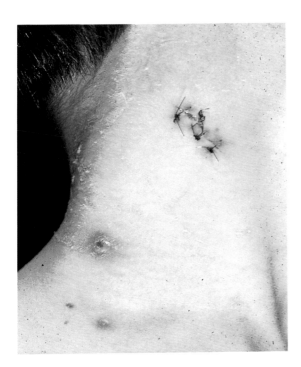

Fig. 7.14 *Cat scratch disease.* Two small ulcerated papules are visible on the neck. There was extensive lymphadenopathy and the surgical scar relates to recent lymph node biopsy (courtesy of Dr G. Lee).

Fig. 7.15 *Lyme disease.* There is an erythema which spreads outwards from the site of the tick bite. In this case the bite was acquired while picnicking in a deer park and the disease was accompanied by myalgia and arthralgia.

The erythema is thus most marked at the advancing edge of the lesion, producing the characteristic appearance of erythema chronicum migrans. There may be associated lymphadenopathy. The cutaneous disease may persist for several months before becoming disseminated.

COMPLICATIONS

1 Neurological: meningitis, mononeuritis multiplex.
2 Cardiac: myocarditis, arrhythmias.
3 Arthritis.
4 Cutaneous: about 10% of patients develop secondary skin lesions (acrodermatitis chronica atrophicans).

DIFFERENTIAL DIAGNOSIS

Other insect (e.g. spider) bites may be difficult to distinguish in the early stages. The diagnosis of Lyme disease is confirmed by positive serology (enzyme-linked immunoadsorbent assay, ELISA).

MANAGEMENT

1 The earlier the antibiotic treatment, the less chance of later serious disease with major organ involvement.
2 Doxycycline for 3 weeks is the optimal treatment, but erythromycin is partially active against the organism.
3 In children Amoxycillin or phenoxymethyl penicillin daily is the preferred regime.

Kawasaki disease (mucocutaneous lymph node syndrome)

DEFINITION

An infection first described in Japan in 1967, characterized by high fever, desquamative rash and lymphadenopathy, which may be associated with serious cardiac sequelae and sudden death.

AETIOLOGY

The causal organism has not been identified, but is thought to act as a superantigen, capable of stimulating massive cytokine release, so inducing a marked immunological response.

CLINICAL FEATURES

Although the disease has been reported most commonly in Japan, it occurs worldwide. It most often affects 3–6-year-olds, but the diagnosis may often be missed. The infection begins with the onset of high fever, lasting an average of 8 days. The eyes become infected and the lips red and cracked. A maculopapular rash follows (Fig. 7.16), and transient, itchy, red plaques may develop. The hands and feet become red and swollen and then desquamate, peeling beginning distally around the

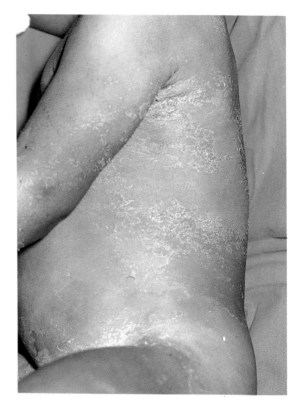

Fig. 7.16 *Kawasaki disease.* Fever, general erythema with desquamation, conjunctival congestion, dry red lips, red swollen palms and soles with cervical lymphadenopathy are features of this disease (courtesy of Professor J. Price).

finger tips and moving proximally. Cervical lymphadenopathy is present in at least 50% of affected children.

COMPLICATIONS

1 Coronary artery aneurysms may develop, which can result in arrhythmias, myocardial ischaemia or sudden death. Coronary artery damage is most frequent in children in whom the fever persists for longer than 2 weeks.
2 Peripheral gangrene may complicate infection in children under the age of 1 year.

DIFFERENTIAL DIAGNOSIS

The rash and conjunctival injection of measles (see p. 87) initially are quite similar to those of Kawasaki disease, but there is no palmoplantar desquamation. In measles there is a relative leucopenia and the platelet count may be low. In contrast, in Kawasaki disease there is a leucocytosis, thrombocytosis and a high erythrocyte sedimentation rate.

MANAGEMENT

1 Rapid recognition of the syndrome, with early administration of intravenous gammaglobulin, reduces the risk of cardiac complications. The optimum regime is still under investigation, but a single 2 g/kg dose appears superior to the 4-day schedules administered in the past.
2 Aspirin should be given to reduce fever, and has not been associated with Reye's syndrome in this context.
3 Echocardiography should be used to monitor coronary artery size at diagnosis and 4 weeks after treatment to assess whether aneurysms have developed.

Tuberculosis

DEFINITION

A granulomatous bacterial infection which may affect a variety of organs, including the skin. It is now less common in westernized countries, but there has been some resurgence of the infection in patients with AIDS.

AETIOLOGY

Mycobacterium tuberculosis or *M. bovis* are the responsible organisms, but the incidence of infection has declined since the advent of bacille Calmette–Guérin (BCG) inoculation. The primary organ infected is usually the lung (in the case of *M. bovis*, the gut) and the disease is spread by droplets. Primary infection of the skin (tuberculous chancre) is rare (Fig. 7.17). Cutaneous infection is normally a secondary phenomenon.

CLINICAL FEATURES

Tuberculosis of the skin is relatively rare and now usually only seen in immigrants or in immunocompromised patients. It may take several forms.

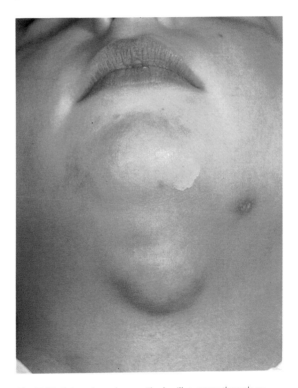

Fig. 7.17 *Tuberculous chancre.* The bacillus enters through an abrasion and produces a red-brown papule and is associated with regional adenitis.

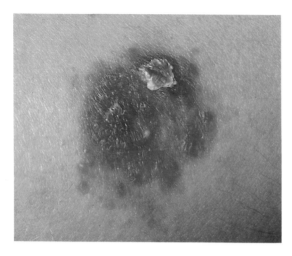

Fig. 7.18 *Lupus vulgaris.* There is a well-defined red-brown plaque, most commonly on the cheek. It is very rare in westernized countries.

1 Lupus vulgaris is caused by secondary infection of the skin. Reddish-brown, gelatinous papules form soft plaques (Fig. 7.18) which may ulcerate. The 'apple-jelly' nodules may be more clearly seen on diascopy (pressing a glass microsope slide against the skin).

2 Scrofuloderma: multiple sinuses can develop within an indurated area of skin as a result of breakdown of an underlying tuberculous lymph gland.

3 Tuberculosis verrucosa cutis: a slowly expanding, purple-brown, warty plaque develops as a result of contact with contaminated sputum in children who are already infected with tuberculosis and therefore have some degree of immunity. It is rare.

4 Erythema nodosum: this is the most common presentation of tuberculosis. Red, tender nodules occur on the legs, especially the shins (Fig. 7.19) and calves. Mycobacterial DNA has been demonstrated in the lesions by the polymerase chain reaction.

5 Tuberculides: these occur as a result of haematogenous spread of the bacillus, secondary to active tuberculosis elsewhere. The histology of the lesions is granulomatous. Indolent inflammatory necrotic

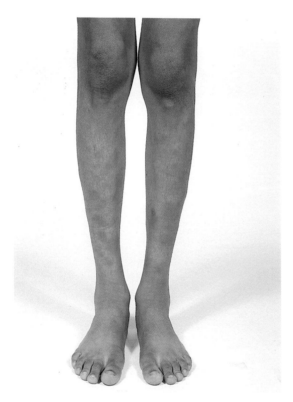

Fig. 7.19 *Erythema nodosum.* Red, tender nodules occur on the lower legs. This 14-year-old Indian boy was found to have consolidation of the middle lobe secondary to tuberculosis.

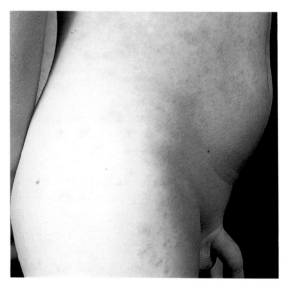

Fig. 7.20 *Lichen scrofulosorum.* Small lichenoid yellow-brown papules occur on the trunk. A skin biopsy showed a granulomatous histology and suggested the diagnosis (courtesy of the Institute of Dermatology).

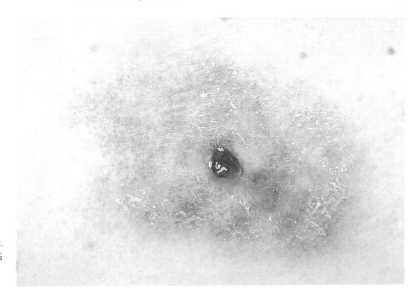

Fig. 7.21 *BCG vaccination granuloma.* This is a common complication of BCG inoculation. It discharges and persists as a sore.

papules may occur on the extremities (papulonecrotic tuberculide) or small lichenoid, often follicular, papules (Fig. 7.20) on the trunk (lichen scrofulosorum). They are very rare in western countries.

MANAGEMENT

1 The diagnosis should be confirmed by identifying acid-fast bacilli in a skin biopsy and subsequent culture.
2 Triple therapy should be given with isoniazid and rifampicin for 6 months, plus pyrazinamide for the initial 2 months. Ethambutol can cause disturbances of colour vision and is better avoided in children.

BCG vaccination granuloma

Persistent purulent ulceration occasionally develops at the site of BCG inoculation (Fig. 7.21). Treatment is the same as for lupus vulgaris, but milder cases may settle with potent topical steroids.

Swimming pool granuloma (fish tank granuloma)

DEFINITION

An atypical mycobacterial infection of the skin.

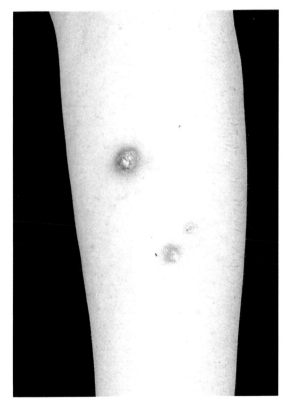

Fig. 7.22 *Fish tank granuloma.* This youth injured himself whilst cleaning out his fish tank. The fish had died from *Mycobacterium marinum* which was inoculated into his skin.

AETIOLOGY

The eruption is caused by *Mycobacterium marinum* and may be acquired through grazing the skin in a contaminated swimming pool or from infected fish in those who keep tropical fish as a hobby.

CLINICAL FEATURES

Indurated erythematous papules slowly enlarge and eventually ulcerate. Infection usually occurs on the feet in swimmers, but the back of the hands or lower arms (Fig. 7.22) in fish-fanciers. The infection may spread proximally along the lymphatics in a sporotrichoid manner.

MANAGEMENT

1 The diagnosis should be confirmed by culture of a skin biopsy at low temperatures (32°C).
2 Co-trimoxazole (or tetracycline in teenagers but not young children) is more effective than standard antituberculous drugs, but the infection can be quite resistant to treatment.
3 If a swimming pool is considered to be the source of infection, the public health authorities must be notified and the chlorination procedure monitored carefully.

Syphilis

DEFINITION

An infection with the spirochaete *Treponema pallidum* which is usually acquired sexually, but can be transmitted transplacentally.

AETIOLOGY

The infection is very rare in childhood, except in cases of childhood prostitution in Third World countries. In countries where serological tests for syphilis are performed routinely during pregnancy, transplacental transmission of maternal infection should not occur, but cases have been reported in the USA in recent years, most in deprived ethnic minorities.

CLINICAL FEATURES

The severity of the congenital syndrome depends at which stage in pregnancy infection occurs, and very early infection may result in spontaneous abortion. Although some infants with congenital syphilis may be asymptomatic at birth, over 50% develop a syphilitic rash by the age of 6 months. The baby is of low birth weight, snuffly, with failure to thrive and hepatosplenomegaly. Non-pruritic copper-red macules and papules develop on the skin, especially in the napkin area and on the palms and soles. The eruption may become bullous. Moist plaques of condyloma lata may develop in the genital area. Later signs of congenital infection include the classical triad of linear fissures around the mouth (rhagades), saddle nose and conical (Hutchinson's) teeth.

Acquired infection is occasionally seen in adolescence. Most cases should be diagnosed in the

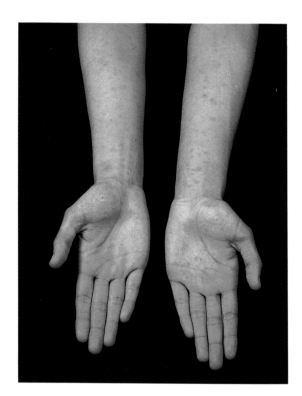

Fig. 7.23 *Secondary syphilis.* The eruption is widespread on the trunk and limbs and is red-brown or copper coloured. It does not itch.

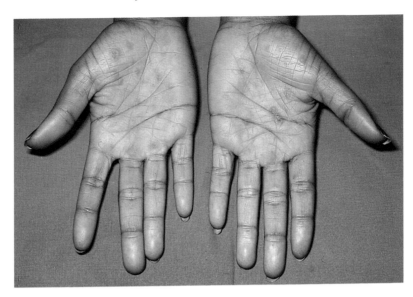

Fig. 7.24 *Secondary syphilis.* The palmar and plantar surfaces are characteristically involved with brown macules as in this 17-year-old.

primary stage of a painless sore or ulcer (chancre) on the genitalia or around the anus, but may occur at any point of cutaneous contact or in the rectum and on the cervix. If the infection is missed, the secondary stage ensues within a couple of months. The patient is unwell, has a fever, generalized lymphadenopathy and a non-pruritic, red-brown macular (Fig. 7.23) or papular rash on the face, genitalia trunk and characteristically on the palms (Fig. 7.24) and soles. Patches in the intertriginous areas of the groin and around the anus (condylomata lata) are moist and eroded and highly infectious. White eroded patches occur in the mouth. Hair loss is common. If untreated, the condition may remit or pass on to the tertiary stage and involve the cardiovascular and central nervous systems.

MANAGEMENT

1 The diagnosis should be confirmed serologically.
2 Treatment is with benzylpenicillin (crystalline penicillin G) 500,000 units/kg IM or IV for 10 days.

Chapter 8
Viral Infections

Exanthems

The acute, epidemic diseases, in which cutaneous lesions are a central part, are termed the exanthems. Most exanthems are viral in origin, but a few bacterial conditions (e.g. scarlet fever) may also have a very characteristic exanthemous rash and are discussed in Chapter 7.

DNA viruses (e.g. the pox virus) replicate within epidermal cells, producing vesicles. For the most part, RNA viruses do not replicate within the skin. Instead, immune complexes formed of viral particles and antibodies circulate in the blood, localizing to

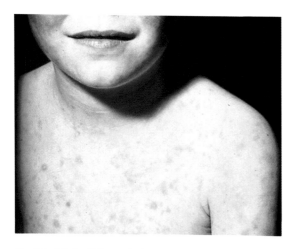

Fig. 8.1 *Rubella.* Pink macules begin on the face and spread caudally, becoming confluent. There is a tender occipitocervical lymphadenopathy (courtesy of Professor D. Candy).

the dermis where they induce an inflammatory reaction, clinically manifest as a maculopapular erythema.

The prodrome, evolution and distribution of the exanthem and presence or absence of accompanying symptoms form the basis of the diagnosis, which in children is virtually always on clinical grounds alone. If the diagnosis is in doubt and confirmation is required, comparing IgM levels in acute and convalescent sera will establish the diagnosis.

The aetiology, incubation period, clinical features and complications for each of the common viral exanthems are outlined below. Treatment of the exanthems is essentially symptomatic, but the isolation period and any specific aspects of management are discussed.

Rubella

AETIOLOGY

The disease is caused by an RNA togavirus, and is spread via droplets. The incubation period is 14–21 days. Congenital infection results from maternal transmission of the rubella virus to the fetus before 20 weeks' gestation.

CLINICAL FEATURES

Often there is no prodromal illness, although mild fever may occur, before the rash appears. Pale, pink macules (Fig. 8.1) begin on the face and spread caudally, becoming confluent over the course of 3 days. The rash is accompanied by tender occipito-cervical lymphadenopathy. Arthritis may occur, but is rare in young children.

MANAGEMENT

1 The patient remains infectious until 5 days after the rash has disappeared.
2 Extreme care should be taken not to expose non-immune pregnant women to the patient.
3 Immunization is available against rubella and is normally offered to toddlers between the ages of 12 and 18 months. All girls should be tested for evidence of rubella antibodies in their teens, and non-immune individuals vaccinated to protect against infection during pregnancy later in life.

Congenital rubella syndrome

The spectrum of the congenital rubella syndrome comprises bluish purple macules on the face and scalp associated with thrombocytopenia, intrauterine growth retardation, and other congenital anomalies (e.g. deafness). The rash, often referred to as 'blueberry muffin' lesions, appears purpuric, but is in fact due to dermal erythropoiesis.

Measles

AETIOLOGY

The infection is caused by an RNA paramyxovirus with droplet spread. The incubation period is 7–14 days.

CLINICAL FEATURES

The rash is preceded by prodromal symptoms of fever, malaise, catarrh, cough and conjunctivitis. Small white Koplick's spots develop on the buccal mucosa 24–48 hours prior to the eruption of the rash. The cutaneous eruption itself develops on the fourth day after the onset of symptoms. Initially there is a bright red erythema, beginning on the forehead, which spreads to the whole face (Fig. 8.2), and becomes more maculopapular in morphology as it descends onto the trunk (Fig. 8.3) and limbs.

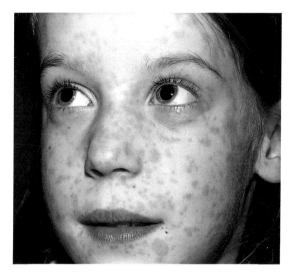

Fig. 8.2 *Measles.* Blotchy erythematous (morbilliform) lesions start on the face on the fourth day of a prodome of fever, malaise, catarrh, cough and conjunctivitis.

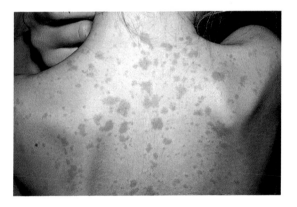

Fig. 8.3 *Measles.* The rash spreads to the trunk and limbs.

COMPLICATIONS

1 Bronchiolitis, pneumonia, otitis media and, rarely, encephalitis may complicate the exanthem.
2 Following measles infection, there is transient T-cell suppression with increased susceptibility to other infections, e.g. tuberculosis.

MANAGEMENT

1 The patient remains contagious for 1 week after the rash develops.
2 Treatment is supportive as there is no specific antiviral therapy.
3 Immunization is available against measles, and in the UK is offered between the ages of 12 and 18 months as part of the measles, mumps and rubella vaccine.

Chickenpox

AETIOLOGY

Chickenpox is caused by the DNA virus varicella zoster and is spread by droplet transmission. The incubation period is 14–21 days.

CLINICAL FEATURES

Following a 1–2-day prodromal period with pyrexia and malaise, erythematous papules develop on the trunk (Fig. 8.4), which progress to form tense, turbid vesicles with a rim of surrounding erythema (Fig. 8.5). As the vesicles resolve, they crust over. Crops of lesions are apparent in different stages of evolution. The scalp and genitalia (Fig. 8.6) are often affected, but the distribution of the eruption is essentially centripetal.

COMPLICATIONS

1 Encephalitis.
2 Pneumonia, especially in older individuals.
3 The infection may be very severe and haemorrhagic in immunosuppressed patients.
4 Localized recurrence of the disease, herpes zoster (see p. 99), may occur later in life.

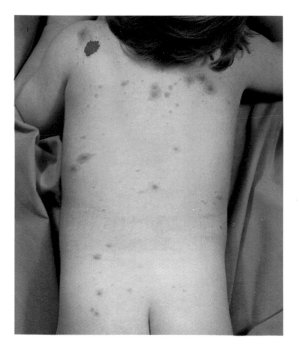

Fig. 8.4 *Chickenpox.* The eruption is predominantly on the trunk. The lesions are at different stages of development, starting as macules and progressing to papules, vesicles and scabs. Note the strawberry haemangioma on this girl's left shoulder.

MANAGEMENT

1 The child should remain off school for 1 week after the rash appears.
2 Therapy with acyclovir may be indicated for severe infections in older or immunocompromised subjects, but is rarely necessary in childhood.
3 Non-immune pregnant women and other vulnerable individuals (e.g. neonates and immunocompromised patients) who are exposed to chicken pox may require specific varicella zoster immunoglobulin. However, this is expensive and needs to be administered on the advice of a microbiologist.

Neonatal varicella

Maternal infection around the time of delivery is associated with a severe infection in the neonate.

The incidence of neonatal varicella is 5/10,000 pregnancies. The severity of disease in the baby depends upon the timing of the infection. If the

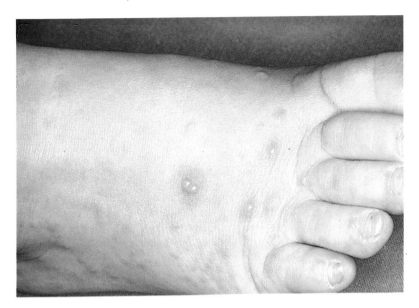

Fig. 8.5 *Chickenpox.* The hallmark of the eruption are the tense vesicles surrounded by erythema.

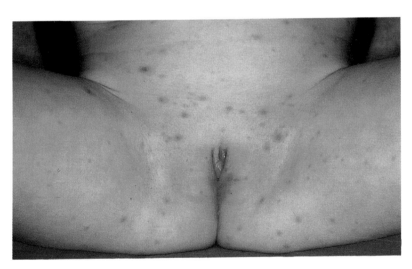

Fig. 8.6 *Chickenpox.* The genitalia are frequently involved. There is a 24–48-hour prodome of fever and malaise before the eruption appears.

mother develops her rash 5 or more days before delivery, then the baby's disease is usually mild. However, if the maternal infection erupts during the period between 4 days before birth to 2 days after delivery, there is a 30% mortality in the baby. The difference in prognosis is accounted for by the degree to which passive transfer of maternal antibodies occurs. The rash of chickenpox in the neonate resembles that of older children, but complications are more frequent.

MANAGEMENT

1 Intramuscular zoster immunoglobulin (ZIG) reduces the severity of infection in the neonate and should be given immediately the maternal diagnosis has been made if it falls during the high-risk period (less than 5 days before, to 2 days after, delivery).
2 Intravenous acyclovir 60 mg/kg/day 8 hourly should be given to all neonates who develop varicella.

Roseola (exanthem subitum)

AETIOLOGY

The infection is due to a DNA virus, human herpes virus type 6 (HHV-6), which is transmitted in saliva. The incubation period is 5–14 days.

CLINICAL FEATURES

Roseola is common and over 75% of infants have antibodies to HHV-6 by the age of 1 year. The infection is characterized by the abrupt onset of a high fever in a child with no other symptoms, which lasts for 3 days. As the pyrexia settles, a fine, generalized, macular erythema appears which is often reticulate in pattern (Fig. 8.7). The rash lasts 48 hours and fades without desquamation. Occipital lymphadenopathy is common.

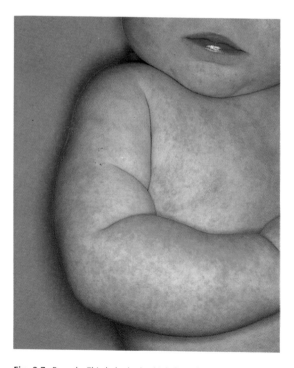

Fig. 8.7 *Roseola.* This baby had a high fever for 3 days which abruptly settled when a fine macular reticulate erythema developed. The rash lasted for 48 hours (courtesy of Mr C. Chandler).

COMPLICATIONS

Febrile convulsions may occur during the period of high fever.

MANAGEMENT

1 The child should be isolated for 1 week.
2 Treatment is symptomatic, but tepid sponging and paracetamol elixir reduce the fever.

Fifth disease (erythema infantum)

AETIOLOGY

The infection is caused by the RNA virus human parvovirus B-19, and is spread by the droplet mode.

CLINICAL FEATURES

The infection occurs in epidemics, mostly in the spring. The incubation period is 7–14 days. There is no prodromal illness. The rash begins on the face, as a hot, bright red erythema simulating a 'slapped cheek' appearance (Fig. 8.8). As the eruption spreads onto the trunk and limbs, it becomes more reticulate (Fig. 8.9a). The palms (Fig. 8.9b) and soles may be affected. The rash fades over the course of a week, but recrudescences are common for several weeks after the initial infection, especially if the child gets hot (after bathing or exercise) or if the child is exposed to sunlight.

COMPLICATIONS

Aplastic crises may occur in children with haemoglobinopathies.

MANAGEMENT

1 The child should remain off school for 1 week.
2 Pregnant women should avoid exposure to parvovirus as transplacental infection is associated with a high incidence of hydrops fetalis and intra-uterine death.

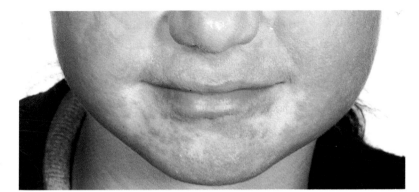

Fig. 8.8 *Fifth disease.* There is a hot, bright-red erythema on the cheeks, almost as if they had been slapped.

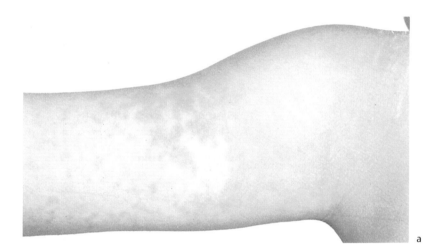

a

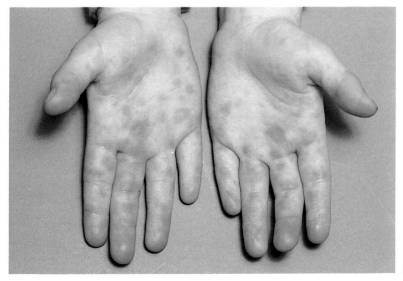

Fig. 8.9 *Fifth disease.* (a) A more diffuse reticulate eruption may be present. (b) There is a patchy erythema over the palms. The infection is caused by human parvovirus B-19.

b

Other viral infections

Warts

DEFINITION

A common papillomavirus infection of the skin or mucous membranes.

AETIOLOGY

Warts are caused by infection with human papillomavirus (HPV). Over 50 different types of HPV have now been identified. Warts in children are most often due to HPV 1, 2 or 4. They may be spread by direct contact or via damp floors in sports changing

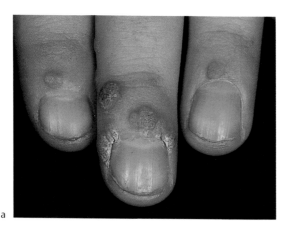

a

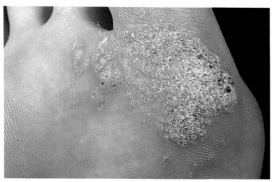

b

Fig. 8.10 (a) *Common warts.* These are well-defined, rough-surfaced papules. Around the nails is a common site of warts in nail-biters. (b) *Plantar warts.* Many warts may coalesce at this site to produce large mosaic plaques.

rooms, but the incubation period appears to be quite prolonged. Trauma and nail-biting facilitates spread, e.g. of periungual warts to the lips.

CLINICAL FEATURES

Warts are unusual in children under 2 years, but thereafter are common, becoming most prevalent during the teen years. They may occur anywhere on the skin, but are most frequent on the dorsum of the fingers (Fig. 8.10a), soles (Fig. 8.10b) and knees. There are various clinical types of wart, e.g. common, plantar, filiform, plane and genital.

Common warts

These are mainly caused by HPV 2. They are thickened papules with a rough horny surface that slowly enlarge to achieve a size of several millimetres in diameter and may coalesce to form large plaques. The fingers and hands are the usual sites (see also Fig. 17.20).

Plantar warts

Pressure from walking prevents exophytic growth of the wart, which forms a painful, thickened plaque on the sole of the foot. Plantar warts often coalesce to form large aggregations (mosaic warts) (Fig. 8.10a). Pinpoint haemorrhages can usually be seen within the wart and clearly distinguish it from a simple corn.

Filiform warts

Fine spicule-like warts are not uncommon on the face in children, especially around the nostrils and lips (Fig. 8.11).

Plane warts

Small, flat, flesh-coloured or pigmented papules may occur on the face and the backs of the hands. These warts sometimes occur in a linear fashion at the site of trauma (the Koebner phenomenon) (Fig. 8.12). Plane warts tend to be more resistant to treatment.

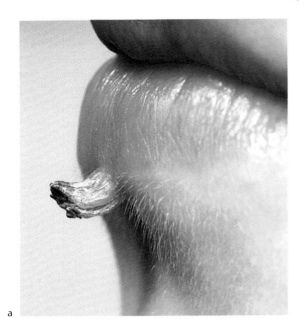

a

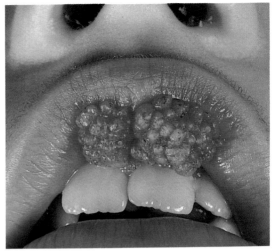

b

Fig. 8.11 (a) *Filiform wart*. Warts on the face in children are often filiform in character. (b) *Oral warts*. Warts may be transferred to the mouth from the fingers.

Genital warts

Anogenital warts are less common in children than adults. Their presence may indicate sexual abuse, but auto-inoculation of hand warts or perinatal transmission of maternal genital warts are other possible explanations.

MANAGEMENT

1 Warts eventually disappear spontaneously, but some may take several years. Overall, 35% of warts resolve within 6 months and a further 20% within 1 year.
2 Wart paints: the application of a topical keratolytic solution may be beneficial especially if it is in a waterproof (collodion) base (e.g. Salatac). The surface of the wart should be pared down or filed to assist penetration of the solution.
3 Cryotherapy: freezing with liquid nitrogen is often the most effective treatment, but is quite painful and not well tolerated by young children. Pretreatment of the area with topical local anaesthetic (e.g. EMLA) may reduce the discomfort.
4 Plane warts can be very persistent, but may respond to cryotherapy or topical Retin-A 0.025%.

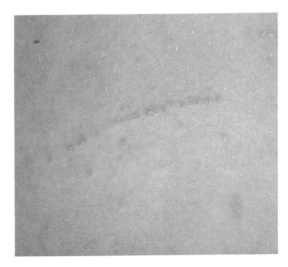

Fig. 8.12 *Plane warts*. These are flat-topped, often pigmented, papules. They may occur in a linear manner (the Koebner phenomenon). They are caused by HPV 3.

Molluscum contagiosum

DEFINITION

A common viral infection, characterized by pearly, umbilicated papules.

AETIOLOGY

Infection is caused by a DNA pox virus. Mollusca are more common in atopic children and those who are immunosuppressed.

CLINICAL FEATURES

Whitish, dome-shaped papules, 1–5 mm in diameter,

develop in clusters (Fig. 8.13). They have an umbilicated centre (Fig. 8.14) which contains a core of molluscum bodies. They persist for several months but eventually resolve spontaneously. The papules often become inflamed (Fig. 8.15) and crusted or develop eczema around them before involuting.

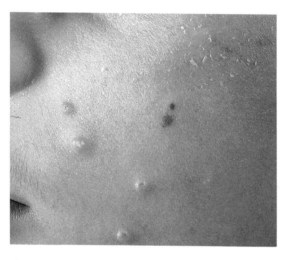

Fig. 8.13 *Molluscum contagiosum.* These are dome-shaped, flesh-coloured papules with an umbilicated centre.

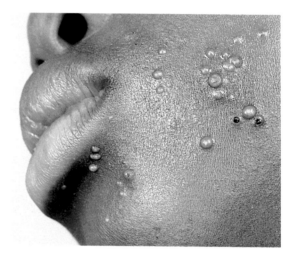

Fig. 8.14 *Molluscum contagiosum.* The lesions persist for many months but eventually resolve spontaneously and do not recur. The face is a common site.

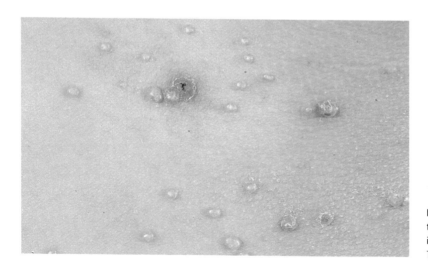

Fig. 8.15 *Molluscum contagiosum.* As the lesions resolve they become inflamed or surrounded by eczema. They are common in atopic children.

MANAGEMENT

1 Since the papules usually resolve within a year, many physicians recommend no treatment.
2 Cryotherapy is effective if it can be tolerated. Prior treatment of the area with topical local anaesthetic (e.g. EMLA®) may facilitate the cryotherapy.
3 Phenol or weak iodine solution may be applied to the centre of the lesion with a sharpened orange stick.

Orf (ecthema contagiosum)

DEFINITION

An acute vesiculopustular infection of the digits, contracted from infected sheep.

AETIOLOGY

The infection is due to a parapox virus. Infection results from direct inoculation from infected animals, but the virus can survive for long periods on inanimate matter such as fences. The infection occurs in rural areas, especially at lambing time.

CLINICAL FEATURES

Following an incubation period of less than 1 week, a solitary, red papule develops; it enlarges, becoming vesicular, haemorrhagic and finally pustular. Lesions most typically occur on the fingers (Fig. 8.16) and there may be accompanying lymphangitis, regional lymphadenopathy and even a short-lived fever.

COMPLICATIONS

1 Erythema multiforme (see p. 184) may follow the acute infection.
2 Secondary bacterial infection may occur.

MANAGEMENT

Spontaneous resolution occurs after a month and the lesion heals without scarring.

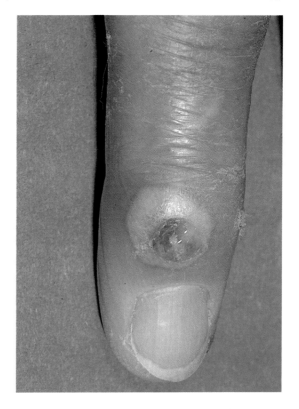

Fig. 8.16 *Orf.* The lesion looks like a target, being red in the centre and then surrounded by white and red peripherally. The condition lasts 35 days.

Hand, foot and mouth disease

DEFINITION

An erythematous infection producing a syndrome with mild fever and vesicles in the mouth and on the extremities.

AETIOLOGY

The infection is caused by Coxsackie A virus (usually type 16), which is spread via droplets or faecal contamination. The incubation period is 7 days.

CLINICAL FEATURES

Vesicles initially develop in the mouth and then ulcerate. Tense blisters, up to 0.5 cm in diameter

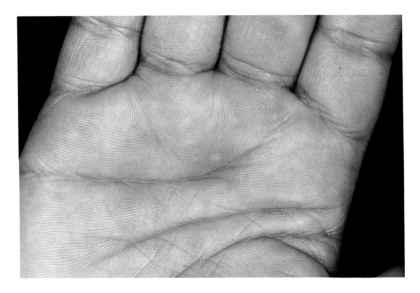

Fig. 8.17 *Hand, foot and mouth disease.* There are vesicles surrounded by an erythema. The palms, soles and mouth are involved.

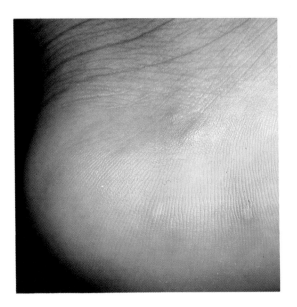

Fig. 8.18 *Hand, foot and mouth disease.* It is caused by a Coxsackie A virus, usually type 16. There is a mild fever.

MANAGEMENT

No treatment is required as the eruption is self-limiting and clears over 7 days.

Herpes simplex

DEFINITION

A common localized vesicular infection, occurring anywhere on the body but especially the face. Following a primary attack, the infection recurs.

AETIOLOGY

The herpes hominis virus (HSV) is spread by direct inoculation. Most infections in children are due to HSV type I, but neonatal infection and occasional cases resulting from sexual abuse may be caused by HSV-II (genital) infection.

CLINICAL FEATURES

Primary infection

The initial episode (Fig. 8.19) most commonly occurs in children between the ages of 2 and 5 years,

with a narrow rim of erythema, occur on the palms (Fig. 8.17) and soles (Fig. 8.18), fading within 3 days. A more widespread maculopapular rash may occur in infants with constitutional upset.

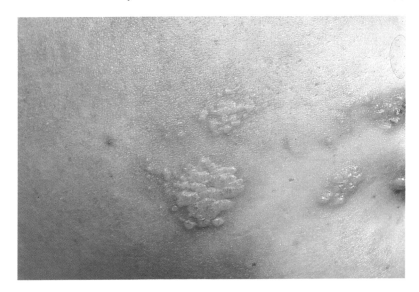

Fig. 8.19 *Herpes simplex.* The initial primary episode is most extensive. There are clusters of vesicles on an erythematous base.

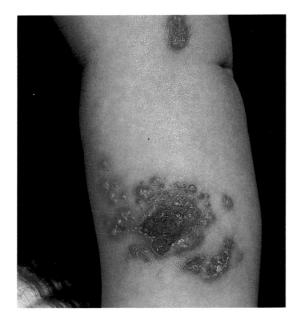

Fig. 8.20 *Herpes simplex.* The virus may affect any area of the body including the arm, as in this infant with a primary infection.

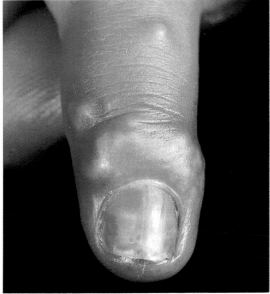

Fig. 8.21 *Herpetic whitlow.* There are a group of tense vesicles occurring around the thumb-nail.

but it may be subclinical. More than 10% of children have been infected by HSV by the age of 9 years. The prevalence of HSV infection correlates with lower social class and the highest incidence occurs in developing countries. In the USA three times as many black children have serological evidence of infection as white children. If overt, the primary infection is usually an acute gingivostomatitis, although any area may be affected (Figs 8.20 and 8.21). Following an incubation period of 2–12 days,

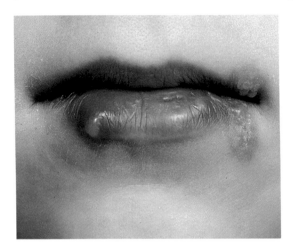

Fig. 8.22 *Herpes simplex.* The lips are the commonest site to be involved.

painful vesicles erupt on the lips and buccal mucosa. The lesions erode and are accompanied by fever and lymphadenopathy. The episode may be so severe that eating and drinking are too painful. The lesions scab over and heal in 10–14 days without scarring.

Recurrent infection

The virus remains latent in the sensory ganglia and periodically causes localized recurrences, typified by the eruption of clusters of vesicles (Fig. 8.22) in the affected area preceded by prodromal discomfort and paraesthesia. Fifty per cent of the population who have had a primary attack will experience an episode of recurrent HSV infection at some point in life. Reactivation may be precipitated by sun exposure, extreme cold, stress or fever. Recurrent disease is always milder than the initial attack.

Eczema herpeticum (see p. 45)

HSV infection may be very extensive in atopic children.

COMPLICATIONS

1 Auto-inoculation (e.g. to produce a herpetic whitlow) may occur.

2 A dendritic ulcer may arise from conjunctival inoculation.
3 Erythema multiforme (see p. 184).
4 Encephalitis is a rare but serious complication of primary infection, due to spread of the virus to the central nervous system via the olfactory nerves.

MANAGEMENT

1 Diagnosis is confirmed by viral smear for electron microscopy and culture. A Giemsa-stained Tzanck smear from the base of a vesicle will show ballooned cells with viral inclusions.
2 Primary stomatitis, if severe, may be treated with oral acyclovir 200 mg (100 mg in children under 2 years) five times a day for 5 days.
3 Recurrent infections are self-limiting and require no treatment in healthy children with mild disease. Topical acyclovir may be used prophylactically as soon as prodromal symptoms occur, if recurrences are troublesome.
4 Immunocompromised patients: oral acyclovir 400 mg should be given five times a day (or 5 mg/kg IV three times a day) for 7 days.

Neonatal herpes simplex infection

AETIOLOGY

The majority of neonatal infections are usually acquired during delivery but intrauterine infection may occur. The likelihood of transmission to the baby is ten times higher from primary maternal infection than from recurrent disease. The parental disease may be asymptomatic in as many as 60% of children infected with neonatal herpes. If the onset of disease is delayed until 2–4 weeks after birth, then the virus is more likely to be HSV-I, acquired from hospital staff or relatives during the neonatal period.

CLINICAL

Intrauterine infections are evident at birth (Fig. 8.23). Peripartum infection does not usually become apparent until a few days later. The syndrome consists of the triad of chorioretinitis, widespread erosions of the skin and mucous membranes and neurological involvement. Clustered vesicles are often visible on the scalp, especially if the inoculation site was at the insertion of a fetal scalp electrode. The disease is much more prevalent in the USA, with an estimated incidence of 1/7000 births compared to 1/50,000 births in the UK.

COMPLICATIONS

The mortality is 40% even with antiviral treatment and there is a high morbidity in survivors. Encephalitis and disseminated infection with multisystem involvement occur. Multiple cutaneous recurrences within the first 6 months are associated with a high incidence of late neurological complications.

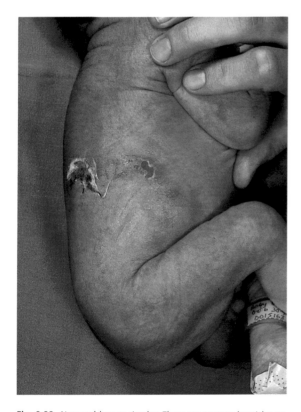

Fig. 8.23 *Neonatal herpes simplex.* There are scattered vesicles on an erythematous base. This was type II herpes simplex contracted from the mother's genital tract.

MANAGEMENT

Neonatal infections should be managed with high-dose IV acyclovir 10 mg/kg for 10 days. Vaginal delivery is contraindicated in mothers with active vesicular genital herpes, and delivery should be by caesarian section.

Herpes zoster (shingles)

DEFINITION

A vesicular viral eruption occurring in a unilateral, dermatomal distribution.

AETIOLOGY

The infection is due to the reactivation of the varicella virus, which has lain dormant in the dorsal nerve root ganglion. There are rare cases of shingles in very young babies, where the initial varicella infection occurred *in utero*.

CLINICAL FEATURES

Herpes zoster is much less common in children than in adults. However, it may be the first indication of infection if the original chicken pox was subclinical. The rash is often preceded by pain within the dermatome, followed by small red papules which evolve to become vesicular and then pustular, finally crusting over to heal in 2–3 weeks. The eruption is unilateral (Fig. 8.24).

COMPLICATIONS

1 The infection may become disseminated and haemorrhagic with necrotic areas in immunosuppressed children, e.g. those with HIV or leukaemia.
2 Postherpetic neuralgia may develop within the affected dermatomes.

MANAGEMENT

1 No treatment other than simple analgesia is required for uncomplicated infection in the healthy child.

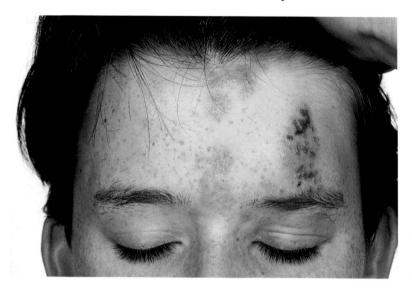

Fig. 8.24 *Herpes zoster.* Shingles is uncommon in children. The eruption is unilateral with groups of vesicles and scabbed lesions involving the ophthalmic branch of the trigeminal nerve in this 14-year-old.

2 In severe infections in ill children, acyclovir 10 mg/kg IV should be given for 7–10 days.

Human immunodeficiency virus (HIV) infection in childern

DEFINITION

A retrovirus infection resulting in multiorgan involvement, characterized by frequent and recurrent opportunistic infections and malignancy.

AETIOLOGY

Infection with HIV in children is thought to occur perinatally in the majority of instances. About one third of babies born to HIV-positive mothers become infected, but it is unknown whether the infection is acquired *in utero* or intrapartum. Older children may become infected through contaminated blood products, as has happened with some haemophiliacs.

CLINICAL FEATURES

The asymptomatic period is shorter in children (mean, 8 months) than it is in adults. Essentially, many features of the disease in children are similar to those of adults, with recurrent infections, chronic seborrhoeic dermatitis and a high incidence of drug reactions. However, there are some unique features of the disease in children. Salivary gland enlargement, interstitial lymphoid pneumonitis and a dysmorphic syndrome with growth retardation and craniofacial abnormalities are specific to the disease in children.

Oral candidiasis (Fig. 8.25) is the most common infection in HIV-positive children, but recurrent bacterial infections (e.g. impetigo and ecthyma) are also common and are more prevalent in children with HIV than in affected adults.

DIFFERENTIAL DIAGNOSIS

Congenital immunodeficiencies (e.g. di George syndrome) can be distinguished because of the polyclonal hypergammaglobulinaemia in children with HIV.

MANAGEMENT

1 Standard HIV testing cannot confirm the diagnosis in an infant because of the transplacental transfer of maternal antibody which persists until the age of 10

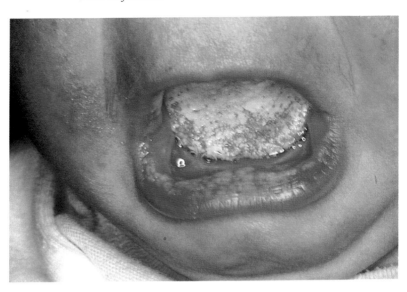

Fig. 8.25 *HIV infection.* Recurrent infections are common, particularly oral candidiasis.

months. Viral DNA may be identified within cells using the polymerase chain reaction, but the test is not available routinely.

2 There is no consensus on the optimum treatment yet, but children with HIV should be cared for in specialist centres to ensure accurate diagnosis, maximize early supportive treatment and allow them to be included in current trials of prophylactic therapy.

3 Aggressive early treatment of opportunistic infections is imperative.

4 The child and family should be provided with adequate support services.

Chapter 9
Fungal Infections, Infestations and Tropical Infections

Fungal infections

Fungal infections may be classified as superficial or deep (Table 9.1). The superficial dermatophyte fungi are classified into three species (*Trichophyton*, *Microsporum* and *Epidermophyton*). They may also be categorized according to their source of origin as anthropophilic (from humans), zoophilic (from an animal reservoir) or geophilic (from soil).

Certain superficial infections are common in children, especially dermatophytes (syn. tinea or 'ringworm') affecting the scalp. However, tinea pedis, tinea unguium (see p. 221) and tinea cruris are rare in children. Only the most common fungal infections will be discussed here. For information on the more rare species and tropical infections, the reader is referred to a specialized text.

Tinea capitis

DEFINITION

A fungal infection of the scalp, caused by a dermatophyte and common in children.

AETIOLOGY

Various species are capable of invading hair. Fungi which invade the hair shaft (e.g. *T. tonsurans*) are termed endothrix infections whereas species which lay spores on the outside of the hair (e.g. *M. audouinii*) are classified as ectothrix infections.

The common causes of tinea capitis in different parts of the world are listed in Table 9.2. Anthropophilic infections (Fig. 9.1) are spread from child to child at school, whereas zoophilic infections are acquired from animals. *Microsporum canis* infection, from puppies and kittens, is the most prevalent cause in the UK, whereas *T. tonsurans* is responsible for 90% of tinea capitis in the USA. The epidemiology of tinea capitis is changing as a result of immigration, and new species are becoming prevalent in the UK and USA, e.g. *T. soudanense*. The multiple use of unsterilized razors for close-cropped hairstyling (Fig. 9.2) has been observed to spread fungal infection, presumably as a result of direct inoculation.

Table 9.1 Classification of fungal infections

Class	Example
Superficial mycoses	
Dermatophyte (hyphal)	*Trichophyton*
	Microsporum
	Epidermophyton
Yeasts	*Candida*
	Pityrosporum
Deep mycoses	
Tropical infections	Sporotrichosis
	Coccidiomycosis
Systemic infection	Systemic candidosis
	Oppurtunistic fungi (e.g. aspergillosis) in immunosuppressed patients

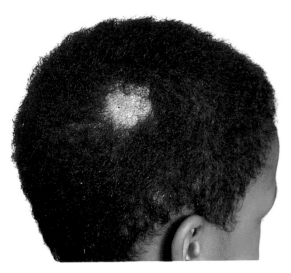

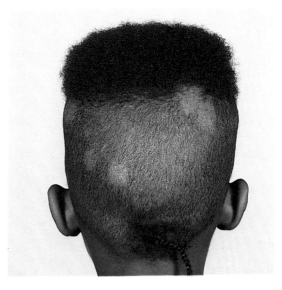

Fig. 9.1 *Tinea capitis.* There is a circumscribed area of hair loss with scaling. The degree of inflammation is least with human (anthropophilic) infection as in this 7-year-old.

Fig. 9.2 *Tinea capitis.* Infection may be spread by unsterilized razors used for close-cropped hairstyles favoured in Afro-Caribbean children.

Table 9.2 Common causes of tinea capitis, worldwide

Species	Classification	Endemic areas	Morphology	Fluorescence*
Microsporum audouinii	Anthropophilic	Worldwide	Small-spore ectothrix	Yes
Microsporum canis	Zoophilic (cats, dogs)	Worldwide	Small-spore ectothrix	Yes
Microsporum ferrugineum	Anthropophilic	Central Africa, Far East, eastern Europe	Small-spore ectothrix	Yes
Trichophyton megninii	Anthropophilic	South-west Europe, north and central Africa	Straight chains of spores, ectothrix	No
Trichophyton schoenleinii (favus)	Anthropophilic	Europe, Middle East, north and south Africa	No spores. Typical airspaces seen within hair	Yes
Trichophyton gourvilii	Anthropophilic	West Africa	Endothrix	No
Trichophyton soudanense	Anthropophilic	Africa	Endothrix	No
Trichophyton tonsurans	Anthropophilic	Worldwide	Endothrix	No
Trichophyton verrucosum	Zoophilic (cattle)	Worldwide	Large-spore ectothrix	No
Trichophyton violaceum	Anthropophilic	Europe, north Africa	Endothrix	No

Anthropophilic, human reservoir; zoophilic, animal infection.
* Fluorescence under Wood's light.

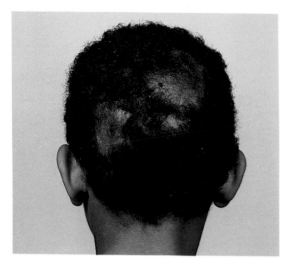

Fig. 9.3 *Tinea capitis*. There are multiple patches of hair loss with inflammation and scaling. The affected hairs are broken and short.

CLINICAL FEATURES

Patches of alopecia (single or multiple) develop, but unlike alopecia areata, the scalp appears inflamed and scaly (Figs 9.3 and 9.4) and there are multiple short, broken hairs. There may be small pustules. The degree of inflammation varies with different species, but is most marked in zoophilic infections. Ectothrix infections may fluoresce green under Wood's light. With the exception of favus (a rare condition which produces patchy alopecia and dry, yellowish crusts on the scalp), endothrix infections never fluoresce.

In the case of infection with certain zoophilic species, e.g. the cattle ringworm *T. verrucosum*, a large, boggy, pustular swelling develops called a kerion (Fig. 9.5), which, unless treated promptly, can result in permanent hair loss.

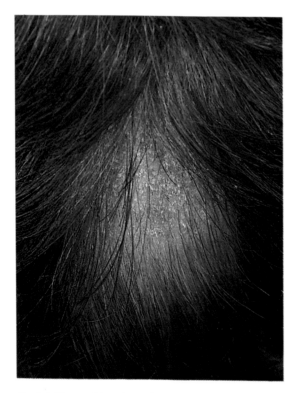

Fig. 9.4 *Tinea capitis*. Anthropophilic infections spread in epidemic form, particularly at school. *Microsporum audouinii* is the most common cause; it fluoresces green under a Wood's light.

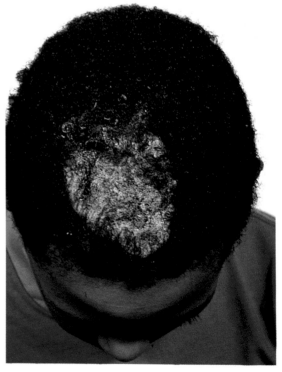

Fig. 9.5 *Kerion*. A boggy, purulent swelling may develop with zoophilic infections.

MANAGEMENT

1 The diagnosis should be confirmed by microscopic examination of plucked hairs on a potassium hydroxide preparation and by culture.

2 Examining the scalp under Wood's light differentiates endothrix and ectothrix infections (see Table 9.2) and can be useful in screening large numbers of children in school epidemics.

3 Since topical antifungals are ineffective in treating tinea capitis, systemic treatment with griseofulvin 10 mg/kg/day for 6 weeks is the current standard treatment. A new fungicidal therapy (terbinafine) is not yet licensed for use in children, but the early results of clinical trials are promising.

4 The use of steroids in kerion to reduce inflammation is controversial and has been superceded by more potent antifungal therapy.

5 Children infected with *T. tonsurans* or *M. audouinii* should remain off school until treatment is completed, but human–human transmission is unusual in infections from zoophilic species.

6 If pets are the source of infection, they should be adequately treated by a veterinary surgeon.

Tinea corporis

DEFINITION

Superficial fungal infection of the skin occurring in a characteristic annular pattern.

AETIOLOGY

Any dermatophyte can produce tinea corporis, but in the UK infection is most often due to *T. rubrum* (acquired from other family members) or *M. canis* (from pets). In rural areas, *T. verrucosum* infection may be contracted from farm animals. Occasionally, tinea corporis in children may be secondary and spread from the scalp.

CLINICAL FEATURES

Well-defined, circular, erythematous and scaly lesions with an active inflammatory border (Fig. 9.6) arise anywhere on the body. The infection spreads slowly outwards in an annular fashion (Fig. 9.7). The border particularly in zoophilic infections may be pustular. Multiple lesions may occur, but

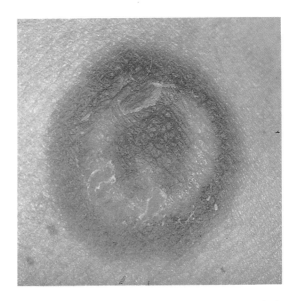

Fig. 9.6 *Tinea corporis.* On the body ringworm is annular, with the inflammation at the periphery. It is most marked in animal infections, in this case from a puppy (*Microsporum canis*).

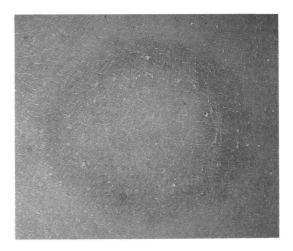

Fig. 9.7 *Tinea corporis.* The redness and scaling is at the periphery of the lesion with a tendency towards central healing. This child had been in contact with the same puppy as her sister shown in Fig. 9.6.

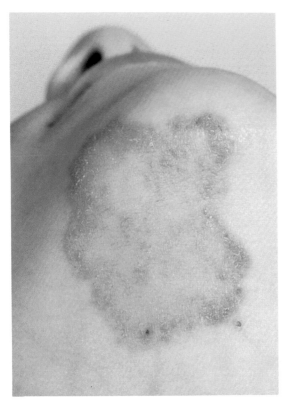

Fig. 9.8 *Tinea facei.* The eruption is annular and asymmetrical. There is a distinct, red, very slightly raised, scaly margin with central healing.

the infection is usually asymmetrical (Fig. 9.8). If the condition is misdiagnosed and treated with topical steroids in error, the signs become modified, the margins less sharply defined and a pustular folliculitis develops: tinea incognito.

DIFFERENTIAL DIAGNOSIS

Psoriasis can be distinguished from tinea corporis by a potassium hydroxide (KOH) preparation which should rapidly demonstrate the hyphae in tinea infection.

MANAGEMENT

1 Infection is confirmed by microscopy and culture of skin scrapings.

2 Most cases will respond to topical treatment with an imidazole twice daily for 2–4 weeks or the newer fungicidal agent terbinafine cream for 2 weeks.

Pityriasis versicolor (tinea versicolor)

DEFINITION

A superficial yeast infection of the trunk, which may result in temporary hypopigmentation of the skin.

AETIOLOGY

Pityriasis versicolor is caused by the organism *Pityrosporum ovale*, previously known as *Malassezia furfur*. Although common in adults, pityriasis versicolor is not often seen in children in temperate climates until the development of functional sebaceous glands during adolescence. When younger children are affected, there is usually a history of an adult member of the household also being affected.

CLINICAL FEATURES

Children account for only 5% of pityriasis versicolor infections. In adolescents and adults the disease is usually confined to the trunk, whereas in children the face is often affected. This is especially true in hot, humid countries, and indeed the face may be the only site of infection. Multiple fawn or pinkish-brown patches (Fig. 9.9) coalesce to produce plaques with a geographic border. Scraping the surface of the lesion produces profuse scale. The eruption is asymptomatic, but affected areas may become hypopigmented (Fig. 9.10). This is most evident in black skin or following tanning, and takes many months to resolve. The patient may be unaware of the original infection and only present at the hypopigmented stage.

DIFFERENTIAL DIAGNOSES

1 Vitiligo tends to be more widely distributed and is not scaly. There is complete loss of pigment in the affected ares, and the eruption tends to be symmetrical.
2 Pityriasis alba (see p. 57) can be differentiated

Fig. 9.9 *Pityriasis versicolor.* The trunk is usually affected in this condition, which is common in adolescence and youth but is rare before the sebaceous glands mature. The macules are fawn-coloured.

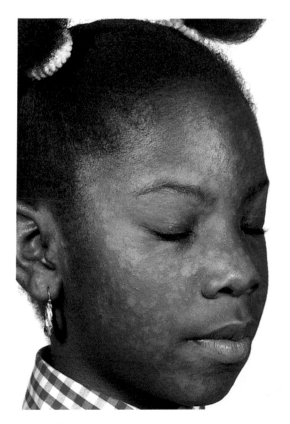

Fig. 9.10 *Pityriasis versicolor.* The face is frequently affected in black children in whom the lesions may be hypopigmented and scaly.

from pityriasis versicolor on the face in children by the absence of fungi on microscopy.

MANAGEMENT

1 Pityriasis versicolor is easy to identify microscopically, since the fungus readily takes up Parker Blue Quink added to the standard KOH preparation of skin scrapings, revealing the characteristic mix of hyphae and yeasts.

2 Applying selenium sulphide 2.5% shampoo to the skin for 8 hours and then washing it off, once or twice a week for 3 weeks, is inexpensive and effective but may cause irritation and has an unpleasant odour.

3 Alternatively, ketoconazole 2% cream or an imidazole cream can be applied topically twice daily for 2 weeks.

4 Chronic infection in adults may be treated with a short course of oral itraconazole, but this is rarely appropriate in children.

Candidiasis (monilia, thrush)

DEFINITION

A superficial yeast infection of the skin and mucous membranes.

AETIOLOGY

Infection is caused by the yeast *Candida albicans*, which has a predilection for warm, moist body sites, such as the mouth and napkin area. If recurrent infection becomes a problem, the gut may be serving as a reservoir of infection. In infants the infection is acquired during delivery. It is rare in older children unless they are on immunosuppressive drugs or have disorders of the immune system.

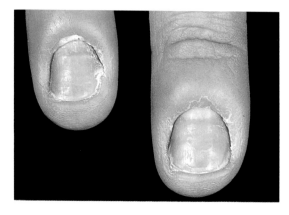

Fig. 9.11 *Candida paronychia.* This is rare in childhood but may occur in adolescence. The proximal nail fold becomes swollen and red, the cuticle is absent and ridging of the nail results.

CLINICAL FEATURES

Oral candidiasis

Small (1–2 mm in diameter) white pustules which become plaques are very common on the buccal mucosa in neonates. The infection is acquired from the maternal genital tract at birth. The white plaques can easily be scraped off with a tongue depressor to reveal the bright red base. Oral candidiasis is rare in older children unless they are immunocompromised. In such patients oral candidiasis is often severe and the infection may become systemic.

Angular cheilitis

Painful, erythematous fissures colonized by *Candida* may develop in children undergoing orthodontic treatment if the wearing of braces causes drooling.

Candida paronychia

The proximal nail fold becomes swollen with loss of the cuticle and ultimately a nail dystrophy develops with ridging of the nail plate (Fig. 9.11). The condition develops in moist, macerated skin and although it is less common than in adults, it may be seen in children who suck their thumbs (or other digits) repeatedly.

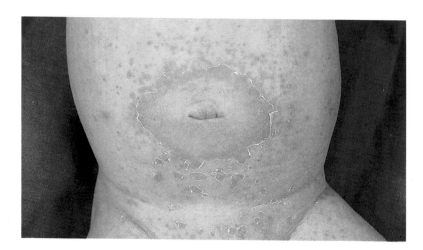

Fig. 9.12 *Candidiasis.* Superficial pustules coalesce and break, leaving behind erosions. Satellite pustules peripheral to the central eruption are characteristic as in this infant with *Candida* under his nappy.

Napkin candidiasis

If napkin dermatitis is neglected, *Candida* will often colonize the macerated skin and infection may become disseminated. Superficial erosions with satellite pustules are characteristic (Fig. 9.12).

MANAGEMENT

1 The organism should be identified from a skin swab, nail clippings or blood cultures as appropriate.
2 Oral infections are treated with nystatin suspension 100,000 iu/ml. In neonates the dosage is 1 ml daily.
3 Superficial infections: topical nystatin or an imidazole cream rapidly eradicates infection.
4 Topical treatment may be applied to *Candida* paronychia in children, but the mainstay of treatment is to try to keep the area dry.

Chronic mucocutaneous candidiasis

DEFINITION

A genetic disorder of immune function characterized by severe, widespread candidosis of the mouth, nails and skin associated with various endocrinopathies.

AETIOLOGY

Usually inherited in an autosomal dominant manner, but autosomal-recessive variants exist.

CLINICAL FEATURES

Persistent, hypertrophic oral thrush (Fig. 9.13) (especially involving the tongue), cutaneous candidiasis and florid nail involvement (Fig. 9.14) are seen from early childhood. The condition is associated with a predisposition to other infections and thyroid, parathyroid and adrenal insufficiency.

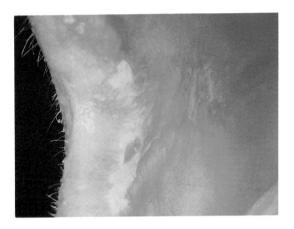

Fig. 9.13 *Chronic mucocutaneous candidiasis.* This girl had persistent oral thrush in addition to chronic nail changes.

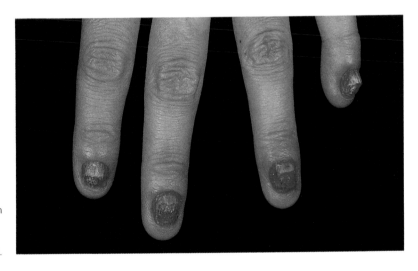

Fig. 9.14 *Chronic mucocutaneous candidiasis.* The nail is thickened and dystrophic. The nail folds are normal in this adolescent who also had chronic hypoparathyroidism. She had tried to disguise the problem with nail varnish.

MANAGEMENT

1 *Candida* can be cultured from swabs/clippings from the affected sites.
2 Since the condition is refractory to topical treatment, oral itraconazole or ketoconazole is indicated. Although this treatment is effective, it is required over a long period, and continuous therapy may be limited by side effects of the drugs.

Systemic fungal infection

DEFINITION

Disseminated fungal infection may occur in immunosuppressed individuals.

AETIOLOGY

Common organisms which are normally confined to the skin, e.g. *Candida*, may cause invasive disease in immunosuppressed individuals. Also, a number of rare fungi have now been described as causing opportunistic infections in immunocompromised patients.

CLINICAL FEATURES

The skin may be involved directly, or through embolic spread from an internal focus (e.g. the heart). Systemic infection may also arise if cutaneous organisms colonize sites of instrumentation (e.g. Hickman lines), and enter the circulation. Embolic foci appear as painless, firm, small red papules (Fig. 9.15) in a severely ill patient.

MANAGEMENT

1 The diagnosis is confirmed by skin biopsy, which should be divided to provide a specimen for histology (including special stains for organisms) and tissue culture to identify the species involved.
2 Systemic treatment is always required.

Infestations

Papular urticaria

DEFINITION

An itchy, erythematous papulovesicular eruption from insect bites.

AETIOLOGY

A variety of arthropods – e.g. bed bugs, cat and dog fleas and certain mites (e.g. *Cheyletiella* in dogs) – can produce this clinical picture. A very florid variant of papular urticaria is produced by contact with the hairs of the caterpillar of the brown-tail moth (Fig. 9.16).

CLINICAL FEATURES

Intensely pruritic urticated papules develop in asymmetrical clusters on exposed parts of the body, e.g. the face, arms and, particularly, the lower legs (Fig. 9.17). A central haemorrhagic punctum may be visible (Fig. 9.18) and the lesions may become bullous. Secondary infection following scratching is common. Often only one child in the family is affected. The eruption usually settles within 1 week, but if the source is not eradicated, new crops of lesions will appear, and further investigation is required.

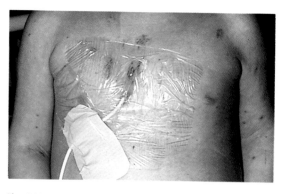

Fig. 9.15 *Systemic candidiasis.* In severely immunocompromised patients, embolic foci of fungus may occur in the skin, as firm red papules seen here on the arms. Skin biopsy is essential for diagnosis.

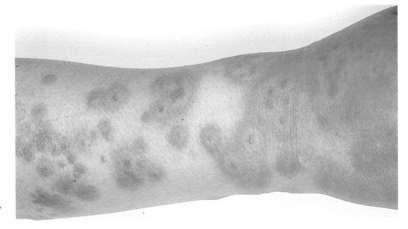

Fig. 9.16 *Caterpillar moth urticaria.* The hairs of the caterpillar of the brown-tail moth produce a striking urticarial eruption on the exposed areas of the skin.

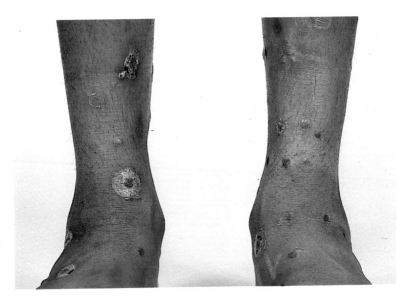

Fig. 9.17 *Papular urticaria.* The lesions are pruritic and urticated papules which crust and become pigmented. The ankles are a common site. They may become bullous.

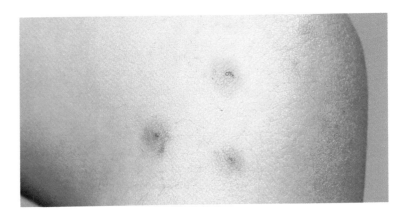

Fig. 9.18 *Papular urticaria.* The lesions are often grouped and a central haemorrhagic punctum may be visible.

MANAGEMENT

1 The source of the problem should be sought and pets (and their brushings) examined carefully for evidence of infestation. It is important to check the animals' bedding as well as the animal itself, as fleas can survive in a pet's basket (or surrounding carpet) for long periods.

2 The source of the flea is not always a domestic pet; wild animals in the garden (e.g. hedgehogs) may be responsible.

3 Investigation by the local environmental health office may be necessary to eradicate some infestations, e.g. pigeon mites from birds nesting in the eaves.

4 Antihistamines and a moderately potent topical steroid provide symptomatic relief.

5 Secondary infection should be treated appropriately.

Scabies

DEFINITION

A pruritic and highly contagious infestation, the clinical hallmark of which is the burrow, in which the female mite lays her eggs.

AETIOLOGY

The rash is caused by infestation with *Sarcoptes scabiei*. The infestation is spread through prolonged physical contact, usually by sharing a bed with an infected person, but the mite may be transmitted in children by close contact and hand-holding.

CLINICAL FEATURES

Scabies is common throughout the world and endemic in some remote island communities. Children are most commonly affected, but the disease spreads rapidly through close family contacts. The adult female mite lays numerous eggs in burrows dug out of the superficial epidermis. After an incubation period of about 1 month, the child begins to itch. This is insidious at first, but becomes intense, especially in bed at night and after a bath. Burrows

(Fig. 9.19) may occur anywhere on the body, but are most prevalent on the soles (Fig. 9.20), wrists, interdigital spaces (Fig. 9.21), thenar eminences (Fig. 9.22) and genitalia. Erythematous papules and

Fig. 9.19 *Scabies.* The serpiginous track, the burrow, is the hallmark of scabies infestations.

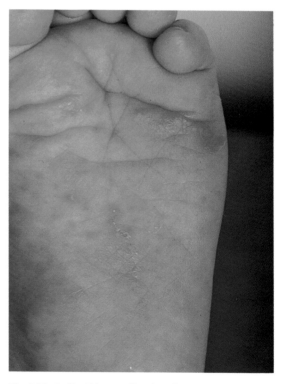

Fig. 9.20 *Scabies.* This may affect the soles particularly in babies. The itching is intense and the child may be seen rubbing its feet together to get relief.

pustules are seen intermingled with the burrows and there are multiple excoriations. The rash tends to be widely disseminated in infants, in whom many of the lesions are vesicular (Fig. 9.23). In males, large inflammatory nodules, which may persist for several months, often occur on the penis and scrotum (Fig. 9.24). They also occur on elbows and axillae (Fig. 9.25) and occasionally are widespread (Fig. 9.26).

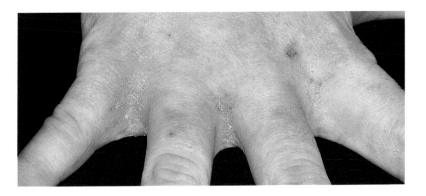

Fig. 9.21 *Scabies.* Papules between the finger webs are characteristic of scabies.

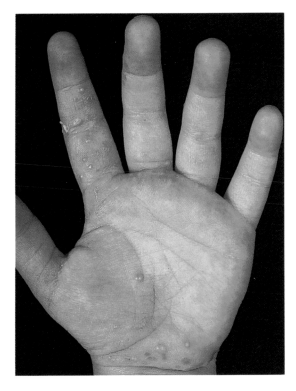

Fig. 9.22 *Scabies.* The wrists, palms, and fingers are the usual sites for burrows.

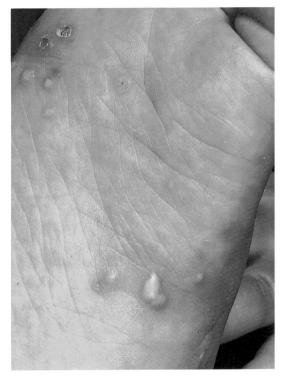

Fig. 9.23 *Scabies.* The burrows may be quite vesicopustular in infants and young children.

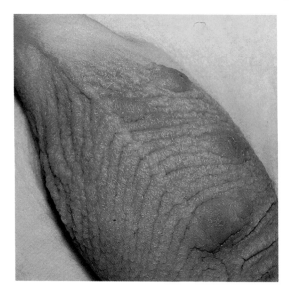

Fig. 9.24 *Scabies.* The scrotum and penis are often involved with inflammatory papules or nodules. The latter may persist.

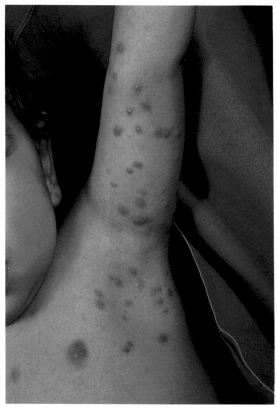

Fig. 9.26 *Scabies.* In some cases, inflammatory nodules are pronounced and will persist for several weeks after the condition has been treated.

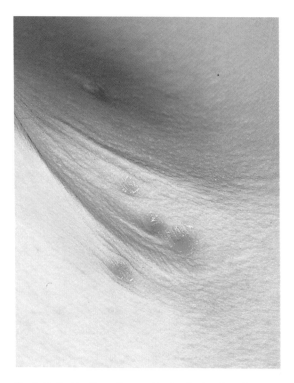

Fig. 9.25 *Scabies.* The axillae are often involved, with small papules occurring.

COMPLICATIONS

1 In immunocompromised patients (e.g. children with AIDS), a particularly heavy infestation may occur, producing a crusted variant of the disease 'Norwegian scabies'. A similar pattern may be seen if the patient is misdiagnosed as having eczema and treated with superpotent topical steroids.

2 Secondary bacterial infection is not uncommon in neglected cases, and this can lead to serious complications such as glomerulonephritis. This is a particular problem in developing countries.

DIFFERENTIAL DIAGNOSES

1 Infantile acropustulosis: this can be difficult to distinguish from scabies, because of the pustules on the palms and soles, except that there are no burrows.

2 Infected eczema (see p. 45): scabies is often misdiagnosed as eczema because of the severe pruritus and excoriations, but the presence of burrows and extraction of a mite is diagnostic.

MANAGEMENT

1 The diagnosis is confirmed by extracting the mite from a burrow using a blunt needle, and identifying the acarus under the microscope.

2 Many scabicides are available, but some can be quite irritant. Neurotoxicity has been reported following systemic absorption of gammabenzene hexachloride (lindane) in infants, and permethrin 5% cream or malathion 0.5% in aqueous solution are often better tolerated. Following a bath, the chosen lotion is carefully and thoroughly applied to the whole body, including the soles and interdigital webs. The head is treated in infants (avoiding the eyes and mouth) but excluded in older children and adults (Table 9.3).

3 All family members and close contacts must be treated simultaneously to avoid reinfection. Clothes and bedding can be adequately treated by machine washing on a hot cycle.

4 The pruritus lessens after treatment but may persist to a degree for several weeks. It is important to ensure that treatment has been adequate, but further applications of scabicides will only produce an irritant dermatitis and exacerbate the pruritus. Crotamiton 2% cream may provide symptomatic relief.

5 Secondary infection should be treated with oral antibiotics.

Pediculosis

DEFINITION

A pruritic infestation of lice affecting the scalp hair, skin or eyelashes.

AETIOLOGY

Three species of lice can affect humans

1 *Pediculus humanus capitis* is responsible for head

Table 9.3 Treatment of scabies

Permethrin 5% cream	1 Change clothes and bedding
	2 Bath
	3 Apply cream all over (including to head in babies)
	4 Wash off after 12 hours
	5 A single application is effective
Malathion 0.5% in aqueous solution	1 Change clothes and bedding
	2 Bath
	3 Apply lotion from the neck down (crotamiton cream to head in babies), and leave on for 24 hours
	4 Wash off
	5 Repeat after 7 days
Lindane 1% lotion	1 Change clothes and bedding
	2 Bath
	3 Apply lotion from the neck down, and leave on for 24 hours
	4 Repeat application the following day

lice. It is spread by head-to-head contact and it is common in children.

2 *P. humanus humanis* is the body louse, which rarely affects children except in conditions of extreme overcrowding and deprivation.

3 *Pthirus pubis* is the crab louse which is usually a sexually transmitted disease of adults, but children may develop infestation of the eyelashes by close contact with infected parents.

CLINICAL FEATURES

The majority of infections in children are due to *Pediculus humanus capitis*. This infestation is common in school children, especially in urban communities, but is far more common in white children. The infestation is characterized by scalp pruritus, scratching and a papular eruption on the back of the neck. The adult louse is about 3 mm in length, white with a long thin body. However, the most visible signs of infection are the numerous empty egg cases (nits) attached to the hair shafts (Fig. 9.27).

DIFFERENTIAL DIAGNOSES

1 Pityriasis amiantacea: this is occasionally confused

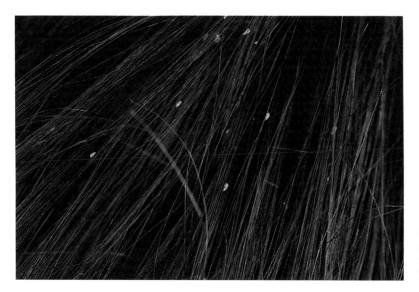

Fig. 9.27 *Pediculosis capitis.* Nits, the egg cases for the louse, are often the most prominent physical sign in scalp infestations.

with head lice, as the thick scales adhere tightly to the hair shaft, mimicking nits.

2 Dandruff: this should rarely cause confusion as the scale is easily dislodged.

MANAGEMENT

1 Malathion 0.5%, carbaryl 0.5% or permethrin 2% lotion are the current treatments of choice, but resistance has been reported.

2 Apply the chosen lotion, leave on for the recommended time and wash off.

3 The nits can be removed by using a fine-toothed metal comb.

Tropical infections

With increasing travel and immigration, more unusual infections are now sometimes seen in western countries.

Cutaneous leishmaniasis

DEFINITION

A chronic, crusted ulcer due to an arthropod-borne infection, most prevalent in Asia (Delhi boil, Oriental sore), the Middle East and South America.

AETIOLOGY

The organism is transmitted by the sandfly. Different species are endemic in different parts of the world, e.g. *Leishmania major* in southern Europe, north Africa and the Middle East and *L. mexicana* in parts of South America (new world leishmaniasis).

CLINICAL FEATURES

The incubation period is often several months and the patient may not remember the insect bite. An indolent pink papule develops at the site of inoculation and then breaks down to form a heavily crusted lesion, 1–3 cm in diameter, with an erythematous margin (Fig. 9.28). When the crust is removed, a deep ulcer with slough at the base is revealed. The lesion may eventually enlarge to a considerable size. Without treatment, the ulcer slowly heals to leave a cribriform scar. In most cases the infection is confined to the skin, but certain species (e.g. *L. braziliensis*) are capable of extensive mucocutaneous destruction.

MANAGEMENT

1 The diagnosis is confirmed by taking a biopsy or smear from the ulcer base, stained with Giemsa to

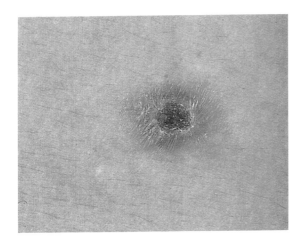

Fig. 9.28 *Cutaneous leishmaniasis.* An indolent red papule develops at the site of the sandfly bite, which ulcerates and crusts.

demonstrate the Donovan bodies (amastigotes within macrophages).
2 Pentavalent antimonials have been the standard treatment in the past, but are painful to administer.
3 Oral itraconazole is effective and less toxic.
4 Topical paromycin is currently under evaluation in trials and appears promising.

Cutaneous larva migrans (creeping eruption)

DEFINITION

A parasitic infection characterized by a pruritic 'creeping' rash caused by larvae migrating within the skin.

AETIOLOGY

Several different species of dog hookworm can cause this eruption, which is prevalent in the Caribbean and Florida. Faeces from an infested dog containing the ova contaminate beaches. When the larvae hatch, they can burrow into the skin of people walking barefoot along a beach.

CLINICAL FEATURES

An itch develops at the site of penetration of the worm. The larva moves through the skin producing a serpiginous eruption (Fig. 9.29). Humans are incidental hosts and as the larvae do not survive for long, the infection subsides after about 4 weeks.

MANAGEMENT

Topical thiabendazole 10% twice daily usually clears the eruption in 7 days.

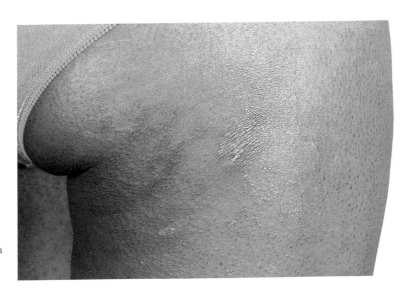

Fig. 9.29 *Cutaneous larva migrans.* The dog hookworm larvae move through the skin producing a serpiginous eruption. The buttock is a common site from sitting on a contaminated beach.

Leprosy (Hansen's disease)

DEFINITION

A chronic mycobacterial infection affecting the skin and peripheral nerves.

AETIOLOGY

The disease is caused by *Mycobacterium leprae* and is endemic in parts of Asia, Africa and the Far East.

CLINICAL FEATURES

The course of the disease depends on the level of host immunity, and may be classified as tuberculoid, borderline or lepromatous leprosy.

1 In tuberculoid leprosy the host immunity is high and few bacilli are detectable within the skin. A hypopigmented, anhidrotic and anaesthetic plaque develops with an erythematous, scaly edge. The sensory nerves close to the affected skin become thickened and palpable and a peripheral neuropathy develops.

2 In lepromatous leprosy the host immunity is low, the bacilli are numerous and the individual is highly contagious. The first symptoms are nasal congestion and discharge. The disease becomes widely disseminated with a multitude of flesh-coloured dermal papules (Fig. 9.30) on the face (particularly the cooler areas such as the ears) and limbs. The lesions coalesce producing widespread infiltration of the skin and exaggerated facial lines (the leonine facies). The disease may be complicated by a peripheral

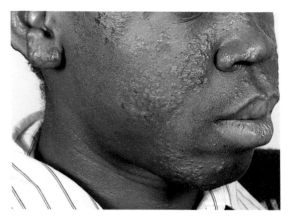

Fig. 9.30 *Leprosy.* The dermal flesh-coloured papules that occur on the face (especially lips, eyebrows and ears) ultimately coalesce, producing furrows in the skin.

neuropathy with subsequent destruction of digits through unappreciated trauma.

3 In borderline leprosy the clinical features form a spectrum between those of the tuberculoid and lepromatous variants of the disease.

MANAGEMENT

1 The specialist advice of a lepromatologist should always be sought.

2 Combination antibiotic therapy with rifampicin and dapsone for 6 months treats tuberculoid leprosy.

3 In lepromatous or borderline leprosy, clofazimine should be added to the regime, and treatment should continue for a total of 2 years.

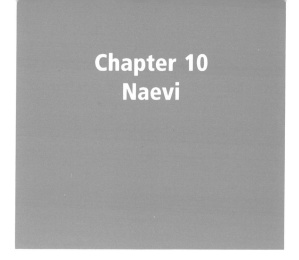
Introduction

A naevus is a benign developmental abnormality, in which there is an excessive aggregation of one of the components of normal skin.

Vascular naevi

Capillary haemangioma (strawberry naevus)

DEFINITION

A benign naevoid vascular proliferation, which characteristically resolves with time.

AETIOLOGY

Strawberry naevi are a developmental defect of capillaries. Mast cell numbers are increased within the lesion and it is postulated that they may secrete factors which promote angiogenesis.

CLINICAL FEATURES

The lesion may not be apparent at birth, but usually develops within the first 4 weeks of life. They are common, and are present in 1 out of 10 infants aged 1 year. They are slightly more common in premature babies and those with the fetal-alcohol syndrome. The lesion may be superficial, deep or mixed. Superficial lesions are the commonest and are well-demarcated, soft, rounded nodules with a bright red, speckled surface (Fig. 10.1). Deeper lesions appear as soft, bluish swellings beneath a normal epidermis. Capillary haemangiomas occur most frequently on the head and neck, but are not uncommon in the napkin area. They may be single or multiple. Initially, the lesion is seen to expand rapidly, reaching a maximum size at about 6 months. It then gradually involutes over the next few years (Figs 10.2–10.4). Over half the naevi have fully resolved by the time the child enters school.

COMPLICATIONS

1 Bleeding: large superficial lesions may bleed copiously when traumatized.

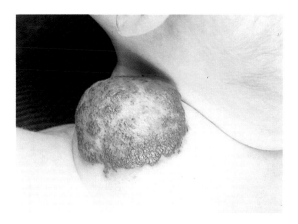

Fig. 10.1 *Strawberry naevus.* The naevus is present at birth or very soon afterwards. By the time the child is aged 4 months, the nodule is well demarcated, soft, rounded and red.

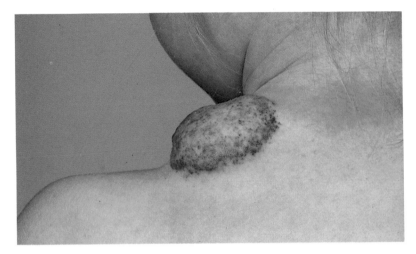

Fig. 10.2

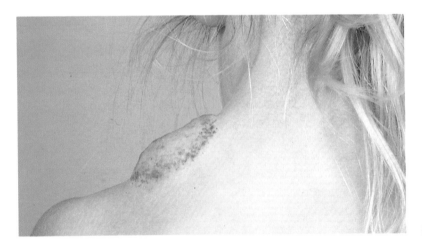

Fig. 10.3

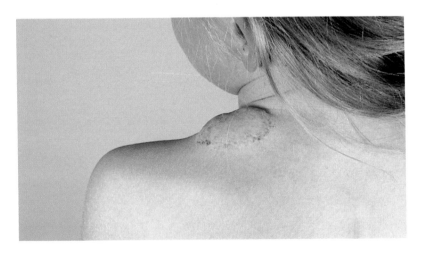

Figs 10.2–10.4 *Strawberry naevus.*
The nodule becomes paler (Fig. 10.2,
aged 2 years) and flatter (Fig. 10.3,
aged 3 years) and smaller (Fig. 10.4,
aged 4 years) as time goes by.

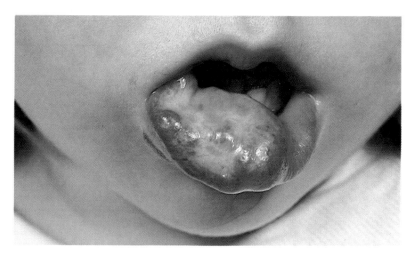

Fig. 10.5 *Strawberry naevus.* Lesions around the mouth may obstruct feeding and breathing but this naevus was asymptomatic.

2 Ulceration: this is not uncommon, especially at a site subject to friction (e.g. the napkin area), and secondary infection may result.

3 Obstruction of vital organs.

    (a) Lesions on the upper eyelid may obliterate the eye and impair visual development.

    (b) Lesions around the mouth (Fig. 10.5) or within the oropharynx may obstruct the airway or lead to difficulties in establishing feeding.

4 Kasabach–Merritt syndrome: platelets may become sequestered within large haemangiomas, resulting in haemorrhage, consumption of clotting factors and, eventually, disseminated intravascular coagulopathy.

MANAGEMENT

1 Reassurance that spontaneous resolution is the norm and that early intervention rarely produces a better, final cosmetic result.

2 If, however, the lesion has a predominantly deep component, early plastic surgery may produce an excellent result, because the tumour acts in effect like a tissue expander. The deep component may therefore be excised through a small linear incision, without epidermal loss, and easy closure of the wound is achieved.

3 Ulcerated lesions may be successfully treated by occlusion under a hydrocolloid dressing (e.g. Granuflex).

4 If vital organ function is threatened (e.g. in the case of large naevi obliterating the eye), then a course of oral prednisolone, 2–4 mg/kg, should be given until shrinkage is achieved (usually 4–6 weeks); the dose should be reduced slowly to zero over the next 2 months. Intralesional steroids may also be effective in reducing the size of the lesion.

5 If resolution is incomplete, or redundant skin remains, then plastic surgery may be required in older children.

6 Lasers are very helpful in treating the superficial component of lesions which persist into adult life. Experience is also showing that they may be useful in treating ulcerated lesions in infants.

Salmon patch (Unna's naevus)

DEFINITION

A common, benign vascular anomaly in which areas of macular telangiectasia are seen, most frequently on the eyelids and nape of the neck.

AETIOLOGY

The lesions represent a vascular malformation in which there are dilated superficial dermal capillaries. They appear to have an inherited basis, and are more common in white children.

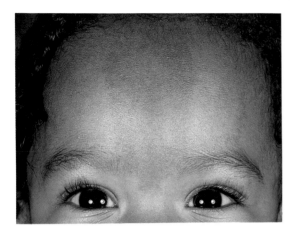

Fig. 10.6 *Salmon patch.* The forehead is a common site for this pink patch which is present at birth and fades by the first year.

AETIOLOGY

The lesions are congenital vascular malformations.

CLINICAL FEATURES

The port-wine stain is present at birth, and although the relative size is constant, it tends to become darker and more prominent with age. The lesion may become raised and develop angiomatous nodules within. They most often occur on the face (Fig. 10.7), and are usually unilateral, with clear demarcaion along the midline. The colour of the lesions is quite variable, ranging from pale pink to deep purple, and they vary in size from a few centimetres to those covering half the face.

CLINICAL FEATURES

Salmon patches are very common, dull-red macular lesions (Fig. 10.6) which are present at birth. It is estimated that up to 40% of neonates have a salmon patch. They may occur anywhere, but are most common in the nuchal area. The glabellum, upper eyelids, nose and upper lip are also frequently affected. Multiple lesions are not uncommon, and the patches may become more prominent during crying episodes.

MANAGEMENT

No treatment is required. The lesions resolve spontaneously, and most of them gradually fade to be imperceptible by the child's first birthday. However, lesions on the nape of the neck may be more persistent, and remain unchanged into adulthood.

Port-wine stain (naevus flammeus)

DEFINITION

A macular, erythematous lesion composed of ectatic dermal capillaries, most characteristically affecting the face, and which persists into adult life. It may be associated with neurological and ophthalmological abnormalities.

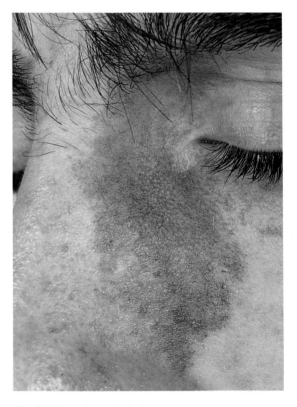

Fig. 10.7 *Port-wine stain.* The lesion is a deep red colour and is present at birth. Glaucoma and the Sturge–Weber syndrome may be associated.

COMPLICATIONS

Glaucoma is an important complication caused by concomitant abnormalities in the ocular vasculature, most commonly a choroidal angioma. The incidence of glaucoma in patients with port-wine stains is around 10%, but is highest in those lesions affecting both the upper and lower eyelids. Children with port-wine stains require regular eye checks, as the onset of glaucoma may be delayed. If it is detected, early treatment is imperative to preserve vision.

MANAGEMENT

1 Cosmetic camouflage may be of benefit, especially for paler lesions.

2 Treatment with the pulsed dye laser or infra-red coagulator can produce excellent permanent benefit. Early treatment is now advocated to reduce the psychological stress associated with large, disfiguring lesions.

Sturge–Weber syndrome

DEFINITION

A congenital abnormality in which a vascular malformation of the leptomeninges is associated with an ipsilateral port-wine stain.

AETIOLOGY

This is a developmental defect.

CLINICAL FEATURES

The naevus flammeus tends to be extensive and nearly always involves the upper eyelid and fore-

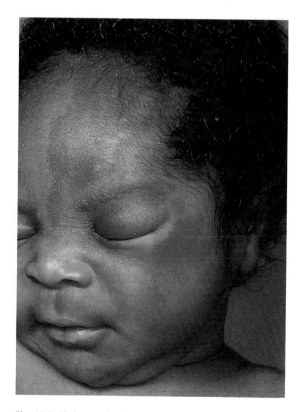

Fig. 10.8 *Phakomatosis pigmentovascularis.* This term refers to the association of an extensive port-wine stain of the Sturge–Weber syndrome with ocular (as shown) or cutaneous melanocytic lesions.

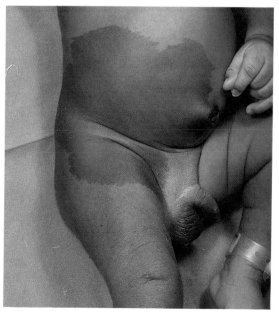

Fig. 10.9 *Phakomatosis pigmentovascularis.* Cutaneous melanocytic lesions.

head, but truncal or limb involvement is not uncommon. Affected children may suffer developmental delay, and 75% will develop epilepsy. When the fits are severe there is often accompanying mental retardation. The Sturge–Weber syndrome may be associated with ocular or cutaneous melanocytic lesions (Figs 10.8 and 10.9), a condition termed phakomatosis pigmentovascularis.

MANAGEMENT

1 The treatment of the naevus flammeus is as already discussed.
2 The extent of intracranial involvement can be assessed by computerized tomography scanning or magnetic resonance imaging.
3 Children who develop fits as part of the syndrome need specialist care by a neurologist from an early age, to maximize the control of the epilepsy and minimalize developmental problems.

Klippel–Trenauney syndrome

DEFINITION

The association of a port-wine stain on a limb with limb hypertrophy.

AETIOLOGY

The underlying developmental malformation may be venous, arteriovenous or mixed venous and lymphatic.

CLINICAL FEATURES

A macular naevus with prominent telangiectasia is seen on the affected limb (Fig. 10.10). It is usually present from birth, and most often the lower limbs are affected. Soft-tissue hypertrophy of the affected limb is virtually always present and there may be associated bony overgrowth. The tissue hypertrophy can extend beyond the limb to involve other areas of the body. The patient may develop venous varicosities within the naevus during late childhood and adolescence.

COMPLICATIONS

1 Angiokeratomas, which can occur within the lesion later in life.
2 Lymphangioma circumscriptum.
3 Other congenital abnormalities may be associated, especially deformities of the digits.

DIFFERENTIAL DIAGNOSES

1 Maffucci's syndrome: cavernous venous malformations are associated with dyschondroplasia and prominent limb hypertrophy.
2 Proteus syndrome: a polymorphic disorder comprising vascular malformations and hypertrophy of many parts of the body, including the epidermis.

MANAGEMENT

1 Attention to any discrepancy in limb length with appropriate correction is important to prevent the development of compensatory scoliosis.
2 Varicosities can be treated surgically.
3 In rare cases, amputation of a grossly deformed limb may be required if function is severely impaired.

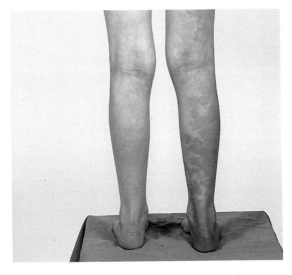

Fig. 10.10 *Klippel–Trenauney syndrome.* There is a diffuse, macular, purple naevus associated with soft tissue and often bony hypertrophy (courtesy of Mr P. Baskerville).

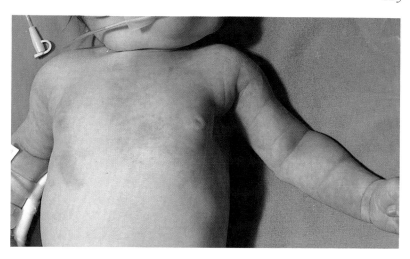

Fig. 10.11 *Reticulate vascular naevus.* Extensive prominent marbling of the skin is present on the limbs and trunk at birth. It ultimately fades.

Cutis marmorata telangiectatica congenita (reticulate vascular naevus)

DEFINITION

An uncommon variant of the port-wine stain, with a characteristic reticular pattern, which tends to fade gradually as the child gets older.

AETIOLOGY

It is a vascular malformation with venous and capillary components. While usually a sporadic occurrence, some cases are familial.

CLINICAL FEATURES

A prominent marbling of the skin is seen in affected areas from birth, due to the network of purplish erythema and telangiectatica (Fig. 10.11). It most frequently affects the limbs, but if it affects the face the naevus may be confluent and resemble an ordinary port-wine stain. It is accentuated by cold, but does not disappear on rewarming. Atrophy may develop within the affected area and ulceration can ensue. There may be associated limb hypoplasia.

DIFFERENTIAL DIAGNOSES

1 Cutis marmorata: the normal physiological response of neonates is a more generalized phenomenon and less florid.
2 Neonatal lupus erythematosus: this is usually bilateral.
3 Congenital livedo: this is rare and associated with other clinical abnormalities.

MANAGEMENT

1 Patients with facial lesions should always be assessed for glaucoma.
2 The naevus tends to fade slowly over time.
3 Ulcerations heal conservatively, but severe atrophy may persist and restrict limb development.

Naevus anaemicus

DEFINITION

A macular area of permanently blanched skin which does not to respond to any normal vasodilatatory stimulus.

AETIOLOGY

There is no microscopically detectable abnormality within the affected area. It is thought that the naevus develops as a result of increased vascular sensitivity to catecholamines and subsequent vasoconstriction in the affected area.

CLINICAL FEATURES

The lesion appears as an irregular area of persistently pale skin, with a scalloped edge (Fig. 10.12). It may occur anywhere on the body, and is always entirely macular. It is usually present from birth, and is often quite subtle, but rubbing the surrounding skin may accentuate the lesion. The abnormal area becomes imperceptible if the surrounding skin is blanched by pressure.

DIFFERENTIAL DIAGNOSIS

In achromic naevus (naevus depigmentosus) there is a hypo- or depigmented area (Fig. 10.13) which may be multiple or whorled. There is a reduction in the numbers of melanocytes in the skin, but normal vasodilatatory responses are preserved.

MANAGEMENT

No treatment is required and the lesion rarely presents a cosmetic problem.

Angiokeratoma circumscriptum

DEFINITION

A rare condition characterized by a hyperkeratotic, vascular plaque.

AETIOLOGY

This is a vascular malformation, in which ectatic vessels within the papillary dermis are associated with overlying acanthosis.

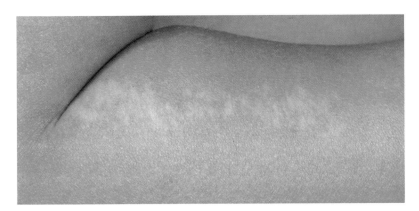

Fig. 10.12 *Naevus anaemicus.* There is an area of permanent pallor on the forearm, with a scalloped margin caused by vasoconstriction.

Fig. 10.13 *Achromic naevus.* There is an area of pale skin, due to low melanocytes.

CLINICAL FEATURES

Hyperkeratotic, purplish papules are present at birth and become larger and wartier with time. They most often affect the lower leg (Fig. 10.14). The larger lesions may bleed if traumatized.

DIFFERENTIAL DIAGNOSES

1 Lymphangioma circumscriptum (see p. 138).
2 Angiokeratoma of Mibelli: a familial disorder that develops in late childhood, particularly in girls.

MANAGEMENT

Depending on the size of the lesion, cauterization, surgical excision or laser ablation may be useful.

Angioma serpiginosum

DEFINITION

A rare naevoid condition of small blood vessels in the skin occurring on the limbs or buttocks.

AETIOLOGY

The cause is unknown. It starts in childhood and predominantly affects girls. It is occasionally inherited as an autosomal dominant.

CLINICAL FEATURES

The lesions are normally unilateral and consist of minute red or purple macules (Fig. 10.15), often on

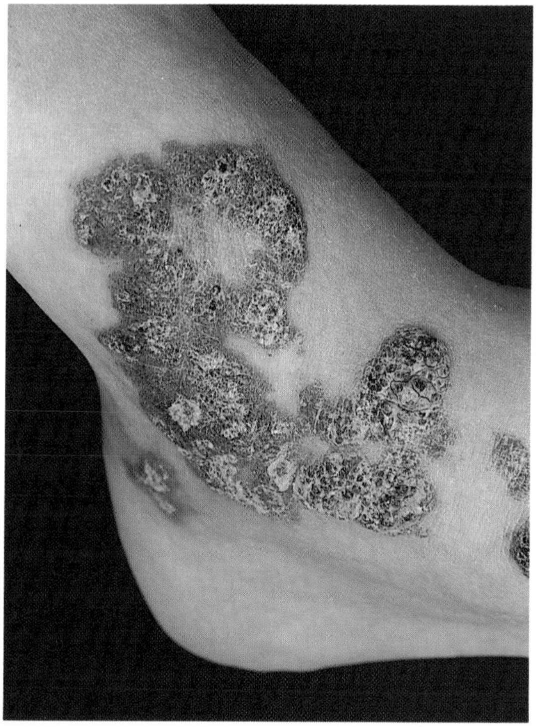

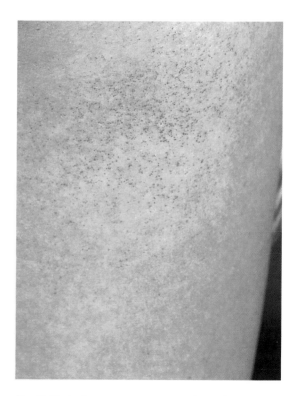

Fig. 10.14 *Angiokeratoma circumscriptum.* Hyperkeratotic, purplish papules and plaques are present at birth and may become larger and wartier with time. They frequently affect the lower leg (courtesy of the Institute of Dermatology).

Fig. 10.15 *Angioma serpiginosum.* Minute deep red or purple macules occur unilaterally over a limb or buttock in childhood. Girls are predominantly affected.

a background of erythema. The condition extends over a period of time but may occasionally disappear in adult life.

MANAGEMENT

There is no specific treatment.

Epidermal naevi

DEFINITION

A congenital lesion comprising warty, pigmented skin, often in a linear distribution. It may be quite inflamed. Several forms of epidermal naevi exist, the clinical features of which will be considered separately.

AETIOLOGY

These hamartomas are thought to arise from a somatic mutation in a single keratinocyte during embryonic development.

Verrucous epidermal naevi

CLINICAL FEATURES

Very warty lesions are present at birth or develop later in childhood (Fig. 10.16). Initially, they may be quite pink and smooth, but with age they gradually become more pigmented with a roughened surface. They may occur anywhere on the body, but tend to be unilateral (Fig. 10.17). They follow the embryonic lines of development (Blaschko's lines),

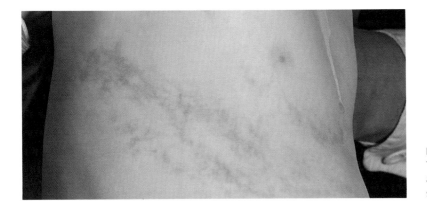

Fig. 10.16 *Verrucous epidermal naevi.* The naevi are linear and often multiple and may be only lightly pigmented and smooth at first.

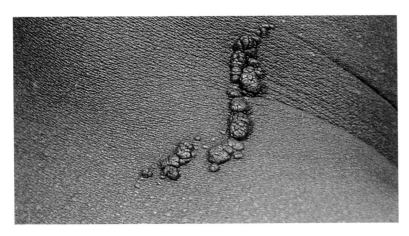

Fig. 10.17 *Epidermal naevus.* This group of warty papules are present in a linear configuration.

so that when they are extensive they produce a whorled pattern (Fig. 10.18).

DIFFERENTIAL DIAGNOSES

1 Lichen striatus: although linear, it is composed of asymptomatic white or pink papules and is not pigmented.
2 Viral warts (see p. 93): a linear arrangement of hyperkeratotic warts occasionally may be seen as a Köebner phenomenon.
3 Incontinentia pigmenti (see p. 28): an X-linked dominant syndrome in which blistering precedes the development of the warty lesions, in girls.
4 Sebaceous naevus (see p. 130): before puberty the typical papilliferous surface may not be as well developed.

MANAGEMENT

1 Cryotherapy may be effective in small lesions.
2 Shave excision is simple, but the naevus may recur.
3 Surgical excision provides a definitive cure, but may not always be feasible.

Inflammatory linear verrucous epidermal naevus (ILVEN)

CLINICAL FEATURES

These intensely pruritic, inflamed lesions (Fig. 10.19) tend to begin early in childhood, often during the first year, and are most common on the leg. They may look eczematous or psoriasiform.

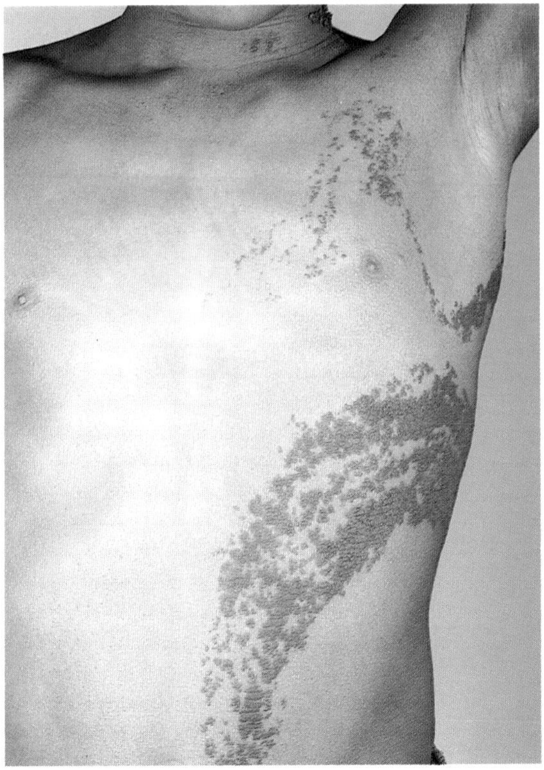

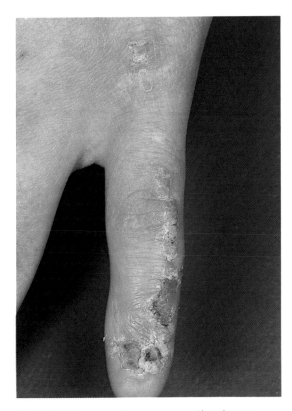

Fig. 10.18 *Verrucous epidermal naevi.* The naevi become more pigmented and warty, as in this 10-year-old boy, and have a whorled pattern.

Fig. 10.19 *Inflammatory linear verrucous epidermal naevus.* Occasionally, there may be an inflammatory margin to a linear epidermal naevus which may therefore be mistaken for eczema.

DIFFERENTIAL DIAGNOSES

1 Naevoid psoriasis: this is less itchy and responds to standard treatments for psoriasis.
2 CHILD syndrome: an inflammatory ichthyosiform naevus occurring in association with congenital hemidysplasia and limb defects.

MANAGEMENT

Treatment of these lesions is often unsatisfactory and the pruritus can present quite a management problem. Spontaneous improvement is rare, but has been documented occasionally.

Sebaceous naevus of Jadassohn

DEFINITION

A common papillomatous hamartoma seen predominantly on the head and neck and composed of sebaceous cells.

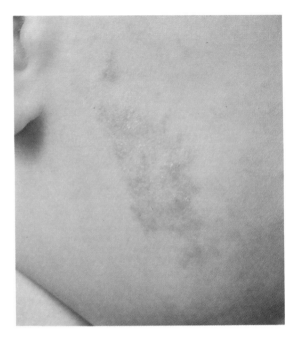

Fig. 10.20 *Naevus sebaceous.* This well-defined, raised, orange-yellow plaque is present on the cheek from birth.

AETIOLOGY

The lesion is considered to arise in the same way as an epidermal naevus.

CLINICAL FEATURES

Sebaceous naevi are common, occurring in three out of 1000 babies. The naevi are well-circumscribed, orange-coloured plaques (Fig. 10.20), especially on the scalp and around the ear (Fig. 10.21). The lesion is hairless and so tends to be more noticeable on the scalp (Fig. 10.22). Initially the surface is quite soft and velvety, but it becomes wartier at puberty when the sebaceous glands mature.

COMPLICATIONS

1 Development of a secondary, benign appendigeal tumour within the lesion, e.g. syringocystadenoma papilliferum – an apocrine tumour.
2 A small proportion of sebaceous naevi will undergo malignant change in later life, e.g. develop a basal cell carcinoma.

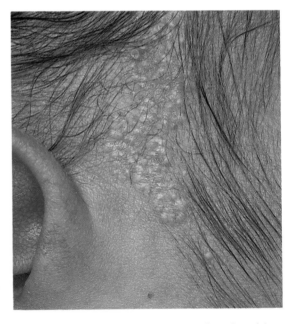

Fig. 10.21 *Naevus sebaceous.* In adolescence the surface of the yellow plaque becomes wartier. There is a significant complication of change to basal cell carcinoma. Excision is therefore advisable.

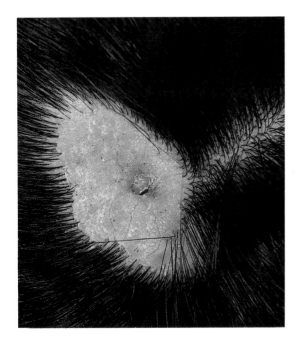

Fig. 10.22 *Naevus sebaceous.* The scalp is the most common site and there is associated hair loss. A basal cell carcinoma is present.

MANAGEMENT

Because of the risk of malignant change these lesions should be excised, if practical, but surgery can be delayed until the child is of an appropriate age.

Epidermal naevus syndrome (Jadassohn's phakomatosis)

Multiple sebaceous naevi may be associated with neurological and other developmental defects. There appears to be a high incidence of internal malignancy in patients with this condition.

Becker's naevus

This variant of an epidermal naevus usually develops in adolescence, but may become apparent in childhood.

DEFINITION

A large, pigmented naevus with associated hypertrichosis, most common in males and typically occurring over the shoulder.

AETIOLOGY

It is a variant of an epidermal naevus, which may be associated with smooth muscle hamartomas and bony abnormalities.

CLINICAL FEATURES

Thickened areas of skin with pigmentation and hypertrichosis develop characteristically in the teens.

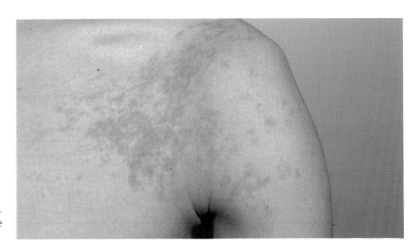

Fig. 10.23 *Becker's naevus.* This pigmented epidermal naevus usually becomes apparent during adolescence. The breast or back of the shoulder are the usual sites.

The lesion is permanent and gradually becomes wartier with time. The front of the upper chest (Fig. 10.23) and back of the shoulder are the most common sites.

MANAGEMENT

The size of the lesion renders excision impractical, but depilation may be offered if the naevus causes embarrassment. Usually no treatment is required, but the Q-switched ruby laser has recently been demonstrated to be effective in ablating the pigmentation.

Pigmented naevi

Melanocytic naevi (moles)

DEFINITION

Melanocytic naevi or moles are common, benign, pigmented lesions consisting of increased numbers of melanocytes within the skin.

AETIOLOGY

They may be congenital or acquired throughout childhood. Melanocytes migrate from the neural crest to the basal layer of the epidermis during fetal life. Some cells may become arrested deep within the dermis, where they clinically take on a bluish hue. Melanocytic naevi are classified as junctional, compound or intradermal, according to the position of the naevus cells in relation to the dermo-epidermal junction.

Congenital naevi

CLINICAL FEATURES

1 Congenital naevi tend to be larger (Fig. 10.24) and more deeply pigmented (Fig. 10.25) than acquired naevi. They may have coarse terminal hairs within. There is a small risk of malignant change in adult life.
2 Giant bathing trunk naevus: this is a rare variant of a congenital naevus, which covers an extensive

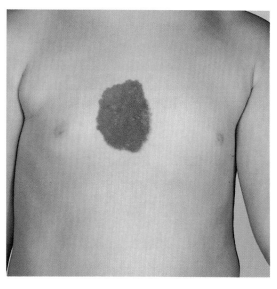

Fig. 10.24 *Congenital pigmented naevus.* Melanocytic naevi present at birth tend to be larger than acquired moles. They should be protected from the sun because there is a small risk of malignant change.

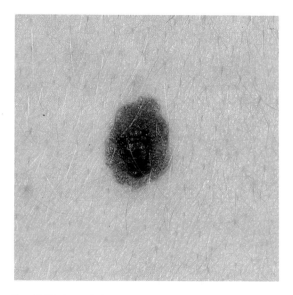

Fig. 10.25 *Congenital pigmented naevus.* These naevi vary in size but are appreciably larger than the average acquired mole. There are two, evenly distributed, shades of pigment in this lesion.

part of the body surface (Fig. 10.26), and is usually confluent over the lower back, buttocks and upper thighs, with individual large pigmented naevi scattered elsewhere. There is a high risk of malignant change within the lesion.

MANAGEMENT

There is no consensus on the best policy in the case of small congenital naevi. Some authorities recommend prophylactic excision, but most consider the risk small enough to follow an expectant policy.

In the case of giant bathing trunk naevi, prophylactic excision is often attempted, but is limited by the extent of the lesion. Grafting is required to cover the defect and can lead to unsightly scarring (Fig. 10.27) and problems with future growth. Sequential treatments may be employed, but they may still be unsatisfactory. An expectant approach may be more reasonable, especially as a melanoma may develop in a non-cutaneous site.

Acquired naevi

CLINICAL FEATURES

1 *Junctional naevi* are small, macular lesions (Fig. 10.28) which are evenly but deeply pigmented in colour.
2 *Compound naevi* are common, slightly raised pigmented lesions (Fig. 10.28) with a junctional and intradermal component.

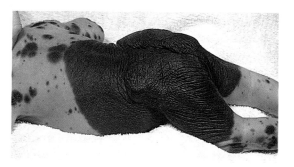

Fig. 10.26 *Bathing trunk naevus.* This is a rare and extensive collection of large naevi that are particularly concentrated on the trunk and buttocks.

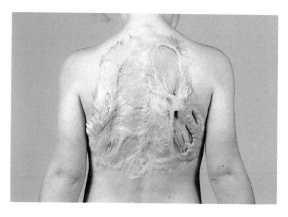

Fig. 10.27 *Bathing trunk naevus.* Although there is a risk of malignant melanoma with this condition, it is uncertain whether extensive surgery is warranted, particularly as cerebral melanoma may develop.

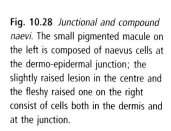

Fig. 10.28 *Junctional and compound naevi.* The small pigmented macule on the left is composed of naevus cells at the dermo-epidermal junction; the slightly raised lesion in the centre and the fleshy raised one on the right consist of cells both in the dermis and at the junction.

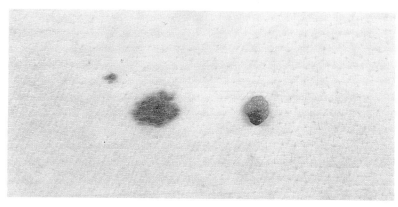

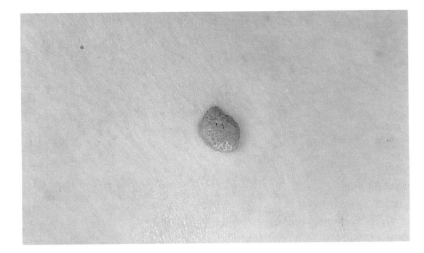

Fig. 10.29 *Intradermal naevus.* This fleshy raised papule with no pigment has naevus cells only within the dermis.

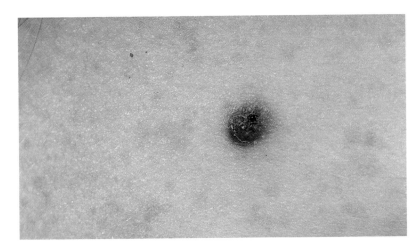

Fig. 10.30 *Blue naevus.* The melanocytes in these acquired naevi are deep within the dermis and reflect a blue rather than a brown colour due to Tindel's effect.

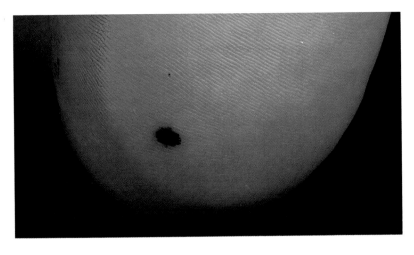

Fig. 10.31 *Trauma.* Haemorrhage into the skin on the foot is usually second to intense physical activity and may simulate a naevus or melanoma.

3 *Intradermal naevi* are often skin-coloured, small-domed lesions (Fig. 10.29), which are particularly prominent on the face. They may be hairy and are more common in adults.

4 *Blue naevi*: melanocytes, deep within the dermis appear blue-black in colour (Fig. 10.30). The lesions are usually small and regular.

DIFFERENTIAL DIAGNOSIS

Trauma (*talon noir*): haemorrhage into the skin (Fig. 10.31) resulting from trauma (usually on the feet) may simulate a junctional naevus or indeed a melanoma.

MANAGEMENT

Simple acquired naevi require no treatment, unless excision is requested for cosmetic reasons. If so, such elective procedures are best delayed until a procedure under local anaesthetic can be tolerated and future growth will not compromise the scar. It is important to appreciate that excision at certain sites, e.g. the anterior chest wall, usually results in unsightly scars, and is therefore best avoided unless absolutely necessary.

Variants of melanocytic naevi

Halo naevus (Sutton's naevus)

DEFINITION

A rim of depigmentation may appear around one or more benign naevi, particularly in adolescence.

AETIOLOGY

The halo naevus is an autoimmune phenomenon. Although it is transient, affected individuals have a slightly increased chance of later developing vitiligo.

CLINICAL FEATURES

Halos of paler skin surrounding and eventually destroying the naevus are not uncommon. Sometimes the process affects a single mole, but more

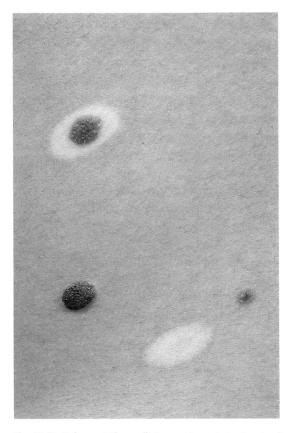

Fig. **10.32** *Halo naevi*. The small pigmented macule is a junctional naevus, the raised papule is a compound naevus. The compound naevus, which is a surrounded by a white halo, will disappear as the mole has done from the completely white area.

often several naevi are affected (Fig. 10.32). The condition is self-limiting, with eventual repigmentation of the skin.

MANAGEMENT

Reassurance and adequate protection from sunburn for the depigmented areas is all that is required.

Mayerson's naevus

DEFINITION

An eczematous reaction around one or more melanocytic naevi.

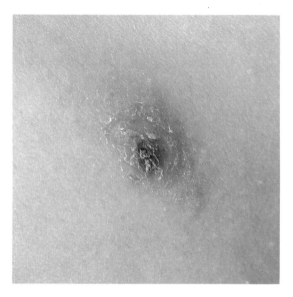

Fig. 10.33 *Mayerson's naevus.* Eczema may occur around a melanocytic naevus. It is a benign phenomenon.

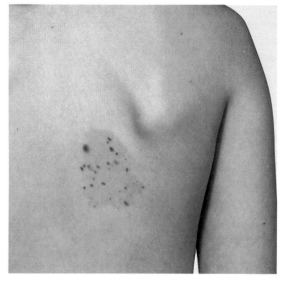

Fig. 10.34 *Naevus spilus.* This is a 'spotty' (spilus) café-au-lait patch which is usually congenital.

AETIOLOGY

This may represent a benign autoimmune phenomenon similar to that of the halo naevus (see p. 135).

CLINICAL FEATURE

Eczema develops around the naevus (Fig. 10.33) which resolves spontaneously.

MANAGEMENT

The eczema will respond to a potent topical steroid.

Naevus spilus

DEFINITION

This is a relatively rare naevus composed of multiple, dark, lentiginous macules scattered over an area of paler background pigmentation.

AETIOLOGY

This is a congenital naevus. There are increased numbers of melanocytes in the background pigmentation, with lentiginous melanocytic hyperplasia in the dark spots.

CLINICAL FEATURES

It is usually macular, but some of the darker areas may be raised. The lesions are often quite large (Fig. 10.34) and may be several centimetres in diameter. It is sometimes associated with neurofibromatosis (see p. 29).

MANAGEMENT

Malignant change has been observed within the lesions and therefore prophylactic excision is often advised.

Spitz naevus (juvenile melanoma)

DEFINITION

A rather vascular pigmented naevus; in children, it is most prevalent on the face. Histologically, it is characterized by bizarre and spindle-shaped cells, with the result that the lesion may appear alarming, but it is benign. The term Spitz naevus is therefore preferred to the older name of juvenile melanoma.

AETIOLOGY

The lesion is essentially a variant of a compound naevus.

CLINICAL FEATURES

The Spitz naevus appears in childhood as a small, solitary, well-circumscribed, reddish-brown nodule (Fig. 10.35), most commonly on the face. The lesion may grow rapidly at first, but then remains static. Occasionally, Spitz naevi may occur in clusters (agminate Spitz naevus).

MANAGEMENT

If the clinical diagnosis is in doubt then local excision may be recommended.

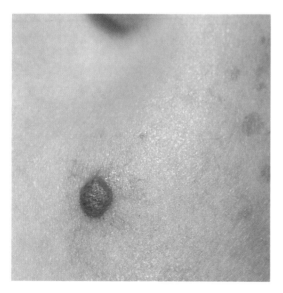

Fig. 10.35 *Spitz naevus.* This benign mole is red-brown in colour and is often on the cheek, as in this case. Pathologically, it may be mistaken for a melanoma, but melanoma is very rare indeed in childhood.

Mongolian blue spot

DEFINITION

A large, benign, macular, pigmented lesion over the lower back, due to melanocytes deep within the dermis, common in Oriental and Afro-Caribbean neonates.

AETIOLOGY

Large numbers of melanocytes collect in the deep dermis during fetal life. It is histologically distinct from an acquired blue naevus as there are no melanophages within the lesion.

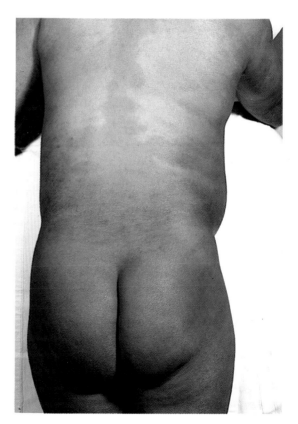

Fig. 10.36 *Mongolian blue spot.* This condition, commonly found on the backs of black and Oriental neonates, disappears spontaneously.

CLINICAL FEATURES

The lesion is present at birth in a high percentage of Oriental children. It appears as a slate-blue pigmented area (Fig. 10.36), particularly over the sacrum. The lesion may darken initially in the neonatal period, but then slowly fades through childhood and finally disappears.

MANAGEMENT

The lesion is a normal occurrence in certain races and requires no treatment.

Naevus of Ota

DEFINITION

A large, speckled naevus of bluish hue occurring in and around the eye, particularly in Oriental people.

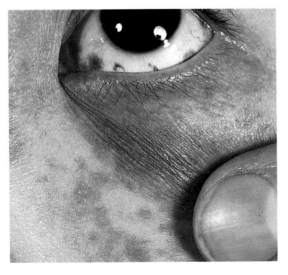

Fig. 10.37 *Naevus of Ota.* This is a common blue naevus of the sclera and the skin around the eye, particularly in Oriental people.

AETIOLOGY

The lesion arises from melanocytes deep within the dermis and sclera.

CLINICAL FEATURES

The lesion is not present at birth, but develops during childhood and persists into adult life. It may have a whorled appearance and can affect a large part of the face and eye unilaterally (Fig. 10.37).

MANAGEMENT

1 The patient can be taught to use cosmetic camouflage if the lesion is considered unsightly.
2 The Q-switched ruby laser can be effective in treating the naevus.

Other naevi

Lymphangioma circumscriptum

DEFINITION

A hamartomatous malformation composed of dilated lymphatic vessels.

AETIOLOGY

Lymphangioma circumscriptum is a developmental anomaly.

CLINICAL FEATURES

The lesion is composed of clustered gelatinous papules and vesicles, some of which may be haemorrhagic (Fig. 10.38). It is usually present at birth, but may develop later in childhood. It may occur anywhere on the skin and can occur intraorally.

MANAGEMENT

Most small lesions are best left alone, as recurrence often occurs after surgical excision.

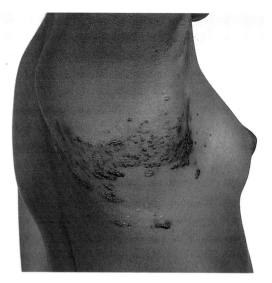

Fig. 10.38 *Lymphangioma circumscriptum.* This 11-year-old girl has a more extensive naevus. The lymphangioma spreads well beyond the obvious clinical margins.

Connective tissue naevus

DEFINITION

A hamartoma of the connective tissue of the skin, especially involving collagen and elastin.

AETIOLOGY

The lesion is a developmental defect. It may occur as a solitary finding or in conjunction with other congenital problems as part of a syndrome.

CLINICAL FEATURES

The lesion, which may be quite subtle, consists of an asymptomatic, irregular plaque of thickened skin, which may be nodular (Fig. 10.39) in places.

COMPLICATIONS

1 Shagreen patch of tuberous sclerosis: this is a type of collagenoma. It is most characteristic over the lower back.
2 Buschke–Ollendorf syndrome: a familial (autosomal-dominant) trait in which connective tissue naevi occur in association with a bony abnormality – osteopoikilosis – identified radiologically.

MANAGEMENT

The lesion itself requires no specific treatment except for the exclusion of any associated anomalies.

Fig. 10.39 *Connective tissue naevi.* A group of flesh-coloured dermal nodules occur particularly on the trunk, producing a thickening of the skin with a corrugated appearance. This naevus may occur in association with tuberous sclerosis.

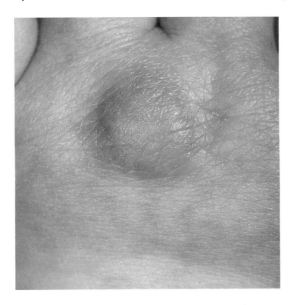

Fig. 10.40 *Mastocytoma.* This nodule appears in infancy but disappears spontaneously within 2 or 3 years.

Mastocytoma

DEFINITION

A solitary, naevoid collection of mast cells.

AETIOLOGY

A developmental accumulation of excess mast cells within the dermis.

CLINICAL FEATURES

The lesion is a small pinkish-brown or flesh-coloured nodule (Fig. 10.40), which urticates (Fig. 10.41), or even blisters, when rubbed.

MANAGEMENT

The lesion often subsides with time.

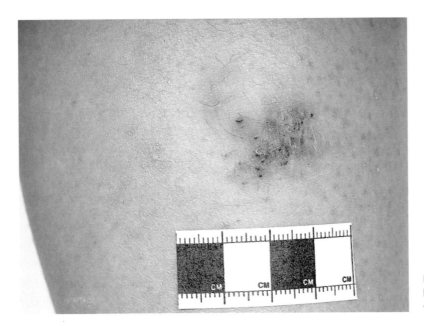

Fig. 10.41 *Mastocytoma.* This is a red-brown nodule, consisting of mast cells, which urticates or blisters with trauma.

Introduction

Tumours may be classified as benign or malignant proliferations of cells. Malignant tumours of the skin are very rare in childhood, and most of this chapter is therefore devoted to the more common benign tumours.

Other benign nodules which might form part of the differential diagnosis of some skin tumours are also included here for clarity, although they are not strictly tumours.

Benign tumours

Juvenile xanthogranuloma

DEFINITION

Single or multiple benign, self-healing nodules composed of lipid-laden histiocytes, common in young children, which resolve spontaneously.

AETIOLOGY

The cause of the lesion is not known, but there is no association with hyperlipidaemia.

CLINICAL FEATURES

The majority of lesions occur in white babies, most frequently as papules or nodules on the head and neck. They are far less common in black children.

Juvenile xanthogranulomas are usually cutaneous, but may also affect internal organs and the eye. They are occasionally associated with neurofibromatosis (see p. 25). A small, rubbery, yellow papule (Fig. 11.1) erupts, which may grow to a size of 1–2 cm. Telangiectasia, particularly around the margin of the tumour, is characteristic. Lesions may be solitary or multiple.

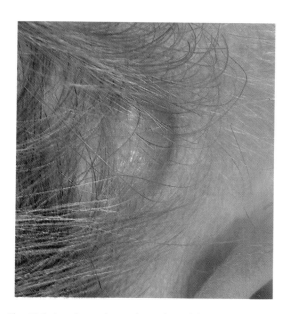

Fig. 11.1 *Juvenile xanthogranuloma.* The nodule is yellow and the scalp is a common site. The lesion regresses within a couple of years of onset.

DIFFERENTIAL DIAGNOSES

1 Eruptive xanthomas: these characteristically involve the extensor sites, and are associated with a hyperlipidaemia.
2 Benign cephalic histiocytosis: multiple erythematous histiocytic papules and larger nodules erupt over the head in infancy. The condition is benign and resolves spontaneously. Histologically, the histiocytes are not foamy, but occasional giant cells may be present.

COMPLICATIONS

Ocular lesions are associated with the development of glaucoma.

MANAGEMENT

1 The diagnosis is clinical and a confirmatory biopsy is rarely required.
2 The lesions regress over 18 months to 2 years.

Dermatofibroma

DEFINITION

A common, very firm, fibrohistiocytic proliferation within the dermis.

AETIOLOGY

Dermatofibromas are thought to arise as a reaction to minor trauma or insect bites.

CLINICAL FEATURES

A small, firm, pea-sized papule (Fig. 11.2) is palpable within the dermis. It is firmly attached to the overlying epidermis, which is often stretched over the surface of the lesion. There is frequently a rim of peripheral pigmentation.

Occasionally the lesions are tender, but more often they are entirely asymptomatic. They are common on the lower legs.

DIFFERENTIAL DIAGNOSES

1 Melanocytic naevi: dermatofibromas are sometimes mistaken for moles, but are much firmer.
2 Keloids (see p. 143): these may achieve a great size, compared with dermatofibromas, and usually occur at sites of obvious trauma.

MANAGEMENT

Surgical excision may produce a disappointing cosmetic result. As the lesions are benign, they are often best left alone.

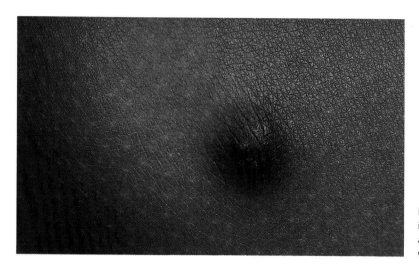

Fig. 11.2 *Dermatofibroma.* The papule is pigmented, smooth and firm. It is attached to the surface but is movable within the skin.

Keloids

DEFINITION

An abnormal hyperproliferative response of connective tissue.

AETIOLOGY

Keloids nearly always arise as a result of trauma (e.g. ear-piercing (Fig. 11.3), burns or surgical incisions), but inflammatory conditions (such as acne or chicken pox) may induce hypertrophic scarring, and occasionally spontaneous lesions occur. There is a familial tendency, and keloids are more common in black skin.

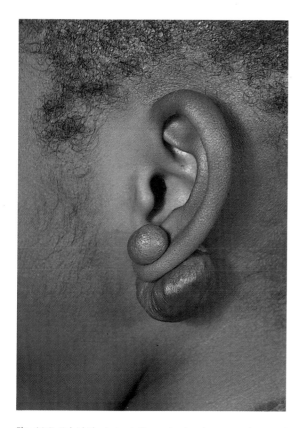

Fig. 11.3 *Keloid.* The lesion is firm or hard and occurs at the site of previous trauma. Ear-piercing is a common cause of the condition especially in black skin.

CLINICAL FEATURES

A keloid may occur anywhere, but they are most common on the head, neck and upper trunk. The lesion begins as a firm, smooth, erythematous plaque, which may become nodular and can achieve a quite massive size. They may be quite a livid colour and in black skin become hyperpigmented.

DIFFERENTIAL DIAGNOSIS

A hypertrophic scar is similar but confined to the margins of the surgical incision, rather than growing outwards in an expansive manner like a keloid.

MANAGEMENT

1 Intralesional steroids or application of superpotent topical steroids under occlusion (flurandrenolone tape) are occasionally helpful in softening early lesions, but may induce hypopigmentation.
2 Small lesions are best left alone, as intervention can exacerbate the problem. If surgical excision is attempted, special pressure dressings (or local radiotherapy in older individuals) are used to try and prevent further fibrocyte proliferation.

Pyogenic granuloma

DEFINITION

A benign eruptive vascular tumour composed of proliferating capillaries, common in childhood.

AETIOLOGY

This condition is believed to arise in response to minor trauma.

CLINICAL FEATURES

A red, glossy papule (Fig. 11.4) develops suddenly, most often on the face (Fig. 11.5) or hand. The lesion enlarges rapidly and often bleeds profusely. The surface is quite friable and often becomes eroded and crusted. There may be a surrounding rim (collarette) of thickened, white skin (Fig. 11.6).

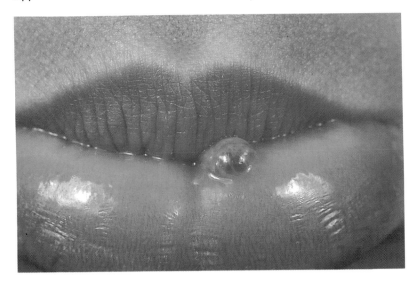

Fig. 11.4 *Pyogenic granuloma.* The lesion grows rapidly, is red and friable and bleeds readily. This lesion was easily removed by curettage and cautery.

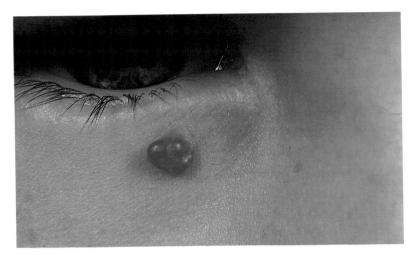

Fig. 11.5 *Pyogenic granuloma.* The face is a common site for this red, vascular papule.

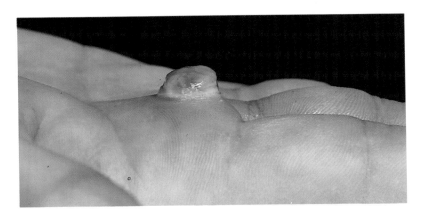

Fig. 11.6 *Pyogenic granuloma.* A well-circumscribed, glistening nodule which is readily traumatized.

MANAGEMENT

The lesion should be removed either by excision or curettage and cautery, depending on the size and site of the lesion.

Spider naevi

DEFINITION

A vascular lesion characterized by a large central arteriole with small feeding vessels in a radial pattern.

AETIOLOGY

In adults the lesions arise in association with hormonal factors or hepatic disease, but in children they are usually spontaneous.

CLINICAL FEATURES

Spider naevi are common in children between the ages of 2 and 6 years, especially on the face. A bright-red papule occurs in association with radiating vessels (Fig. 11.7), and the whole lesion usually blanches on pressure. They may be single or multiple.

MANAGEMENT

1 Spider naevi in children often regress spontaneously after puberty, without scarring.
2 If the lesion is causing embarrassment, then ablation of the central vessel with cold-point cautery, hyfrecater or laser is helpful.

Pilomatrixoma (calcifying epithelioma of Malherbe)

DEFINITION

A hamartoma originating from the hair follicle, which frequently calcifies (Fig. 11.8).

AETIOLOGY

The lesion is derived from the hair matrix.

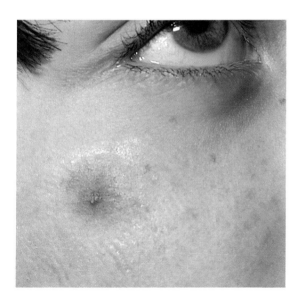

Fig. 11.7 *Spider naevus.* Fine blood vessels radiate from a tiny, central, red papule. Childhood lesions often resolve spontaneously.

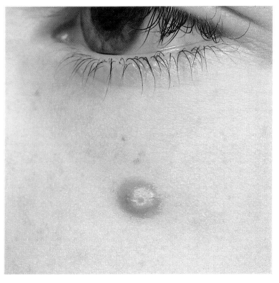

Fig. 11.8 *Calcifying epithelioma of Malherbe.* This lesion, which is solitary, hard and cream-coloured, is commonly sited on the face.

CLINICAL FEATURES

This is the most common appendage tumour in childhood. The lesion arises as a hard, solitary subcutaneous nodule, on the upper body, especially the face (Fig. 11.8). The overlying skin is normal, but a bluish hue may be perceptible. Pilomatrixomas may attain a considerable size.

DIFFERENTIAL DIAGNOSES

1 Epidermoid cyst: these are softer than pilomatrixomas, with an obvious central punctum, but are uncommon in childhood.
2 Calcinosis cutis: the lesions are smaller, papular and more superficial. Dystrophic mineralization may complicate benign cysts, inflammatory conditions such as acne or injury (e.g. burns, neonatal heal pricks).

MANAGEMENT

The lesion is treated by local excision.

Syringoma

DEFINITION

A benign proliferation of the sweat gland apparatus, which are usually multiple, especially around the eyelids.

AETIOLOGY

The lesions are derived from eccrine ducts. They may be familial, and occur with increased frequency in Down's syndrome.

CLINICAL FEATURES

Syringomata most commonly erupt in adolescence and are more common in girls. Multiple small, flat, pale yellow or flesh-coloured papules develop in clusters, symmetrically on the upper cheeks and eyelids (Fig. 11.9). The lesions have a characteristic histology, with multiple comma-shaped ducts in the upper dermis.

DIFFERENTIAL DIAGNOSES

1 Milia are firmer and white rather than pale yellow. They are rarely as numerous.
2 Xanthelasma are most often seen in the inner canthus and are larger plaques, rather than papules, and of a waxy yellow hue.
3 Other appendage tumours can be differentiated histologically.

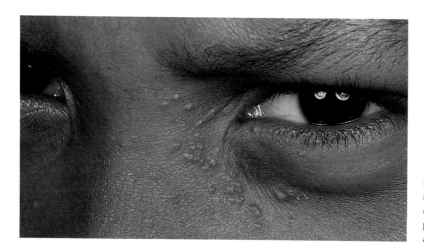

Fig. 11.9 *Syringomata.* These are multiple, often symmetrical, flesh-coloured, small papules which particularly occur around the eyes and are derived from the sweat glands.

MANAGEMENT

The lesions may be cauterized if of cosmetic concern.

Trichoepithelioma (Brooke's tumour)

DEFINITION

A tumour of the pilosebaceous unit, which occurs on the face and is genetic in origin.

AETIOLOGY

The lesions are familial and are inherited as an autosomal-dominant condition. It is quite distinct from the solitary, non-familial lesion of the same name which occur in older individuals.

CLINICAL FEATURES

The tumours usually develop at puberty on the middle aspect of the face particularly the eyelids and nasolabial folds (Fig. 11.10). They are multiple, flesh-coloured, rather translucent firm papules, which may be associated with telangiectasia.

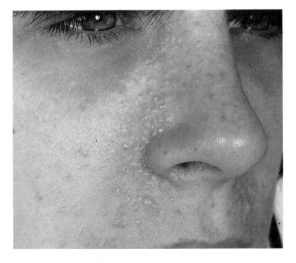

Fig. 11.10 *Trichoepitheliomata.* These multiple, flesh-coloured papules occur around the nose. They are inherited as an autosomal-dominant trait.

DIFFERENTIAL DIAGNOSES

1 Syringomata: the two tumours are easily distinguished histologically.
2 Adenoma sebaceum: the size, site and morphology of the lesions is very similar, but other features of tuberose sclerosis are usually apparent.

MANAGEMENT

1 Removal may be desirable for cosmetic reasons, but there is a high rate of recurrence following excision.
2 The lesions may be removed quite successfully by curettage and cautery.

Milia

DEFINITION

A small, firm, keratin cyst, commonly seen on the face.

AETIOLOGY

Milia develop as keratin retention cysts. They can develop following epidermal damage, e.g. in epidermolysis bullosa (see p. 132), or as an eruptive phenomenon, in which case they arise from sweat ducts or vellus hair follicles.

CLINICAL FEATURES

Minute (1–2 mm in diameter), superficial firm, creamy-white domed papules may develop at any site in damaged skin. Eruptive and solitary lesions are most often confined to the face, especially around the eyes (Fig. 11.11) and cheeks. Milia can occur at any age, but eruptive lesions most commonly develop in the teens. In neonates, milia may resolve spontaneously (see p. 8), but in older individuals the lesions tend to persist.

DIFFERENTIAL DIAGNOSES

1 Syringomata: the lesions may be numerous and occur in a very similar distribution below the eye,

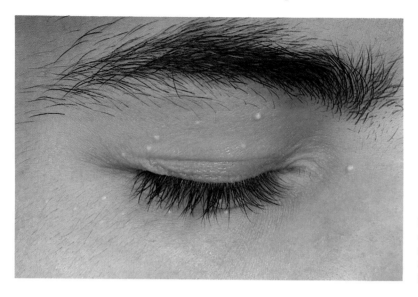

Fig. 11.11 *Milia.* Tiny white papules occur, particularly on the face. These are usually idiopathic but may be the result of acne and may also be caused by sun damage in adolescence.

but tend to be flat-topped rather than domed, and are not so white.

2 Closed acne comedones appear very similar, but the follicular orifice (punctum) is usually just discernible.

MANAGEMENT

1 No treatment is necessary; when milia arise within scars they are best left alone.

2 Solitary or eruptive milia may be gently removed by breaking the surface of the overlying epidermis with the tip of a green (21-gauge) needle and lifting out the cyst.

Lipoma

DEFINITION

A dermal aggregation of fat cells.

AETIOLOGY

It has been postulated that lipomas may arise from a regulatory defect of glycolysis.

CLINICAL FEATURES

Lipomas are soft mobile swellings (Fig. 11.12) within

the dermis; they vary in size but are usually of the order of 3–4 cm in diameter. The epidermis can be readily moved over the surface of the lesion. They are common in adults and may arise in adolescence, but are not usually seen in young children.

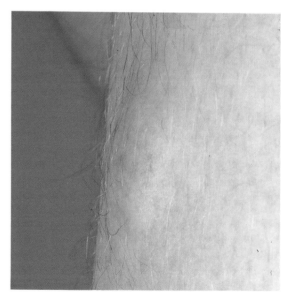

Fig. 11.12 *Lipoma.* This flesh-coloured, subcutaneous nodule, which can be multiple, may be a familial condition.

DIFFERENTIAL DIAGNOSIS

Angiolipomas are clinically identical to lipomas, with the exception that they are painful and tend to occur at a younger age.

MANAGEMENT

1 Local excision under local anaesthetic.
2 It is often impractical to try and excise multiple lesions.

Epidermoid cyst

DEFINITION

A tense dermal cyst containing macerated keratin, most common on the head and neck.

AETIOLOGY

The cyst arises around a dilated or damaged pilo-sebaceous unit and may arise in isolation or as a complication of severe acne. Multiple lesions may be part of an inherited disorder, Gardner's syndrome, associated with intestinal polyposis.

CLINICAL FEATURES

Epidermoid cysts are less common in children than adults, but are not unusual in adolescents. They consist of a firm nodule (Fig. 11.13), adherent to the epidermis, with a prominent central punctum, through which a foul, cream-coloured material may discharge. Lesions on the scalp are referred to as pilar cysts.

COMPLICATIONS

The contents may become infected, producing inflammation and eventually a painful abscess.

MANAGEMENT

The lesions may be excised either for cosmetic purposes or if they become inflamed.

Malignant tumours

Cutaneous malignancies are rare in childhood. When they arise it is mostly within developmental defects (e.g. giant melanocytic naevi), as part of a hereditary syndrome (e.g. Gorlin's syndrome) or by local extension from a soft tissue tumour (e.g. rhabdomyosarcoma).

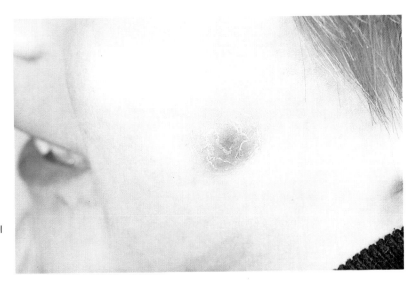

Fig. 11.13 *Epidermoid cyst.* The cyst consists of a firm nodule with a central punctum through which a cheese-like material may discharge. This cyst had recently become inflammed.

Malignant melanoma

DEFINITION

A malignant proliferation of melanocytes.

AETIOLOGY

In children, a malignant melanoma virtually always arises in a congenital naevus, especially the giant bathing-trunk type (see p. 133). It may also com-

plicate xeroderma pigmentosum (see p. 150) Individuals from families with the dysplastic naevi syndrome have a high risk of developing malignant melanomas in their teens and early adult life. Very rarely, malignant melanoma may arise *de novo* in childhood, and over 20 such cases have been reported over a 10-year period from one tertiary referral centre in the UK.

Although still rare, malignant melanoma does sometimes develop in adolescence. Solar damage is the most important aetiological factor.

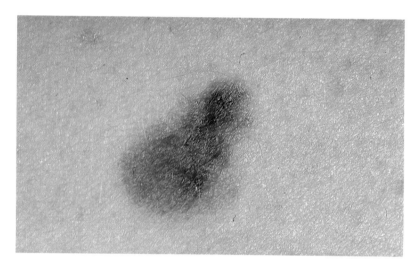

Fig. 11.14 *In situ malignant melanoma.* Malignant melanomas are being seen more frequently in adolescence. This flat patch is irregular in outline and in shades of pigment. It was an in situ melanoma in a 17-year-old.

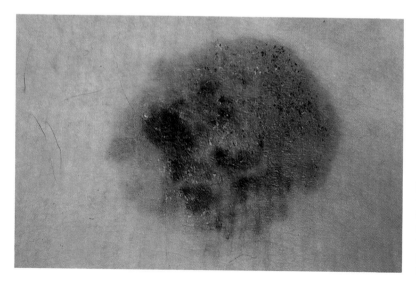

Fig. 11.15 *Superficial spreading malignant melanoma.* This melanoma, which developed in a congenital naevus on the dorsum of the foot of a 16-year-old, has many shades of pigment, including black. It metastasized.

CLINICAL FEATURES

Malignant melanomas are very rare before puberty. When it occurs, it is usually as a deeply, and somewhat unevenly, pigmented nodule within a pre-existing naevus, which is rapidly enlarging and may ulcerate. The estimated risk of developing malignant melanoma within a giant congenital naevus in the first 15 years of life is 8.5%. At least half of those patients who develop malignant change will do so between the ages of 3 and 5 years.

In contrast, malignant melanomas arising in the absence of a pre-existing naevus are rare, but they may appear quite vascular. In children under 5 years of age, this type of malignant melanoma has a predilection for the head and neck, and may be quite difficult to distinguish from Spitz naevi.

In situ (Fig. 11.14) and superficial spreading melanomas (Fig. 11.15) are becoming more common in adolescence. The outline is irregular and there is a variation of pigment in the lesion.

MANAGEMENT

1 Adequate local excision of the tumour, which may require closure with a skin graft.
2 Close follow-up for evidence of secondary spread.
3 Advice on sun protection should be given.

Rhabdomyosarcoma

DEFINITION

A rare malignant tumour of striated muscle.

AETIOLOGY

The tumour is thought to be embryonic in origin.

CLINICAL FEATURES

Although it is rare, rhabdomyosarcoma is the most common soft tissue tumour of childhood. The lesion develops as a rapidly enlarging subcutaneous swelling, which may ulcerate. The tumour (Fig. 11.16)

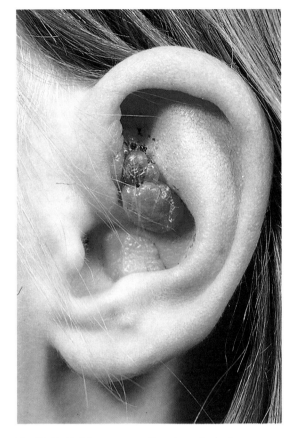

Fig. 11.16 *Rhabdomyosarcoma.* There is a red subcutaneous swelling in the ear. The nose, eye and ear are most often affected by this rare tumour (courtesy of Dr N. Burrows).

most often affects the head and neck. Metastasis occurs via the lymph nodes.

MANAGEMENT

1 The diagnosis is confirmed by biopsy and characteristic histopathology, showing small cell sarcoma with multiple mitoses.
2 Wide surgical excision of the tumour is required, but local recurrence is common.
3 The tumour is radiosensitive, and radiotherapy may be used in conjunction with surgery, but overall the disease carries a poor prognosis.

Chapter 12
Disorders of
Pigmentation

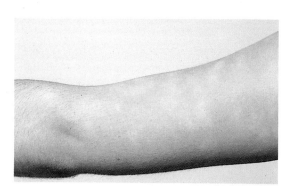

Fig. 12.1 *Postinflammatory hypopigmentation.* Temporary loss of pigment occurs after inflammatory disorders such as in this girl with psoriasis. It is most obvious in sun-tanned and pigmented skins.

Introduction

Abnormalities of cutaneous pigmentation may be congenital or acquired, and localized or generalized. They may represent loss of pigmentation or excess pigmentation. Both disorders may commonly occur as temporary phenomena following resolution of inflammation, e.g. after eczema, psoriasis (Fig. 12.1) and lichen planus (Figs 12.2 and 12.3) (which is known as postinflammatory hyper- or hypopigmentation.

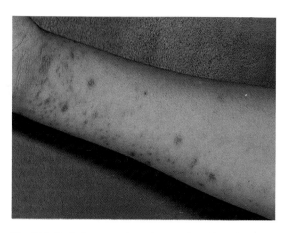

Fig. 12.2 *Postinflammatory hyperpigmentation.* Lichen planus is always followed by hyperpigmentation of the skin which in black skins may take years to fade.

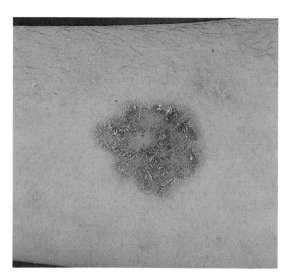

Fig. 12.3 *Postinflammatory hyperpigmentation.* Active flattopped papules are still visible surrounding the healed macular area of pigmentation in this 17-year-old with an annular form of lichen planus.

Congenital disorders of pigmentation

Many pigmentary changes in children are naevoid in origin (e.g. Mongolian blue spot) and are discussed in Chapter 10. Others may be part of a more generalized syndrome (e.g. neurofibromatosis) and are discussed more fully in Chapter 3.

Albinism

DEFINITION

An inherited disorder affecting the eyes and skin, in which there is a failure of melanin synthesis.

AETIOLOGY

There are many variants of albinism, but the majority are inherited as autosomal-recessive conditions. Albinism may affect the eyes alone (ocular albinism) or the eyes and skin (oculocutaneous albinism). The latter may be subdivided into tyrosinase-negative disease and tyrosinase-positive albinism, which is more common. In both forms melanocytes are present in the skin, but there is an abnormality in melanin synthesis, resulting in an absence or reduced levels of melanin.

CLINICAL FEATURES

The incidence of albinism in the UK is 1:20,000 births. It is found all over the world, but the incidence varies in different races. Ocular development is very susceptible to disorders of melanin pigmentation, and extreme photophobia and nystagmus develop early in all types of albinism. Horizontal or rotatory nystagmus is usually evident at birth, but in tyrosinase-positive patients this may become less marked with age.

In tyrosinase-negative albinism the skin is pale, the hair white and the iris red. In contrast, although tyrosinase-positive patients are very fair, they have some degree of pigmentation in the skin, hair (which is pale blonde) and eyes (Fig. 12.4). Patchy freckling may develop with age in sites of sun exposure in Afro-Caribbean patients with tyrosinase-positive albinism.

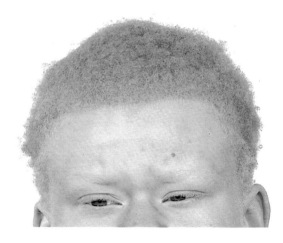

Fig. 12.4 *Albinism.* This boy has white skin, blue eyes and yellow hair with ocular and cutaneous photosensitivity. In the yellow mutant and tyrosinase-positive forms, some pigmentation develops with age.

DIFFERENTIAL DIAGNOSES

1 Chediak–Higashi syndrome: this is a rare abnormality in which a deficiency of oculocutaneous pigmentation is associated with an increased susceptibility to infection and a shortened life expectancy.
2 Phenylketonuria: affected children have pale skin, very fair hair and pale blue eyes, but no nystagmus. Without appropriate dietary restriction mental retardation develops. Infants are screened routinely for the disorder at birth in the UK.

MANAGEMENT

1 No specific treatment is possible, but prevention of complications is critical.
2 The classification is usually made clinically, but the diagnosis may be confirmed by means of incubation of plucked hair bulbs in the presence of tyrosinase. In tyrosinase-positive individuals, some pigment will be produced. In tyrosinase-negative patients, no pigment synthesis is observed.
3 Stringent photoprotection is essential from an early age, because of the vulnerability to skin cancer.
4 Regular ophthalmic follow-up is advised. The condition is disastrous in the topics because fatal squamous cell carcinomas and melanomas may ensue.

Piebaldism

DEFINITION

A congenital localized absence of pigmentation in a patchy distribution affecting the skin and hair, most often manifest as a white forelock.

AETIOLOGY

The condition is inherited as an autosomal-dominant trait. There is usually complete absence of melanocytes in the affected areas.

CLINICAL FEATURES

Irregular, macular areas of depigmentation are present from birth and remain constant throughout life. The cutaneous lesions may be bilateral (Fig. 12.5), but are often asymmetrical. Islands of normal skin or hyperpigmentation are present within the abnormal areas. Depigmented areas are found on the trunk, from the mid upper arm to the wrist and from the mid thighs to the shins or calves. A clump of white hairs in the midline frontal region (poliosis) is common (see also Fig. 16.12), and may be the only feature.

DIFFERENTIAL DIAGNOSES

1 Vitiligo: the depigmentation is acquired.
2 Waardenburg's syndrome: cutaneous lesions identical to those of piebaldism occur, but they are in association with congenital facial anomalies and deafness.

MANAGEMENT

1 No curative treatment is available.
2 The pale areas should be adequately protected from exposure to the sun.
3 Cosmetic camouflage can be useful.

Hypomelanosis of Ito (incontinentia pigmenti achromians)

DEFINITION

A congenital naevoid disorder with streaks of hypopigmentation occurring in a whorled pattern.

AETIOLOGY

Inheritance is via an autosomal-dominant trait.

CLINICAL FEATURES

Multiple, swirled areas of hypopigmentation are present in linear streaks from birth (Fig. 12.6). These areas may be unilateral or symmetrical, but are most often found on the trunk, and follow Blaschko's developmental lines, producing the characteristic whorled appearance of the disorder. The areas of involvement may gradually extend over the years, but occasionally repigment in later life. Rarely, there may be associated congenital defects of the central nervous system.

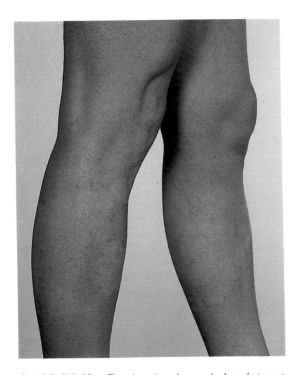

Fig. 12.5 *Piebaldism.* There is an irregular macular loss of pigment with areas of hyperpigmentation present within the affected area. This patient had a white forelock (see Fig. 16.12).

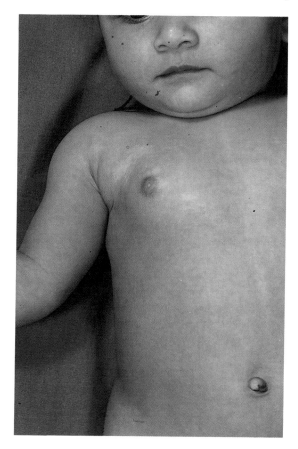

Fig. 12.6 *Hypomelanosis of Ito.* Unilateral or symmetrical linear and whorled areas of loss of pigment are present at birth. There may be other ectodermal and central nervous system defects.

DIFFERENTIAL DIAGNOSES

1 Incontinentia pigmenti (see p. 28): the late hypopigmented stage of incontinentia pigmenti may appear very similar, but the evolution of the lesions through their inflammatory, vesicular and hyperpigmented stages is characteristic and allows the condition to be distinguished from hypomelanosis of Ito.
2 Focal dermal hyperplasia: in this condition, the hypopigmented areas occur in association with dermal atrophy. It is usually lethal in males, so virtually all cases occur in females.

MANAGEMENT

There is no specific treatment.

Café-au-lait macules

DEFINITION

Large, evenly coloured hyperpigmented macules on the skin.

AETIOLOGY

Café-au-lait macules may occur as isolated lesions which are usually present at birth, or as part of an inherited syndrome (e.g. neurofibromatosis or Albright's syndrome), in which case they may become more numerous with time.

CLINICAL FEATURES

Ovoid, macular areas of hyperpigmentation may develop anywhere on the body, but especially the trunk. They may be segmental. They are usually light brown and evenly pigmented and may achieve several centimetres in diameter. Café-au-lait macules are found in 10% of the normal population, but if they are particularly extensive (greater than six in number), an underlying syndrome should be considered.

MANAGEMENT

1 The number and size of the macules should easily identify whether these are an isolated finding or part of a syndrome.
2 No treatment is required and isolated lesions rarely present any cosmetic problem.

Peutz–Jeghers syndrome

DEFINITION

Multiple, perioral (and occasional acral) palmar and plantar, lentigines occur in association with intestinal polyposis.

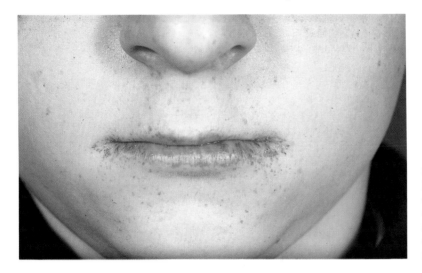

Fig. 12.7 *Peutz–Jeghers syndrome.* Multiple, small, pigmented macules occur on the face, especially the lips, oral mucosa and extremities in association with intestinal polyps. The oral macules are permanent but the rest may fade at puberty.

AETIOLOGY

Inheritance is autosomal dominant, but many patients have no family history and the condition appears to arise as a result of spontaneous mutations.

CLINICAL FEATURES

Multiple pigmented macules, up to 0.5 cm in size, develop on the lips (Fig. 12.7) and surrounding facial skin from infancy. The oral mucosa is nearly always extensively involved. Macules may be round or ovoid and vary in colour from mid-brown to almost black. They may occur on the hands and feet, including the palms and soles. There is a strong association with hamartomatous polyps of the gastro-intestinal tract (especially the small intestine), which may undergo malignant transformation. Female patients with the syndrome have an increased risk of developing ovarian tumours later in life.

MANAGEMENT

Patients should be followed up by a gastroenterologist with periodic endoscopy or radiological examination to exclude any malignant change.

Acquired disorders of pigmentation

A wide variety of drugs may cause pigmentary changes in the skin (e.g. amiodarone, phenothiazines and heavy metals), but they are rarely administered to children or adolescents. However, minocycline may induce a blue-black pigmentation (Fig. 12.8) of the skin and nails when given in high dosage for long periods to treat acne. Such changes are not due to melanin pigmentation, but to the deposition of various compounds related to the drug's metabolism.

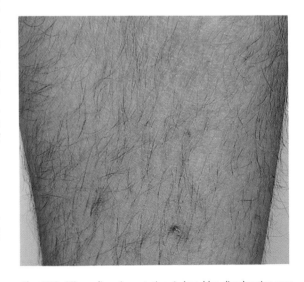

Fig. 12.8 *Minocycline pigmentation.* A deep blue discoloration very occasionally occurs with minocycline, when used to treat acne. It is dose- and time-related.

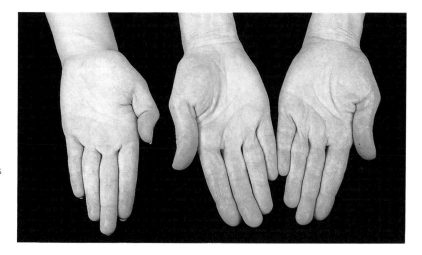

Fig. 12.9 *Carotenaemia.* An orange-yellow discoloration of the skin occurs in those who eat excess amounts of carrots or oranges. There is a striking difference between a normal hand (left) and the pair of affected hands (right).

Additionally, the excess ingestion of dietary substances rich in carotene (e.g. carrots and oranges) may produce a striking orange pigmentation of the skin, most marked on the palms (Fig. 12.9) and soles. Such carotenaemia may be seen in adolescent girls following food fads in an attempt to diet.

Finally, pigmentary disturbance may occur in endocrine disease, such as Addison's disease and hypopituitarism.

Vitiligo

DEFINITION

An autoimmune disorder producing extensive macular depigmentation of the skin (Fig. 12.10).

AETIOLOGY

The exact cause of vitiligo is unknown, but there is a strong hereditary basis for the disorder, with up to 40% of patients having a positive family history. There is an association with autoimmune disease, especially thyroid disorders. Halo naevi (see p. 135) are more common in patients with vitiligo.

CLINICAL FEATURES

Vitiligo may occur at any age and in any race. Over half the cases begin during the first two decades of life and there is a female preponderance. The disorder appears to be more common in pigmented skin.

Vitiligo usually begins on the face (often around the mouth) and frequently affects the axillae, groin and genitalia. Any body site may be affected and the extent of the depigmentation may be more obvious under Wood's light. The macular areas of depigmentation usually develop in a symmetrical fashion, but the incidence of segmental vitiligo in children is

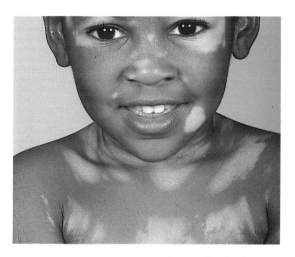

Fig. 12.10 *Vitiligo.* Melanocytes are absent so that the skin is completely depigmented and white. However, in black skins, some areas may be hypopigmented.

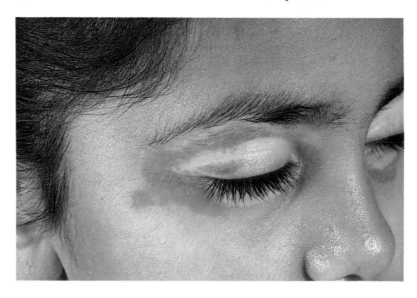

Fig. 12.11 *Vitiligo.* An irregular geographic and hyperpigmented outline surrounding the loss of pigmentation is not uncommon.

higher than in adults. Individual patches have an irregular geographic outline which may be hyper-pigmented (Fig. 12.11). There may be partial or complete loss of pigment in any one area, and varying shades of pigment within one area may produce a trichrome appearance. Lesions often localize to sites of friction as an isomorphic (Koebner) phenomenon. The hairs within long-standing patches of vitiligo also eventually lose their pigmentation. In severe instances, the vitiligo may be virtually total, but a few islands of pigmented skin always persist. Spontaneous repigmentation is reported in up to 20% of patients, and younger individuals have a better prognosis. When repigmentation occurs, it begins in a perifollicular fashion and is often patchy.

DIFFERENTIAL DIAGNOSES

1 Idiopathic guttate hypomelanosis: small, regular, completely amelanotic macules are seen, especially on the limbs. They are acquired and thought to be related to age and exposure to the sun and are therefore more common in adults.
2 Vogt–Koyanagi–Harada syndrome: this is a rare condition. Vitiligo, alopecia areata and poliosis, (the latter often limited to the eyebrows and lashes) develop following an acute febrile illness with meningism and uveitis.

MANAGEMENT

1 The disorder may present a considerable cosmetic problem and in certain cultures may lead to ostraciz-ation because of historical associations between hypopigmentation and leprosy. Counselling is available in several countries through the vitiligo patient support groups.
2 The prognosis is best in patients with pigmented skins and in those with isolated facial involvement. Recovery is less likely in white patients, in cases where there is widespread disease or in patients whose mucosae, fingers and toes are affected (the lip–tip syndrome).
3 Total protection from the sun with a high-factor sun block is essential, as the areas of vitiligo will not tan, have no natural protection against the sun and therefore may burn. The use of sun blocks also helps to limit the contrast between the tanned areas of normal skin and vitiligo.
4 A short trial of a superpotent topical steroid may be worthwhile in lesions of recent onset as repig-mentation may be induced, particularly on the face (Figs 12.12 and 12.13). It is of little value in estab-lished lesions.
5 Photochemotherapy (PUVA) with psoralens – either applied as a paint or given systemically as 8 methoxypsoralens – followed by exposure to

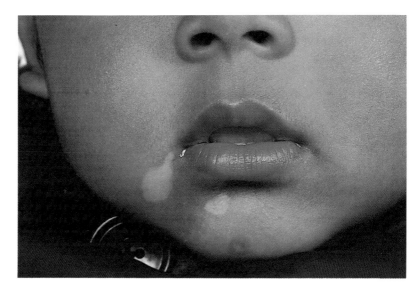

Fig. 12.12 *Vitiligo.* The condition responds poorly to treatment. However, partial repigmentation may occur on the face.

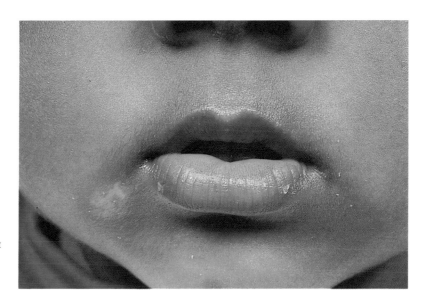

Fig. 12.13 *Vitiligo.* The child in Fig. 12.12 was treated with a superpotent topical steroid for 6 weeks and there has been some degree of repigmentation.

longwave ultraviolet light (UVA) is often tried. However the treatment required is prolonged (up to 200 exposures). The results are often disappointing, with limited and very patchy repigmentation and there are the associated risks of side effects; from burning in particular and the development of cutaneous carcinogenesis many years later.

6 Cosmetic camouflage taught by a skilled beautician can be very helpful in disguising vitiligo in exposed areas such as the face and hands, and may boost the patient's confidence.

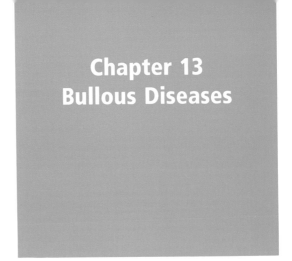

Chapter 13
Bullous Diseases

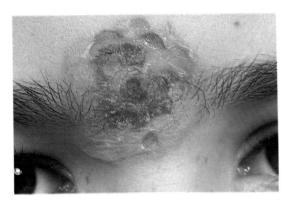

Fig. 13.1 *Bullous impetigo.* Staphylococcal infections of the skin may start as a blister containing purulent material which subsequently becomes crusted.

Introduction

Most of the bullous diseases that can occur in children are serious, but rare. However, they need to be clearly distinguished from the more common causes of blistering such as impetigo (Fig. 13.1), viral infections (see Chapter 8), acute eczema (see Fig. 5.15) including phytophotodermatitis (see Fig. 14.11) and insect bites (Fig. 13.2) (see p. 110).

Epidermolysis bullosa

This is the term given to a group of inherited disorders characterized by florid blistering in response to minor trauma. There are several variants of the

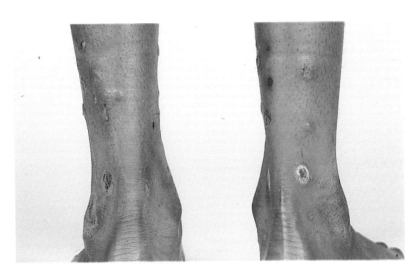

Fig. 13.2 *Insect bites.* Insect bites may be bullous as well as urticarial. This is a common cause of blistering on the lower legs.

condition, ranging in severity from localized blistering of the extremities to life-threatening disease affecting the skin and mucous membranes. Classification of the different entities is based upon the level of the split in the skin and is determined by electron microscopy.

Epidermolysis bullosa simplex (Weber–Cockayne type)

DEFINITION

A familial disorder characterized by localized bullae on the hands and feet, which heal without scarring.

AETIOLOGY

The condition is inherited as an autosomal-dominant trait, but male members of the pedigree tend to be more severely affected than females. On electron microscopy, the level of the split occurs between the basal and suprabasal cells of the epidermis, and on routine histology, basal cell cytolysis is seen.

CLINICAL FEATURES

Large, tense, non-haemorrhagic bullae (Fig. 13.3) form on the hands and feet (especially the soles) in response to minor frictional trauma (Fig. 13.4). The

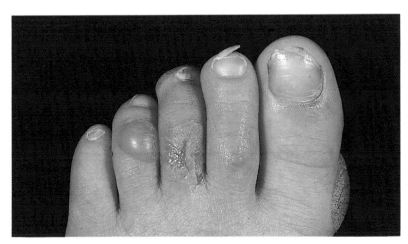

Fig. 13.3 *Epidermolysis bullosa simplex.* Large tense, non-haemorrhagic blisters form in response to minor frictional trauma, particularly on the hands and feet. The splitting occurs just above the dermo-epidermal junction through the basal cells.

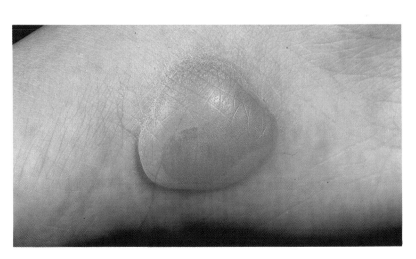

Fig. 13.4 *Epidermolysis bullosa simplex.* The feet are a common site as in this 2-year-old. It is exacerbated by footwear and sweating and is more common in the summer.

condition usually begins in childhood, but some mild cases do not begin until the teens. The condition is exacerbated by sweating and tends to be worse during the summer months. Friction from heavy footwear also encourages blister formation. The individual lesions last 1–2 weeks and heal without scarring. A more generalized form of the condition (the Koebner variant) may also occur, in which the extensive blistering is prone to secondary infection.

DIFFERENTIAL DIAGNOSES

1 Pompholyx (see p. 54): the lesions are composed of multilocular, small (vesicular) blisters, and pruritus is often pronounced. There is no family history.
2 Tinea pedis (see p. 102): this may occasionally be bullous, but is usually unilateral. The fungal elements can clearly be seen on direct microscopy of scrapings from the deroofed blisters.
3 Papular urticaria: although often localized to the lower limbs, the lesions tend to be smaller, urticated and intensely pruritic.
4 Sucking blisters: large, clear blisters on the fingers may occasionally be present at birth. They are thought to arise from the trauma of vigorous sucking *in utero* and are most common on the thumb. They are transient and will heal without scarring.

MANAGEMENT

1 The diagnosis is usually staightforward on the basis of the limited clinical involvement and the positive family history.
2 When bullae form, they can be made more comfortable by teaching the parents (or older patient) to aspirate the blister fluid using a sterile syringe and 21-gauge needle.
3 The skin should be protected from undue friction. Vigorous exercise is unwise. Light, open-style shoes are less abrasive and antiperspirant preparations on the feet (e.g. aluminium hydroxide 20%) reduce excessive sweating.

Lethal junctional epidermolysis bullosa (Herlitz syndrome)

DEFINITION

A very rare congenital syndrome characterized by severe blistering of the skin with extensive involvement of mucous membranes.

AETIOLOGY

The disease is inherited as an autosomal-recessive condition. The disorder is thought to arise from an abnormality in the hemidesmosomes, resulting in a split within the lamina lucida.

CLINICAL FEATURES

The skin is usually abnormal at birth, with generalized blistering and superficial erosions which are slow to heal (Fig. 13.5). The face, trunk and limbs are all involved, but the extremities (including the nails) may be spared. Blisters are usually present around the mouth and the oropharyngeal mucosa is often affected. The baby may have a hoarse cry, indicating laryngeal involvement.

DIFFERENTIAL DIAGNOSES

1 Recessive dystrophic epidermolysis bullosa (see p. 163): the two conditions are distinguished by electron microscopy of a skin biopsy to differentiate the level of the split. However, in the dystrophic-recessive form, erosions heal with scarring and milia formation, whereas in junctional epidermolysis bullosa scarring is rare unless there is secondary infection.
2 Neonatal pemphigoid gestationis: rarely, placental transfer of antigen may result in transient blistering and urticaria in the baby of a woman with pemphigoid gestationis. The maternal diagnosis should suggest the true diagnosis and prevent any confusion.

MANAGEMENT

1 This diagnosis carries a poor prognosis. The baby should be referred to a specialist centre for accurate diagnosis and specialized management.

2 Death from overwhelming infection usually occurs in early infancy.

Recessive dystrophic epidermolysis bullosa (Hallopeau–Siemens type)

DEFINITION

A rare congenital syndrome characterized by severe recurrent blisters which heal with scarring and milia formation.

AETIOLOGY

The condition is inherited as an autosomal-recessive trait. There is now evidence that recessive epidermolysis bullosa is linked to the HLA-DR4 and HLA-DQw3 loci. The bullae are subepidermal and the ultrastructural level of cleavage is below the lamina densa. The basic defect is an abnormality of type VII collagen, resulting in defective anchoring fibrils.

CLINICAL FEATURES

Large, flaccid, haemorrhagic bullae (Fig. 13.6a) are present at or shortly after birth. Lesions may arise spontaneously, but are exacerbated by trauma (Fig. 13.6b). The child is often considerably distressed and involvement of the mucous membranes may make feeding difficult. The blisters heal with atrophic

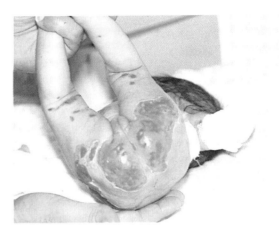

Fig. 13.5 *Junctional (Herlitz) epidermolysis bullosa.* Extensive blistering and erosions on the lower legs and buttocks, in a child who only survived for a few months (courtesy of Dr R. Russel Jones).

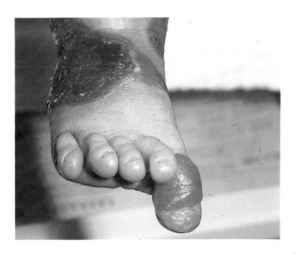

Fig. 13.6a *Dystrophic epidermolysis bullosa.* Large flaccid haemorrhagic bullae are present at birth, following trauma.

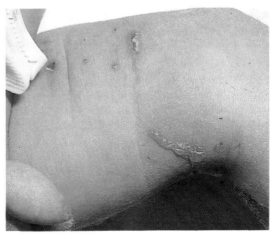

Fig. 13.6b *Dystrophic epidermolysis bullosa.* The blistering may arise spontaneously, but is usually explained by minimal external trauma, such as handling.

scarring (Figs 13.7 and 13.8) and milia formation. With time, the digits may become fused together by scar tissue, ultimately resulting in a useless clubbed fist or foot. The nails are dystrophic, the hair sparse and the dentition abnormal. Corneal erosions may lead to severe scarring and impaired vision. Intellectual development is normal.

COMPLICATIONS

1 Refractory anaemia is common.
2 Recurrent oesophageal blistering may result in stricture formation.
3 Squamous carcinoma of the skin, oropharynx and oesophagus is a late but serious complication of the chronic scarring.

DIFFERENTIAL DIAGNOSES

1 Incontinentia pigmenti (see p. 28): this occurs in girls. The initial small blisters are linear and followed by hyperkeratosis and streaky pigmentation.

2 Lethal junctional epidermolysis bullosa: the blisters usually heal without scarring. The ultimate distinction is made on the basis of electron microscopy of the skin.
3 Dominant dystrophic epidermolysis bullosa: the onset of bullae may be delayed and the lesions tend to be localized to the limbs, especially the pretibial surface. The nails are spared.
4 Congenital bullous ichthyosiform erythroderma (see p. 21): although flaccid bullae are present, the erythroderma and hyperkeratosis are the most striking features.

MANAGEMENT

1 Referral to a specialist centre for confirmation of the diagnosis and expert advice is essential.
2 The child is likely to be severely disabled and need specialist support and schooling. Treatment is largely supportive, but plastic surgery may be required to release fused fingers.
3 The family should be put in contact with the appropriate national support group.
4 Cultured keratinocytes are now being used to cover large defects and prevent scarring, but their use is still confined to research centres.
5 Affected families may be offered prenatal diagnosis by skin biopsy via fetoscopy in subsequent pregnancies.

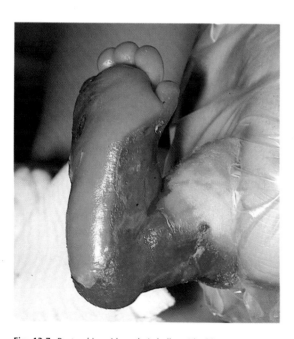

Fig. 13.7 *Dystrophic epidermolysis bullosa.* The blisters eventually heal with scarring and milia formation. In time the digits may become fused, resulting in a useless clubbed foot.

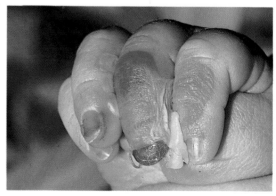

Fig. 13.8 *Dystrophic epidermolysis bullosa.* The blistering occurs below the lamina densa due to defective anchoring fibrils as a result of abnormal type VII collagen.

Chronic bullous dermatosis of childhood

DEFINITION

A rare, self-limiting bullous disease occurring in an orogenital distribution in young children.

AETIOLOGY

The disease is acquired and immunologically mediated. There is a linear band of IgA deposition at the basement membrane zone of the skin of affected patients. There is an association with the HLA-B8 locus. There are many similarities between this disorder and linear IgA disease of adults, and it has now been suggested that it is the childhood variant of the adult disease.

CLINICAL FEATURES

The condition most often begins around the age of 5 years. Large, mildly pruritic blisters develop on normal skin, especially around the genitalia (Fig. 13.9), buttocks and inner thighs. The scalp and perioral region are also frequently involved and there may be intraoral lesions as well. Blisters are usually serous, but occasionally may become haemorrhagic. New lesions may develop in annular clusters mimicking a 'string of pearls'.

DIFFERENTIAL DIAGNOSES

1 Papular urticaria (see p. 110): this is usually seen on the limbs, and the lesions are more urticated.
2 Pemphigus: this is very rare in childhood and adolescence but intraoral and genital blistering occur in addition to cutaneous blisters and erosions (Fig. 13.10). It may be distinguished by histopathology which shows that the blistering is intra-epidermal, and immunofluorescence, in which IgG is deposited intercellularly in a characteristic chicken-wire pattern.
3 Childhood pemphigoid: this is also very rare, but can also be distinguished by direct immunofluorescence. IgG and C3 are deposited along the basement membrane in bullous pemphigoid. The blisters of bullous pemphigoid tend to occur in a more generalized distribution and, in contrast to chronic bullous dermatosis of childhood, may be found on the palms and soles.

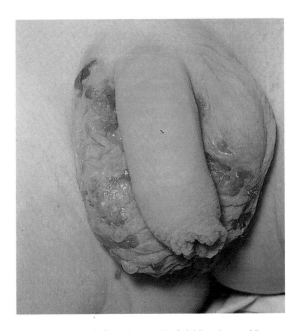

Fig. 13.9 *Chronic bullous dermatosis of childhood.* Large blisters occur in annular clusters around the genitalia, buttocks and inner thighs (courtesy of Dr F. Wojnarowska).

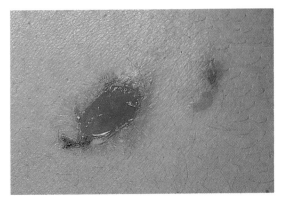

Fig. 13.10 *Pemphigus.* This is very rare, but intra-epidermal blistering and erosions of the skin and mucous membranes occur as a result of auto-antibodies directed towards the desmosomes which connect epidermal cells together.

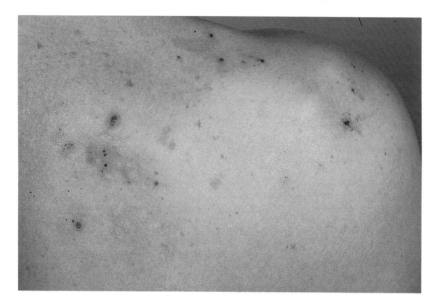

Fig. 13.11 *Dermatitis herpetiformis.* Very itchy vesicles occur symmetrically. The buttocks, elbows, knees, shoulders and scalp are also affected. The condition is associated with a glutensensitive enteropathy.

4 Dermatitis herpetiformis: this usually affects young adults; it may very occasionally occur in children, but rarely before the age of 6 years. Although immunofluorescence of uninvolved skin shows IgA deposition, it is in a granular rather than linear pattern (see below).

5 Epidermolysis bullosa acquisita: this is not as uncommon as previously thought in childhood. The diagnosis requires confirmation by performing direct immunofluorescence on salt-split skin, where the immunoreactants are seen to localize to the floor (dermal side) of the blister.

6 Bullous lupus erythematosus: this is rare, but may occur in childhood. Widespread subepidermal blisters occur, but the presence of a circulating antinuclear factor should suggest the diagnosis.

MANAGEMENT

1 The condition tends to be self-limiting, with resolution over the course of 3–4 years. Attacks during this time are intermittent, but rarely as severe as the initial episode.

2 Dapsone 20–125 mg (or sulphapyridine as an alternative) usually controls the disease, but the dosage needs to be reviewed regularly and titrated according to symptoms. The patient should be

monitored closely for evidence of haemolysis, and the drug is contraindicated in patients with G6PD deficiency.

3 Rarely, oral corticosteroids may be required in addition to the above, but their use should be restricted as much as possible because of the side effects in children.

Dermatitis herpetiformis

DEFINITION

An intensely pruritic symmetrical vesicular eruption affecting primarily the elbows, knees, buttocks and scalp, associated with gluten sensitivity.

AETIOLOGY

All patients have changes in the small bowel consistent with gluten-sensitive enteropathy. The gastrointestinal disturbance is often asymptomatic although occasionally a patient may be seen with established coeliac disease who subsequently develops the cutaneous eruption of dermatitis herpetiformis. It is most common in those of Irish ancestry and there is an association with HLA-A1, HLA-B8 and HLA-DR3 and other autoimmune disorders,

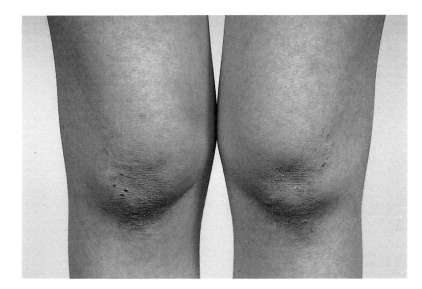

Fig. 13.12 *Dermatitis herpetiformis.* The condition is intensely pruritic. Grouped excoriated erythematous papules may be the most prominent physical signs on examination.

such as Graves' disease and pernicious anaemia. All patients have deposits of IgA in the dermal papillae of uninvolved skin. It may occur at any age, including childhood, but is most common in adult life. There is a limited risk of small bowel lymphoma after a number of years.

CLINICAL FEATURES

The complaint is of intense irritation of the skin. There are small, often excoriated urticated papules (Fig. 13.11) or vesicles which occur in groups on extensor sites, especially the buttocks, just below the elbows and knees (Fig. 13.12), and the shoulders and scalp.

MANAGEMENT

1 The diagnosis is confirmed by biopsy of the skin. A neutrophilic abscess in the dermal papillae is characteristic, but the finding of deposits of IgA in the dermal papillae of normal skin is definitive. The deposition is granular rather than linear as in chronic bullous dermatosis of childhood.
2 The pruritus ceases and the lesions heal within a day or two of instituting therapy with dapsone. However, although not particularly palatable, after a few months of a gluten-free diet, the disorder remits without the need for dapsone, a drug which occasionally causes haemolytic anaemia and significant methaemoglobinaemia.

Chapter 14
Photosensitivity

Introduction

Ultraviolet (UV) radiation may be natural (from the sun) or artificial (e.g. from sunlamps). The important wavelengths of light capable of inducing cutaneous disease are UVC (100–280 nm), UVB (280–315 nm) and UVA (315–400 nm). Visible light has a wavelength of 400–700 nm. Photosensitivity in children may be genetic or acquired.

Inherited disorders

Xeroderma pigmentosum (XP)

DEFINITION

A rare inherited disorder comprising photosensitivity, excessive freckling, premature ageing and malignancy of the skin due to UV-induced mutagenesis.

AETIOLOGY

Xeroderma pigmentosum is inherited as an autosomal-recessive trait. The primary abnormality responsible for the varied clinical features is an abnormality of DNA repair. Fibroblasts from affected individuals are unable to carry out the normal excision repair of the thyomine dimers that are formed after exposure to ultraviolet light and damage to the DNA. Several different subtypes of XP have now been distinguished, labelled types A–G.

CLINICAL FEATURES

The affected child appears normal at birth, but characteristically experiences exaggerated sunburn reactions (Fig. 14.1) with minimal sun exposure from an early age. Freckling and dryness of the skin begin to be noticed in the majority of patients by the age of 3 years. The skin changes are most obvious on the parts exposed to light, e.g. the face and backs of the hands (Fig. 14.2), but freckling may also be seen on mucosal surfaces, e.g. conjunctiva and lips. Ectropion is common. The freckles become more

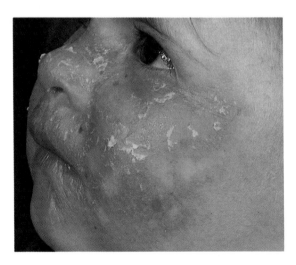

Fig. 14.1 *Xeroderma pigmentosum.* This child is inordinately sensitive to ultraviolet irradiation and, therefore, exposed areas of skin burn. One or two freckles are just visible.

168

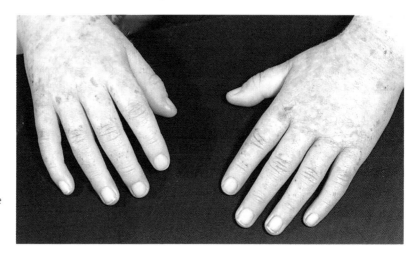

Fig. 14.2 *Xeroderma pigmentosum.* All exposed areas of skin are vulnerable particularly the face, neck, backs of hands, forearms and legs. This is the same child as in Fig. 14.3.

numerous with age and coalesce to form larger, permanent, pigmented macules. The skin is fragile, and superficial ulcers readily form which are slow to heal.

Actinic keratoses and small telangiectasias are numerous from an early age. Malignant tumours, e.g. keratoacanthomas, basal cell carcinomas, squamous cell carcinomas (Fig. 14.3) and malignant melanomas, may form in childhood. Two thirds of patients die before the age of 20, mostly from metastatic malignancy, but also as a result of an increased susceptibility to infection.

Certain subtypes of XP (e.g. A and D) are associated with neurological complications (mental retardation, ataxia and deafness).

MANAGEMENT

1 The diagnosis is usually clinical, based on photosensitivity from birth and the early development of pigmented macules and skin cancers, but may be confirmed by demonstrating abnormal DNA repair in cultured fibroblasts which have been irradiated by ultraviolet light.
2 As soon as the diagnosis is suspected, scrupulous sun protection should be implemented. The patient should stay indoors as far as possible during daylight hours, and when outside should keep the limbs covered, wear a broad-brimmed hat, wrap-around sunglasses and total sunblock.

3 The patient should be under regular follow-up for surveillance of the skin to monitor any development of skin tumours and arrange prompt excision.
4 Long-term oral retinoids have been shown to reduce the incidence of skin cancer in some of these patients.
5 Prenatal diagnosis by amniocentesis is now possible in affected families.

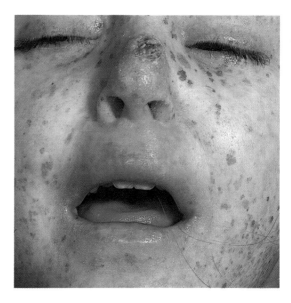

Fig. 14.3 *Xeroderma pigmentosa.* Permanent larger pigmented macules develop and ultimately cutaneous malignant disease; in this case a squamous cell carcinoma has developed on the nose.

Rothmund–Thomson syndrome (poikiloderma congenitale)

DEFINITION

A rare inherited disorder characterized by photo-sensitivity, facial telangiectasia, skin cancer, cataracts and small stature.

AETIOLOGY

This syndrome is an autosomal-recessive disorder, but is expressed more commonly in girls. There is considerable variation in the clinical features described in different pedigrees, suggesting a degree of genetic heterogenicity.

CLINICAL FEATURES

Plaques of erythema and oedema develop on the cheeks of children from the age of 3–6 months. As these subside, prominent telangiectasia with atrophic areas and reticulate pigmentary changes (poikiloderma) appear (Fig. 14.4). The cutaneous

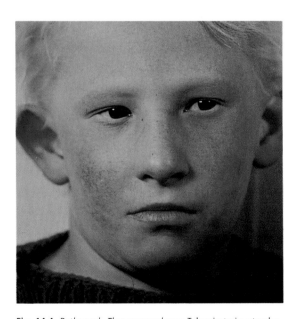

Fig. 14.4 *Rothmund–Thomson syndrome.* Telangiectasia, atrophy and reticulate pigmentation occur over the cheeks.

signs are most marked in the malar region, but may extend onto the trunk and limbs. Photosensitivity is often severe and bullous reactions to light exposure are common. Multiple keratoses develop on light-exposed skin as a result, and may progress to squamous cell carcinomas. Patients are of short stature with small, beak-like noses and normal mental function. Other features which may occur in this syndrome include hypogonadism, sparse hair and cataract formation.

DIFFERENTIAL DIAGNOSES

1 Dyskeratosis congenita: reticulate telangiectasia is also a feature but the changes appear later in child-hood and are associated with abnormal nails and oral leucoplakia, which may progress to malignant change.
2 Bloom's syndrome: this autosomal-recessive condition is also characterized by short stature, an atypical facies, facial telangiectasia and photosensitivity, but there is no poikiloderma. Patients with Bloom's syndrome have an increased risk of developing leukaemia in adult life.
3 Cockayne's syndrome: short stature, facial erythema and photosensitivity are all features of this rare syndrome, but without poikiloderma. Children with Cockayne's syndrome have abnormally large hands, feet and ears, age prematurely and have gross mental retardation.

MANAGEMENT

The diagnosis is made on clinical grounds and sub-sequent management consists of adequate sun protection.

The porphyrias

The porphyrias are a group of disorders arising from abnormalities in the haem-biosynthetic pathway (Fig. 14.5), with consequent accumulation of porphyrins, many of which induce light sensitivity. Childhood forms are genetically inherited, whereas the commonest porphyria in adults (porphyrias cutanea tarda) is usually induced by alcohol misuse or drugs.

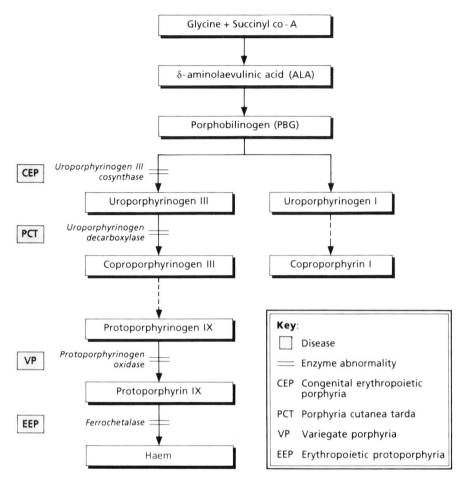

Fig. 14.5 Haem biosynthesis.

Congenital erythropoietic porphyria (Gunther's disease)

DEFINITION

A rare inherited syndrome resulting in severe mutilating photosensitivity.

AETIOLOGY

The condition is autosomal recessive, and consanguinity is frequent in affected pedigrees. The primary defect is a deficiency of the enzyme uroporphyrinogen III cosynthase in the bone marrow, with resultant accumulation of type I porphyrins, which are then distributed around the body, where they produce their clinical effects.

CLINICAL FEATURES

Severe photosensitivity is present from birth, with erythema and blistering on exposed sites. The blistered areas heal slowly, with scarring (Fig. 14.6), and recurrent episodes result in severe deformity of the ears, nose and digits. Keratoconjunctivitis and ectropion are common. Scarring alopecia (Fig. 14.7), hypertrichosis and mottled pigmentation develop later. The urine appears deep red, and pink staining of the nappies may be one of the first signs noted in babies. The teeth fluoresce under Wood's light.

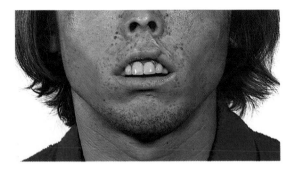

Fig. 14.6 *Congenital erythropoietic porphyria.* The cheeks and around the mouth show considerable scarring. Scabs from previous blisters are apparent.

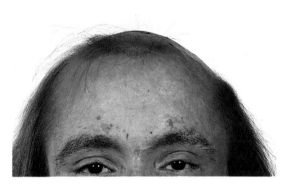

Fig. 14.7 *Congenital erythropoietic porphyria.* Blistering occurs on exposed skin and heals slowly with scarring and, on the scalp, with alopecia as in this 16-year-old.

There is often an accompanying haemolytic anaemia with splenomegaly.

MANAGEMENT

1 The diagnosis is confirmed by the finding of elevated uroporphyrin I in the urine and red blood cells, and coproporphyrin in the faeces.
2 Treatment is essentially symptomatic with life-long sun protection.
3 Beta-carotene may confer some degree of tolerance, but is not as effective as in erythropoietic protoporphyria (see below).
4 Repeated transfusions may suppress erythropoiesis and so reduce porphyrin production, but iron over-load may result in haemochromatosis and must be guarded against.
5 Bone-marrow transplantation may provide a possible treatment in the future.

Erythropoietic protoporphyria

DEFINITION

This is the most common of the erythropoietic porphyrias, characterized by extreme photosensitivity in childhood with consequent pock-like facial scarring.

AETIOLOGY

Inheritance of the condition is autosomal dominant with variable penetrance. The enzyme abnormality is a reduced activity of ferrochelatase in erythrocytes.

The activating wavelengths of light in erythropoietic protoporphyria are around the yellow-green part of the visible spectrum, and so light penetrating through glass may provoke symptoms.

CLINICAL FEATURES

Severe light sensitivity develops within minutes of sun exposure in childhood. The mean age of onset is 4 years. Initially, a pricking sensation and burning develop in light-exposed parts and affected children may scream with pain on sun exposure. Erythema (Fig. 14.8) is sometimes evident and, later on, small pitted scars develop over the nose and cheeks, but bullae are rare. Hepatic involvement is usually, but not always, mild with a slight elevation of serum transaminases, but gallstones are common.

DIFFERENTIAL DIAGNOSIS

Hydroa vacciniforme can be excluded on the basis of porphyrin screening.

MANAGEMENT

1 Sun avoidance and the use of a total sunblock are imperative.
2 Prolonged ingestion of high-dosage β-carotene

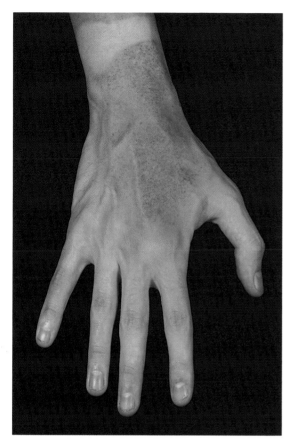

Fig. 14.8 *Erythropoietic protoporphyria.* Affected children are acutely distressed within minutes of sun exposure. The physical signs may be minimal, although erythema may be present and subsequently small pitted scars.

may confer a degree of photoprotection in some patients, but produces an orange discoloration of the skin.

3 Specific H_1-antagonists, e.g. terfenadine, may confer some benefit.

4 Liver transplantation may be necessary.

Porphyria cutanea tarda (PCT)

DEFINITION

The most common variant of porphyria in which photosensitivity results from abnormal hepatic uroporphyrinogen decarboxylase activity.

AETIOLOGY

Porphyria cutanea tarda may be acquired in adults (80%), but in children it is familial (20%) due to an autosomal-dominant trait.

CLINICAL FEATURES

Familial PCT usually presents in childhood, with vesicles and bullae (Fig. 14.9) on light-exposed skin particularly the backs of the hands (Fig. 14.10), during spring and summer. The skin is fragile and breaks easily in response to the mildest trauma. The lesions and erosions which result are slow to heal. Scarring is common, often with associated milia formation. The skin gradually becomes coarse and hyperpigmented with hypertrichosis. The signs are limited to the skin, but patients with PCT have an increased risk of developing hepatocellular carcinoma.

DIFFERENTIAL DIAGNOSIS

Variegate porphyria: This is a rare variant of porphyria which normally presents after puberty. There is a high incidence amongst South Africans of Dutch descent. The cutaneous lesions are identical to those of PCT, but acute attacks (e.g. of abdominal pain) similar to those of acute intermittent porphyria also occur. The definitive diagnosis is made by the demonstration of elevated faecal porphyrins pathognomonic of variegate porphyria.

MANAGEMENT

1 The diagnosis is confirmed on porphyrin screening of urine, blood and faeces. Full screening is essential to differentiate variegate porphyria and PCT.

2 Patients should avoid solar exposure and wear protective clothing, a hat and a total sunblock.

3 Patients should avoid known precipitants of PCT in later life, especially alcohol and the combined oral contraceptive pill.

4 Intermittent venesection to deplete iron stores is the mainstay of treatment.

5 Low-dosage antimalarials have also been shown to be effective treatment in severe cases, but their use is more controversial in children.

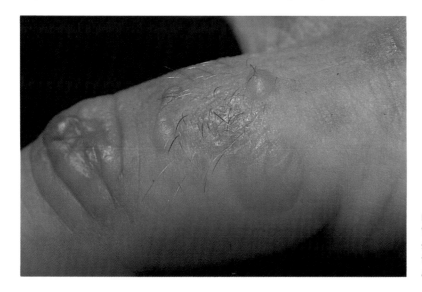

Fig. 14.9 *Porphyria cutanea tarda.* Vesicles and bullae occur in exposed skin, particularly the backs of the fingers and hands. The skin is fragile and breaks easily.

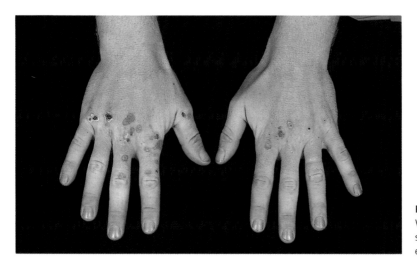

Fig. 14.10 *Porphyria cutanea tarda.* Vesicles, blisters and haemorrhagic scabs occur on light exposure, especially on the backs of the hands.

Acquired disorders

Contact with certain plant substances may induce a transient phototoxic reaction, phytophotodermatitis, with a prominent bullous reaction in linear streaks (Fig. 14.11), which heals to leave considerable postinflammatory pigmentation. Additionally, ingestion of certain drugs (e.g. tetracyclines) may induce a photosensitive dermatitis on light-exposed parts (Fig. 14.12). Although druginduced photo-sensitivity tends to be a greater problem in adults than in children, it may be relevant to teenagers taking demethylchlortetracycline or vibramycin for acne.

Juvenile spring eruption

DEFINITION

An intermittent, pruritic, papulovesicular eruption occurring on the ears of young boys during the spring months.

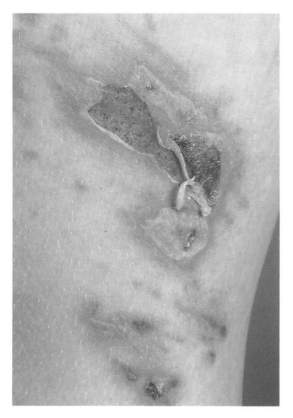

Fig. 14.11 *Phytophotodermatitis.* Blisters followed by erosions and, subsequently, pigmentation occur in a linear streaky pattern due to contact with phototoxic psoralen producing wheals.

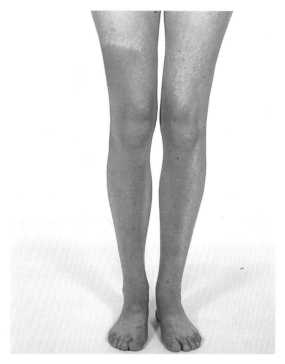

Fig. 14.12 *Drug-induced photosensitivity.* Tetracyclines, especially demethylchlortetracycline and vibramycin, prescribed for acne occasionally cause a phototoxic eruption.

AETIOLOGY

The condition appears to be a localized form of the more generalized polymorphic light eruption, more commonly seen in young adults. It results from a hypersensitivity to UVA (and to a lesser extent UVB) and may occur in epidemics during the spring months. The condition is virtually confined to boys, possibly because their shorter hairstyles expose the ears. There is a familial tendency to develop the eruption.

CLINICAL FEATURES

Erythematous, pruritic papules and vesicles develop on the helices of boys' ears (Fig. 14.13) during the

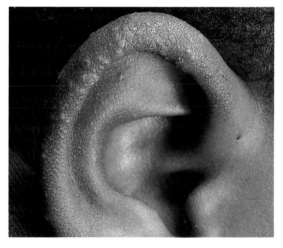

Fig. 14.13 *Juvenile spring eruption.* The ears are covered in papulovesicles. It is most common in boys, probably because the ears are not covered by hair. It lasts about a week and may be associated with cervical adenitis.

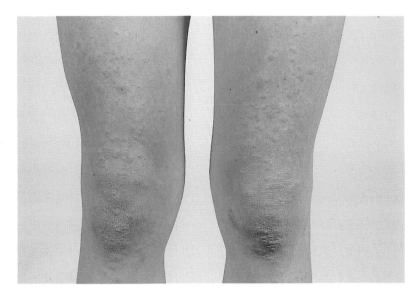

Fig. 14.14 *Polymorphic light eruption.* Red itchy papules or papulovesicles, which may coalesce into plaques, occur on exposed skin, although not always the face (courtesy of Dr M. Clement).

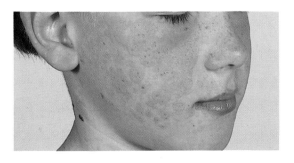

Fig. 14.15 *Polymorphic light eruption.* There is an erythematous papular eruption on the cheeks and nose. It coincided with the first bright sunshine of late spring.

first weeks of fine weather. The condition is self-limiting, lasting for a week or so, but tends to recur each spring for a number of years.

DIFFERENTIAL DIAGNOSES

1 Polymorphic light eruption: this is a more widespread erythematous papulovesicular eruption (Figs 14.14 and 14.15) occurring following initial exposure to strong sunlight often just after the winter is over. The limbs are predominantly affected, the body to a lesser extent but the face is usually not involved.

Vesicles are less prominent than in juvenile spring eruption, but the two conditions may coexist.
2 Recurrent herpes simplex infection: this may look similar, and may be precipitated by sunlight, but tends to be unilateral rather than bilateral and does not commonly involve the ears. Definitive diagnosis is made by confirming the presence of the organism on virology.

MANAGEMENT

1 A moderate topical steroid helps to settle the acute reaction.
2 Subsequently, the affected individual should use a high-protection sunscreen to achieve graduated sun exposure.

Hydroa vacciniforme

DEFINITION

A rare, bullous photodermatosis which begins in childhood and heals with scarring.

AETIOLOGY

The cause of the condition is unknown, but it has been considered a severe variant of polymorphic

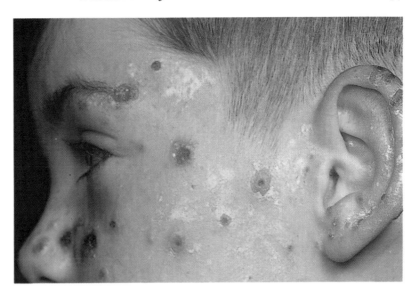

Fig. 14.16 *Hydroa vacciniforme.* Painful symmetrical umbilicated erythematous papules and vesicles occur on light-exposed skin.

light eruption. The condition is provoked by summer sunshine and may be induced by exposure to broad-spectrum artificial radiation.

CLINICAL FEATURES

The condition begins in childhood, and affects both sexes, but is more common in boys. Painful, symmetrical erythematous lesions appear on light-exposed skin, typically the face and hands, within hours of sun exposure, becoming papular and then bullous and occasionally haemorrhagic. The lesions may be umbilicated (Fig. 14.16) and heal with crusting over the course of 2–4 weeks to leave pock-like scars. Systemic symptoms of malaise and fever may accompany severe attacks. The condition usually remits spontaneously in the late teens.

DIFFERENTIAL DIAGNOSIS

The porphyrias are excluded by means of porphyrin screening of blood, urine and faeces.

MANAGEMENT

1 The diagnosis is usually clinical, but may be confirmed by monochromator testing in a specialist photobiology unit.

2 Sun protection is the mainstay of treatment.
3 Antimalarials have been effective in severe cases.

Actinic prurigo

DEFINITION

A rare, itchy, papulonodular eruption of sun-exposed skin, characterized by widespread deep excoriations.

AETIOLOGY

The cause of the condition is not known, and although it may be induced by UVB exposure, UVA is more commonly implicated. In 50% of cases there is a positive family history. There is a particularly high familial incidence among native Americans.

CLINICAL FEATURES

The eruption usually begins in the first decade and is more common in girls. The rash is worse in the summer months, but may persist at other times of the year. Sun-exposed sites develop intensely pruritic erythematous papules, which become excoriated (Fig. 14.17) and crust over, producing a chronic dermatitis. The eruption is most marked on the face, and cheilitis may be severe.

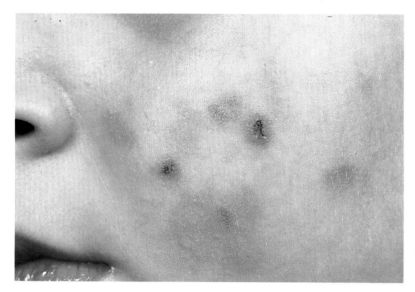

Fig. 14.17 *Actinic prurigo.* Intensely itchy red papules which are readily excoriated occur on light-exposed skin.

DIFFERENTIAL DIAGNOSIS

In young children actinic prurigo may easily be mistaken for atopic dermatitis, but a careful history should elucidate that the exacerbations are associated with sun exposure.

MANAGEMENT

1 The diagnosis is confirmed by specialist light testing.

2 Sunblocks are often ineffective in protecting the patient.

3 Sun exposure should therefore be limited as far as possible.

4 Topical steroids and antihistamines are helpful in the acute phase.

5 Thalidomide has been found to be effective.

6 Gradual increments of exposure to UVB may be of benefit in preventing the eruption in chronic cases. Psoralens and UVA (PUVA) therapy is best avoided because of the real risk of carcinogenesis.

Chapter 15
Reactive Disorders

Introduction

This chapter covers those inflammatory skin diseases which occur as a reactive phenomenon to an antigenic stimulus. In some cases the cause is identifiable and in others it remains unknown. However, most of the diseases to be discussed are mediated through immunological mechanisms.

Drug reactions

Drugs are one of the most common causes of cutaneous reactions. Drug reactions may take many forms. They can be classified as listed in Table 15.1 and are discussed under the individual headings.

Urticaria

DEFINITION

An acquired type I hypersensitivity reaction, in which

acute, well-circumscribed, erythematous wheals develop, each of which may last up to 24 hours.

AETIOLOGY

The disease is a type I allergic reaction mediated via IgE. Urticaria may be classified as:
1 acute;
2 chronic;
3 physical.

An identifiable cause is more likely to be found in children than in adults. Over 75% of cases of urticaria in children are acute. In infants under 6 months of age, the most common precipitant is food allergy, usually cow's milk protein. In older children, over half the acute cases are secondary to either drugs (e.g. aspirin and amoxycillin) or infection (mostly viral) or both. In tropical countries worm infestations may be responsible.

In the small percentage of children who develop chronic urticaria (that is, the disease lasts longer than 6 weeks), the cause is harder to identify, but physical agents (e.g. cold or pressure) may be responsible. Children with chronic urticaria are more likely to have a history of atopy than those with acute disease.

Exercise-induced (cholinergic) urticaria is not uncommon in adolescence, and is characterized by multiple small wheals developing on exertion.

Many young children develop a transient contact urticaria in the perioral region on eating certain foods, especially beef extract spreads such as Marmite® or tomatoes.

Table 15.1 Classification of drug reactions

1 Urticaria
2 Toxic erythema
3 Erythema nodosum
4 Erythema multiforme
5 Photosensitivity*
6 Fixed drug eruption

* See Chapter 14.

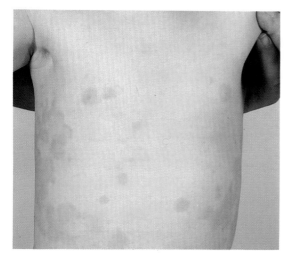

Fig. 15.1 *Urticaria.* Multiple transient, erythematous swellings develop. Each wheal lasts a number of hours and then fades without trace.

CLINICAL FEATURES

Multiple, transient, erythematous wheals (Fig. 15.1) develop suddenly in a widespread distribution. The eruption is dynamic, with individual lesions fading after a few hours, but new lesions appear in crops over several successive days. Unlike urticaria in adults, the childhood condition is not always pruritic. Lesions often occur in an annular pattern (Fig. 15.2) and may be haemorrhagic. Subcutaneous oedema (angio-oedema) occurs in a high percentage (60%), mostly affecting the face (Fig. 15.3). Although often a cause of alarm to the parents, it is rarely serious, and true laryngeal oedema is rare.

DIFFERENTIAL DIAGNOSES

1 Papular urticaria is a reaction to insect bites and tends to be localized to the lower legs and ankles. It is always itchy and is often vesicular and may be bullous.
2 Erythema multiforme (see p. 184): the lesions may be urticated but are of longer duration (usually at least three weeks), and particularly target-like in morphology.
3 Still's disease: a rare fleeting, annular, urticarial eruption may sometimes be seen in children with juvenile arthritis.

Fig. 15.2 *Urticaria.* The lesions are itchy, pink and various shapes and sizes and often annular.

4 C1 esterase deficiency: patients with recurrent angio-oedema should be screened for this rare disorder.

MANAGEMENT

1 The eruption is often self-limiting, but can be distressing, especially when associated with angio-oedema. Reassurance is essential.
2 The cause can usually be suspected in over two thirds of childhood cases on the basis of a careful history and simple screening investigations.
3 Antihistamines will help control the eruption. In children over the age of 3 years, the more specific H_1-antagonist terfenadine may be used, but it is not licensed for use in young children, in whom chlorpheniramine is preferred.

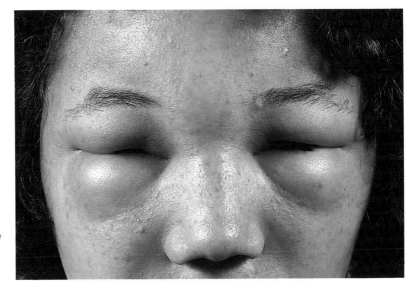

Fig. 15.3 *Angio-oedema.* Subcutaneous oedema may particularly affect the face, hands or feet. It is occasionally associated with laryngeal oedema.

Toxic erythema

DEFINITION

A non-specific descriptive term applied to a generalized macular or maculopapular erythema seen in association with acute infections and drug reactions.

AETIOLOGY

Some erythemas associated with infections are so characteristic as to be termed the exanthems (see Chapter 8), e.g. scarlatina and measles. The less specific eruptions may be grouped together as toxic erythemas and are usually viral in origin. Many drugs, especially antibiotics and anti-epileptics, can induce a toxic erythema. The eruption may not begin until some days after the course of antibiotics has finished and will continue for over a week.

CLINICAL FEATURES

Bright red pruritic macules develop suddenly, and may become urticated or papular in places (Fig. 15.4). The eruption usually begins on the trunk, but rapidly becomes generalized (Fig. 15.5). There

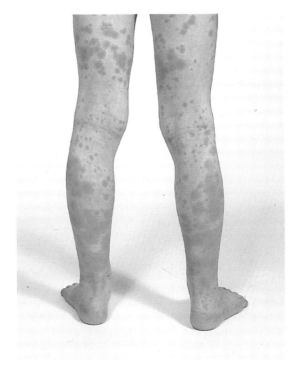

Fig. 15.4 *Toxic erythema.* Bright red pruritic macules develop all over the body. They may become papular or urticarial. Drugs, viruses or bacteria (a streptococcus in this child) are usually responsible.

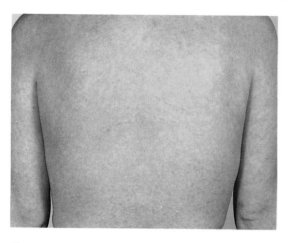

Fig. 15.5 *Toxic erythema.* There is a generalized macular, papular eruption on the trunk. A drug, particularly an antibiotic, is a common cause.

may be fever and malaise in the acute stage. Resolution takes 7–10 days, often with clearance by desquamation.

MANAGEMENT

1 The diagnosis is clinical and a careful history should be taken to elucidate any responsible drug, which should be withdrawn immediately. If a drug is implicated, the patient must be advised to avoid that product in the future and the medical records amended accordingly.
2 When an infective cause is suspected, investigations are directed towards isolating the organism by throat swab, midstream urine specimen, streptococcal titres, blood cultures and viral serology.
3 Treatment is essentially symptomatic. Topical emollients, calamine lotion and oral antihistamines may help relieve the pruritus.

Annular erythema

DEFINITION

A term used to describe a chronic, slowly enlarging, annular eruption, most often localized to the lower limbs, where the cause cannot be identified.

AETIOLOGY

The cause, by definition, is not known. It needs to be distinguished from conditions such as neonatal lupus erythematosus and the more specific annular eruptions which occur with some infections, e.g. Lyme disease (see p. 79).

CLINICAL FEATURES

The eruption may occur at any age, but is most common in young adults. The lesion begins as a small erythematous papule which slowly expands in a centrifugal fashion, finally producing a circular lesion (Fig. 15.6) up to 10 cm in diameter, with a raised, non-scaly, erythematous margin. It may be mildly pruritic and may occur anywhere but most often affects the thighs and buttocks. The eruption occurs in crops over several months, each individual lesion lasting 1–2 weeks.

DIFFERENTIAL DIAGNOSES

1 Tinea corporis (see p. 105): fungal infections may be annular, but have a scaly border. Fungal hyphae can be identified on direct microscopy.
2 Erythema chronicum migrans (see p. 80): in the characteristic annular eruption of Lyme disease there is usually evidence of the original tick bite. Serological tests for *Borrelia burgdorferi* confirm the diagnosis.
3 Erythema marginatum: the annular eruption associated with acute rheumatic fever is now rare. The annular lesions are multiple, of short duration and associated with fever and evidence of cardiac involvement.
4 Granuloma annulare (see p. 261): the raised, beaded border of the lesion is characteristic.

MANAGEMENT

1 The diagnosis is clinical. Skin biopsy reveals a mild, non-specific, perivascular lymphocytic infiltrate.
2 There is no specific treatment.

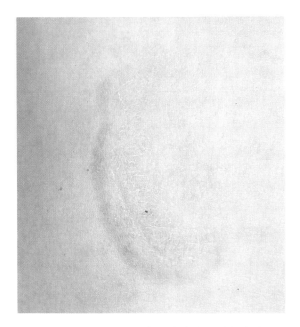

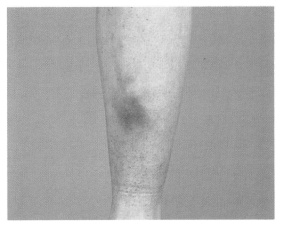

Fig. 15.7 *Erythema nodosum.* Tender, hot, red nodules occur in crops on the lower limbs, particularly the shins. These developed after a throat infection. A streptococcus was isolated.

Fig. 15.6 *Annular erythema.* Red annular lesions with raised margins appear in crops anywhere on the body and last a couple of weeks. They ultimately subside spontaneously.

Erythema nodosum

DEFINITION

Painful, red subcutaneous nodules, especially on the lower legs, caused by an acute reactive panniculitis.

AETIOLOGY

The eruption is an immunologically mediated reaction to a variety of stimuli, in particular streptococcal infection. It may also be seen in association with other infections (e.g. tuberculosis), drug reactions, inflammatory bowel disease and sarcoid.

CLINICAL FEATURES

Erythema nodosum is rare in childhood, but not uncommon in adolescence. Hot, red, tender, firmly indurated nodules, 2–6 cm in diameter (Fig. 15.7), develop on the lower limbs. Lesions may occur anywhere on the arms or legs, but have a predilection for the shins. On the calves (Fig. 15.8) tuberculosis

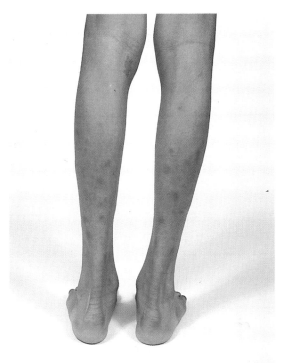

Fig. 15.8 *Erythema nodosum.* These painful nodules were erupting both on the shins and on the backs of the calves. The latter site suggests tuberculosis, which this 14-year-old was found to have in the lung.

may be the cause (erythema induratum). Histologically, there is a florid septal panniculitis (inflammation in the subcutaneous fat). The cutaneous eruption may be accompanied by an arthralgia. The skin lesions resolve over 2–6 weeks, leaving bruise-like markings which gradually fade.

MANAGEMENT

1 Investigations should be directed at elucidating the cause of the eruption by means of a full history, examination, full blood count, viral titres, anti-streptolysin-O titre and chest X-ray.
2 Treatment depends upon the underlying cause. The discomfort is managed symptomatically with simple analgesia or a non-steroidal anti-inflammatory drug.
3 In severe cases, in which pain is limiting mobility, a short course of oral prednisolone may be indicated.

Erythema multiforme

DEFINITION

A polymorphic eruption often composed of distinctive target-like lesions, particularly on the extremities, which may be associated with ulceration of the mucous membranes.

Table 15.2 Some causes of erythema multiforme and Stevens–Johnson syndrome

Infections	Herpes simplex
	Orf
	Infectious mononucleosis
	Hepatitis B
	Mycoplasma
	Histoplasmosis
	Rickettsiae
Drugs/therapy	Sulphonamides
	Penicillin
	Barbiturates
	Salicylates
	Radiotherapy
Systemic disease	Lupus erythematosus
	Polyarteritis nodosa
	Malignancy

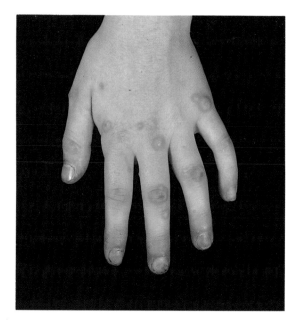

Fig. 15.9 *Erythema multiforme.* Well-defined ring-shaped lesions recur on the extremities. Herpes simplex is the most common known cause.

AETIOLOGY

The eruption is a reactive phenomenon which may occur in response to a wide range of stimuli (Table 15.2), most commonly viral infections or drugs. The most common cause of erythema multiforme in the UK is herpes simplex, which precedes the erythema multiforme by several days. However, in over 50% of cases the cause of the eruption is never identified. The exact mechanism of the reaction is unknown, but it is thought to be immune-complex mediated.

CLINICAL FEATURES

There is a spectrum of severity, from mild localized cutaneous disease to a severe mucocutaneous bullous eruption termed Stevens–Johnson syndrome.

Erythema multiforme may occur at any age, but the more severe bullous forms occur particularly in children and teenagers, especially boys. Round, well-circumscribed, cutaneous papules and plaques develop anywhere on the body, but are most frequent on the extremities (Fig. 15.9). The lesions are

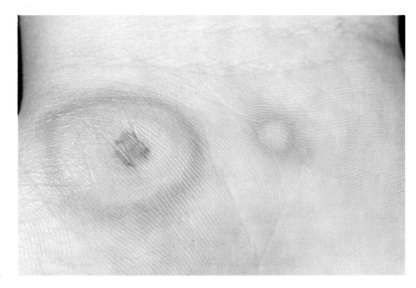

Fig. 15.10 *Erythema multiforme.* There is a concentric ring with a red margin surrounding a bulla with a purpuric centre. This is a target lesion.

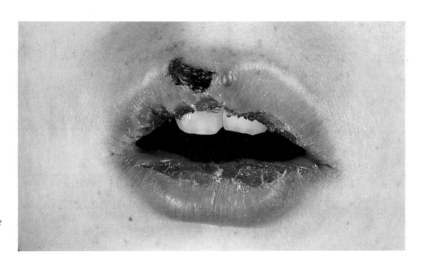

Fig. 15.11 *Erythema multiforme.* Blistering and ulceration of lips, oral mucosa and genitalia may occur in the severe variant known as Stevens–Johnson syndrome.

composed of characteristic concentric rings, with a purpuric centre, forming the so-called target lesion (Fig. 15.10). The lesions may become oedematous and frankly bullous. Simple erythema multiforme fades over the course of 3 weeks, but may be recurrent, especially in cases associated with herpes simplex.

In extreme cases, there is fever and severe blistering with ulceration of the lips (Fig. 15.11), oral mucosa and genitalia. In addition, there may be multisystem involvement in Stevens–Johnson syndrome with arthritis, gastrointestinal symptoms and nephritis. *Toxic epidermal necrolysis* should be considered the most severe end of the spectrum of erythema multiforme. The mucosae (Fig. 15.12) are severely affected with an acutely tender erythema and blistering (Fig. 15.13) that sheets off, leaving a raw, red, denuded surface (Fig. 15.14) like a burn. Drugs are the most common cause.

MANAGEMENT

1 Localized cutaneous forms of erythema multiforme require symptomatic treatment only.

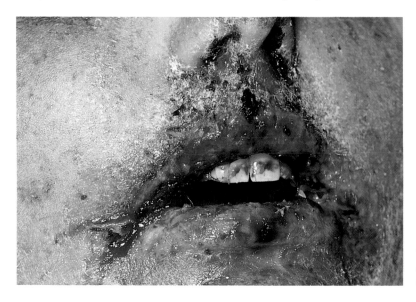

Fig. 15.12 *Toxic epidermal necrolysis.* The eyes, nose, mouth and genitalia are usually involved before the skin eruption develops.

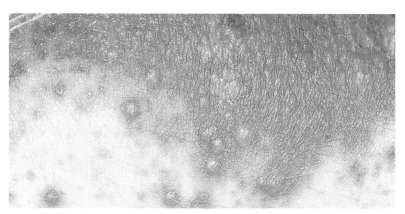

Fig. 15.13 *Toxic epidermal necrolysis.* The skin is exquisitely tender, bright red and covered with vesicles or flaccid bullae. This is the same teenager as in Figs 15.12 and 15.14.

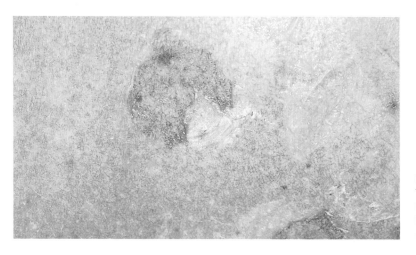

Fig. 15.14 *Toxic epidermal necrolysis.* The surface of the blisters sheet off, leaving raw, oozing, denuded skin. Drugs are the usual cause. The mortality is significant.

2 In cases associated with herpes simplex, recurrent episodes may be suppressed by prophylactic treatment with topical acyclovir, at the onset of symptoms of the cold sore. In frequently recurring cases, long-term oral acyclovir may be justified. Therapy with azathioprine has also been successful in suppressing severe recurrent erythema multiforme, but is usually reserved for older patients.

3 Patients with Stevens–Johnson syndrome may be seriously ill and require careful evaluation with supportive nursing. However, the place of oral steroids in management is controversial, but recently cyclosporin has been suggested to be of benefit. Prevention of secondary infections is paramount.

Fixed drug eruption

DEFINITION

A reaction that recurs in the same place each time the allergen is ingested.

AETIOLOGY

The cause is unknown. Phenolphthalein in laxatives, barbiturates, sulphonamides, tetracyclines, griseofulvin and phenacetin are among the more common causes. Over-the-counter products may be responsible but are often difficult to identify.

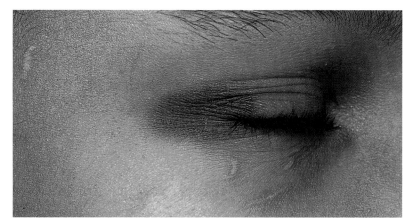

Fig. 15.15 *Fixed drug eruption.* Initially there is erythema and oedema followed by a distinctive round postinflammatory hyperpigmentation. A single patch on the face, genitalia, hand or mouth is characteristic.

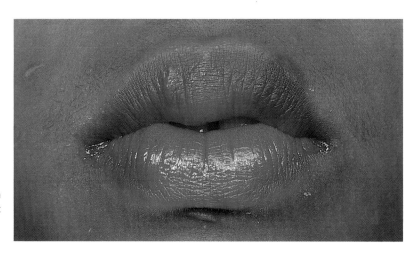

Fig. 15.16 *Fixed drug eruption.* The reaction occurs in the same place each time the offending agent is ingested. It leaves a pigmented patch behind. The lip is a characteristic site.

CLINICAL FEATURES

A red-brown swelling occurs a few hours after the drug has been taken. It subsides, leaving behind a round, deeply pigmented patch. The swelling will recur in the same site if the agent is ingested again and may blister. The face (Fig. 15.15), lips (Fig. 15.16), genitalia, back of the hands and limbs are the usual sites.

MANAGEMENT

The condition ceases once the drug is identified and withdrawn, but the pigmentation remains for a long time.

Henoch–Schönlein purpura (HSP) (anaphylactoid purpura)

DEFINITION

A vasculitic eruption affecting the lower part of the body, which may be associated with arthritis, abdominal pain and glomerulonephritis.

AETIOLOGY

Henoch–Schönlein purpura is an immune-complex mediated disease. C3 and IgA are deposited in the small vessels of the skin and other organs and initiate inflammation through activation of the complement cascade. The end result is a leucocytoclastic vasculitis with fibrinoid necrosis of the vessel wall and extra-vasation of red blood cells. The antigen responsible for the vasculitic response is not always identifiable, but HSP is most often associated with infections, especially by β-haemolytic streptococci.

CLINICAL FEATURES

The most common cause of vasculitis in young people is HSP. The majority of cases occur in children under 7 years, with a mean age of 4 years. The eruption is slightly more common in boys. Although many different organs may be involved in this reactive vasculitis, the purpuric skin lesions are the most common manifestation and are the present-ing feature in over 50% of cases. The eruption is composed of numerous small, purple, maculopapular lesions scattered over the buttocks and legs (Fig. 15.17). The centre of the lesion is purpuric, and often raised. Some of the lesions may be rather urticated. Although the dependent areas of the body are primarily involved, the eruption may extend to the trunk and upper limbs. Fever is common.

Occasionally, the characteristic palpable purpura may be preceded by scrotal erythema and oedema in boys. Facial oedema may also be prominent. Other organs which may be affected include the joints, gastrointestinal tract and kidneys. Arthritis is common and most often affects the ankles and knees. Nausea, vomiting and colicky abdominal pain occur in over 75% of patients. Renal disease is less common, but more serious. Glomerulonephritis usually

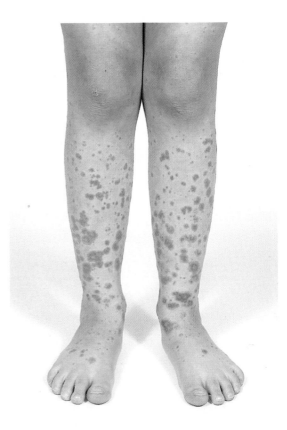

Fig. 15.17 *Henoch–Schönlein purpura.* Purpuric papules occur on the lower limbs and buttocks. It is a leucocytoclastic vasculitis, often caused by a streptococcus in children.

presents as microscopic haematuria, but may progress to nephrotic syndrome and renal failure.

MANAGEMENT

1 The cutaneous lesions resolve over 1–3 weeks. The diagnosis is confirmed by means of a skin biopsy, but no specific treatment is required for the skin.
2 The cause of the eruption should be sought by means of a throat swab, antistreptolysin-O titre and viral titres. If a streptococcal infection is isolated, it should be treated accordingly.
3 Careful evaluation of renal function is imperative. The urine should be tested for blood and protein. If renal involvement is detected, it should be monitored closely in conjunction with the paediatricians and nephrologists as therapy with prednisolone may be indicated.

Pigmented purpuric dermatosis (Schamberg's disease)

DEFINITION

An asymptomatic purpuric eruption affecting the lower legs, with a characteristic orange-brown discoloration.

AETIOLOGY

The disorder is thought to be due to a capillaritis with extravasation of red cells into the skin, but the precise aetiology is unknown.

CLINICAL FEATURES

The eruption may occur anywhere on the body, but it most frequently affects the lower limbs. It may develop at any age, but is more common in childhood, especially in boys. Irregular macular patches of pinpoint purpura (Fig. 15.18) suddenly appear on the lower leg and extend to involve most of the limb. Some lesions may have a scaly surface, but most are macular. The initial lesions may be quite red, but soon fade to an orange-brown colour producing the so-called cayenne pepper appearance. Although it is occasionally itchy, most cases are asymptomatic. The eruption fades over several months and rarely recurs.

MANAGEMENT

1 There is no treatment.
2 The family may be reassured that the disorder is benign and self-limiting and does not represent any abnormality of clotting.

Fig. 15.18 *Pigmented purpuric dermatitis.* Irregular flat patches made up of pinpoint purpura (petechiae) and brown haemosiderin staining occur, particularly on the limbs.

Papular acrodermatitis of childhood

DEFINITION

A benign self-limiting eruption of the extremities occurring as a reactive phenomenon after certain viral infections.

AETIOLOGY

The disorder was originally described following acute anicteric hepatitis B infection in Italian children (Gianotti-Crosti syndrome), but in countries where the prevalence of hepatitis is lower, the causative role of hepatitis B has rarely been demonstrated. It is now clear that this cutaneous reaction may follow infection by a number of viruses, e.g. hepatitis A, Epstein–Barr virus, cytomegalovirus, Coxsackie virus, echovirus and respiratory syncytial virus.

CLINICAL FEATURES

Most reports of the disorder have originated from Europe and Japan and the disease would appear to be rare in North America. However, the incidence has been declining in all regions over the last decade. The eruption has been reported to occur at any age from 6 months to 12 years, but the mean age is 2 years. In keeping with the viral aetiology, it occurs most commonly in spring and autumn. The cutaneous signs appear suddenly and there may be no prior symptoms of a viral illness. Firm, monomorphic, red or flesh-coloured papules 1–5 mm in diameter (Fig. 15.19) are distributed in a symmetrical fashion on the limbs, buttocks and occasionally the face, with a rather characteristic sparing of the trunk (Fig. 15.20). They are most numerous on the extensor surfaces of the limbs. The mucous membranes are not involved. There may be mild constitutional upset (malaise and fever) depending

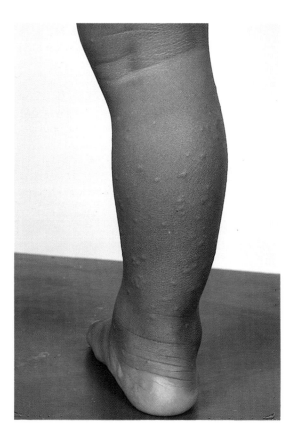

Fig. 15.19 *Papular acrodermatitis of childhood.* Well-defined, asymptomatic, symmetrical red firm papules are present on the arms and legs. There may or may not be mild malaise, fever and lymphadenopathy.

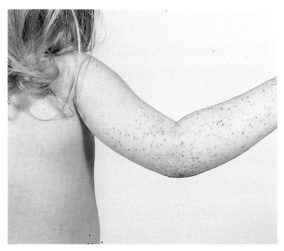

Fig. 15.20 *Papular acrodermatitis of childhood.* Firm, monomorphic, red papules occur on the limbs with remarkable sparing of the torso. Occasionally it is secondary to hepatitis B (Gianotti–Crosti syndrome).

on the nature of the underlying infection, with lymphadenopathy and hepatomegaly in hepaotitic cases. However, the cutaneous lesions, although often dramatic in appearance, are usually asymptomatic.

MANAGEMENT

1 The diagnosis is clinical.
2 The child should be screened for infection by means of a full blood count, hepatitis serology and viral titres.
3 No specific treatment is required for the skin. The eruption resolves spontaneously over 2–4 weeks and recurrences are rare.
4 Follow-up is only indicated if hepatitis B is diagnosed, in which case the child should be referred to a paediatrician.

Graft-versus-host disease

DEFINITION

A multisystem reaction to the transfer of immuno-competent cells from a donor to an immunocom-promised host.

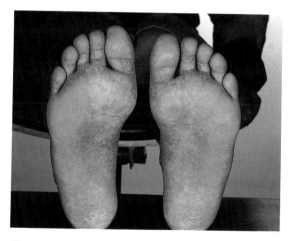

Fig. 15.21 *Graft-versus-host reaction.* A diffuse mauve maculopapular reaction occurs on the palms, soles and face, often with hepatitis and diarrhoea.

AETIOLOGY

The disease was originally described following allogenic bone-marrow transplants, but has now been recognized to complicate liver transplantation, the transfusion of non-irradiated blood products and even up to 10% of autologous bone-marrow transplants.

CLINICAL FEATURES

The disease may be acute or chronic. Acute graft-versus-host disease most commonly begins 1–2 weeks after transplantation, but can develop any time up to 2 months after. The cutaneous eruption is frequently the first evidence of the disease. A faint maculopapular eruption begins, usually on the face and acral areas, including the palms and soles (Fig. 15.21), and is accompanied by fever. The rash spreads to the trunk, becoming more pronounced as it becomes established, and desquamation is common. Severe forms may become bullous. There may be multiorgan involvement, with a florid hepatitis and bloody diarrhoea. Skin biopsy shows solitary epidermal cell necrosis and a mononuclear cell inflammatory infiltrate.

Chronic graft-versus-host disease usually follows the acute disease within 3 months of the transplant. A lichenoid eruption which later becomes sclerotic initially involves the face, palms and soles but may become more generalised.

MANAGEMENT

1 A skin biopsy allows rapid confirmation of the diagnosis.
2 The acute disease is treated with high-dose pulse methylprednisolone. Chronic disease is managed with lower doses of long-term immunosuppressive therapy.
3 UVB has been found to be very helpful in treating graft-versus-host disease.
4 There is a significant mortality with both forms of the disease.

Chapter 16
Hair and Scalp Disorders

Introduction

Rudimentary hair follicles begin to develop in the embryo at the age of 9 weeks. By 28 weeks the scalp hairs have usually completed the first growth cycle and some may be shed (telogen phase) *in utero*. This telogen phase may be delayed in a band of hairs in the occipital region, which are often not shed until 2–3 months after birth (see Fig. 16.24). The normal cyclical pattern of hair growth (Table 16.1) is fully established by the end of the first year of life.

Vellous hairs are the short, soft, fine, unmedullated hairs which cover most of the body. In contrast, scalp hairs are longer, thicker, coarser and pigmented. These are known as terminal hairs. At puberty, androgenic influences promote the change from vellous to terminal hair in the axillae and pubic regions (and the beard area in boys).

Abnormalities of the hair most commonly present as hair loss, and may be congenital or acquired. One of the most common causes of acquired hair loss in children is tinea capitis (Fig. 16.1), which is discussed fully in Chapter 9.

Congenital hair disorders

The congenital absence of scalp skin, aplasia cutis (Fig. 16.2), which may present as a localized patch of alopecia, is discussed in Chapter 3.

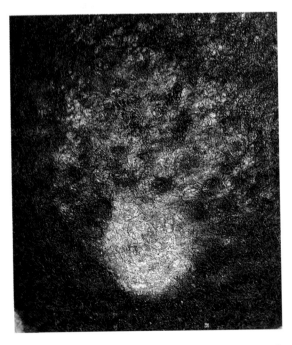

Fig. 16.1 *Tinea capitis.* This is one of the most common causes of acquired hair loss in children. There are one or several patches of alopecia with inflammation and scaling of the scalp.

Table 16.1 The scalp hair cycle

Phase	Function	Scalp hairs (%)	Average duration
Anagen	Growth period	80–90	Up to 3 years
Catagen	Degeneration and transition	2–5	2 weeks
Telogen	Resting period	10–20	3 months

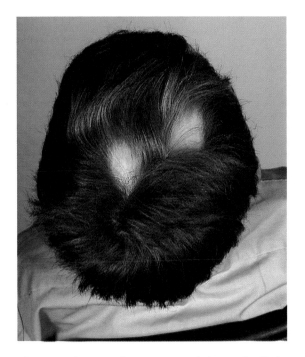

Fig. 16.2 *Aplasia cutis.* There is a congenital absence of scalp skin to a variable degree which presents as one or several localized patches of hair loss (courtesy of Dr M. Clement).

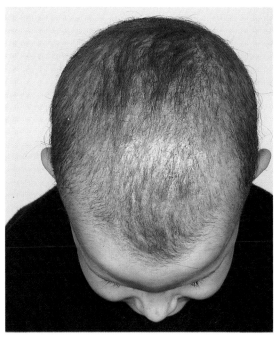

Fig. 16.3 *Monilethrix.* Shortly after birth the normal hairs are replaced by multiple short beaded hairs, resulting in a sparse appearance.

Sparse or absent hair may be a prominent component of many of the genodermatoses, e.g. anhidrotic ectodermal dysplasia and Rothmund–Thomson syndrome (see p. 170). Those inherited conditions which primarily present with abnormalities of the hair are discussed below.

Monilethrix

DEFINITION

A rare congenital abnormality featuring sparse, beaded hair which may be associated with keratosis pilaris and koilonychia.

AETIOLOGY

The condition is normally inherited as an autosomal-dominant disorder with variable penetrance, but occasionally as a recessive trait.

CLINICAL FEATURES

The hair is usually normal at birth, but over the next few months it is replaced by dry, brittle hairs, resulting in a sparse appearance of multiple, short, broken hairs (Fig. 16.3). The hair shaft is of variable thickness along its length, producing a beaded (moniliform) appearance (Fig. 16.4).

Follicles are often plugged by scale, especially at the nape of the neck (Fig. 16.5). The abnormalities are not always confined to the scalp, and hair at other body sites may be abnormal. The nails may show a concave curvature (koilonychia; see p. 213). Monilethrix usually occurs in isolation, but occasionally ocular, dental or mental defects may be associated.

DIFFERENTIAL DIAGNOSES

1 Pili torti: the hair is normal at birth but a few

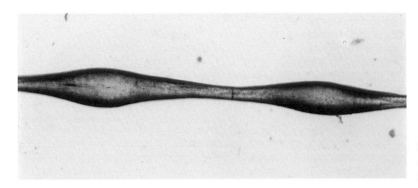

Fig. 16.4 *Monilethrix.* The hair shaft is of variable thickness along its length, producing a beaded appearance.

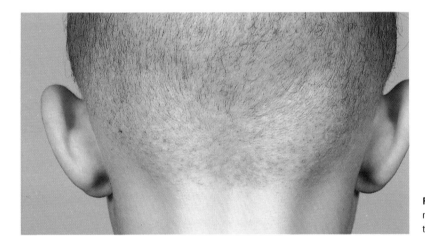

Fig. 16.5 *Monilethrix.* The hair follicles may be plugged by scale especially at the back of the neck.

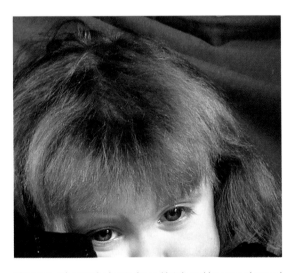

Fig. 16.6 *Pili torti.* The hair is dry and brittle and becomes abnormal a few months after birth. In reflected light it appears spangled.

months later it becomes dry and brittle. It has a spangled appearance (Fig. 16.6) in reflected light due to rotation of the hair through 180° (Fig. 16.7).

2 Other hair shaft abnormalities, e.g. pili torti (twisted hair) or trichorrhexis nodosa: these can be excluded by light or electron microscopy of the hair shaft.

3 Menkes' kinkey hair syndrome: this is a rare X-linked recessive disorder, in which copper deficiency results in pale twisted hairs, abnormal blood vessels, growth retardation and severe neurological abnormalities.

MANAGEMENT

1 The diagnosis is confirmed by the characteristic (beaded) appearance of the hair shaft on light microscopy.

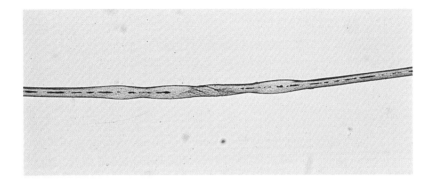

Fig. 16.7 *Pili torti.* Under the light microscope, the hair is seen to be rotated 180° through its long axis.

2 The condition usually persists, but partial or total regression may occur at puberty.

3 Topical retinoids have been used in conjunction with minoxidil with limited success.

Trichorrhexis nodosa

DEFINITION

A disruption of cuticular walls such that they splay out forming nodes, most often as a result of injury to the hair, but occasionally occurring as a congenital defect.

AETIOLOGY

Excessive combing, washing, swimming and sun exposure are the commonest explanations of injury to the hair shaft. However, it may also occur in Netherton's syndrome, argininosuccinic aciduria, pseudomonilethrix and as an isolated familial defect of hair.

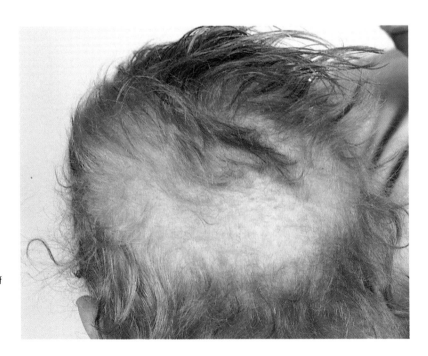

Fig. 16.8 *Trichorrhexis nodosa.* In congenital forms, quite large areas of alopecia are visible. The hairs are broken off, leaving stumps. Light microscopy of the shaft reveals the frayed cortical fibres.

CLINICAL FEATURES

In the congenital forms the hair breaks very easily and areas of the scalp are affected by quite marked hair loss (Fig. 16.8) due to the fractured hair shafts.

MANAGEMENT

The diagnosis is confirmed by identifying the splayed-out nature of the cortical cells on light microscopy. There is no treatment for the congenital forms.

Trichothiodystrophy

DEFINITION

An inherited disorder in which the hairs are sulphur-deficient and break easily.

AETIOLOGY

The brittle hair is inherited as an autosomal-recessive trait and may be associated with a variety of other developmental defects including intellectual impairment, decreased fertility and short stature (known as BIDS). BIDS with ichthyosis (IBIDS) and IBIDS with photosensitivity (PIBIDS) are other related syndromes.

CLINICAL FEATURES

The condition is rare. The hair is sparse, dry and breaks easily from birth (Fig. 16.9). Transverse fractures through the hair shaft (trichoschisis) can be demonstrated on light microscopy. On electron microscopy the cuticle is seen to be absent.

Amino acid analysis of the hair reveals a very low cysteine content. The condition may be associated with other neuroectodermal defects, neutropenia, mental retardation, subfertility and photosensitivity.

MANAGEMENT

1 The metabolic abnormality cannot be corrected.
2 The coexistence of neutropenia with associated risk of repeated infection should be excluded.

Trichorrhexis invaginata

DEFINITION

A specific abnormality of the hair shaft occurring as part of the familial disorder, Netherton's syndrome.

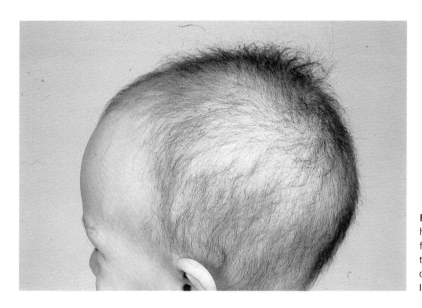

Fig. 16.9 *Trichothiodystrophy.* The hair is sparse, dry and breaks easily from birth. Transverse fractures occur through the hair shaft due to a deficient cuticle (courtesy of the Institute of Dermatology).

The inheritance of Netherton's syndrome (see p. 32) is autosomal recessive with variable penetrance, but the expression is higher in girls.

CLINICAL FEATURES

The hair is short, dry, sparse and brittle from birth (see Fig. 3.30). The hairs refract light unevenly and may appear spangled. Sections of the hair become invaginated into the more proximal hair shaft to produce the characteristic 'bamboo hair' which is visible on scanning electron microscopy. A florid dermatitis, ichthyosis linearis circumflexa, persists from the neonatal period, and may initially be mistaken for eczema.

MANAGEMENT

There is no treatment for the hair shaft abnormalities.

Uncombable hair ('cheveux incoiffables')

DEFINITION

A structural abnormality in which the hair is short and unmanageable.

AETIOLOGY

The cause is unknown, but there is no apparent familial basis.

CLINICAL FEATURES

The hair may be sparse or normal at birth. It subsequently becomes pale and coarse and grows in a disordered fashion (Fig. 16.10). The hair cannot be made to lie flat against the scalp and often appears to have been artificially 'crimped'. There are no other associated developmental defects.

MANAGEMENT

1 The hair appears normal under light microscopy,

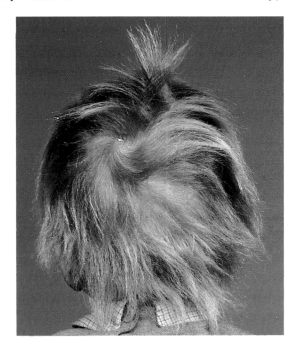

Fig. 16.10 *Uncombable hair.* This little girl's hair is rather spangled and will not lie flat, especially at the back of the head (courtesy of Dr R. Staughton, 1988. *The Colour Atlas of Hair and Scalp Disorders.* Upjohn and Wolfe Publishing Ltd, London).

but scanning electron microscopy reveals longitudinal grooves in the hair shaft.
2 No treatment is effective.

Woolly hair

DEFINITION

Tightly coiled hair occurring in individuals who are not of black African extraction.

AETIOLOGY

The condition is familial. Both autosomal-dominant and autosomal-recessive patterns of inheritance have been described.

CLINICAL FEATURES

From birth the scalp hair is tightly curled (Fig.

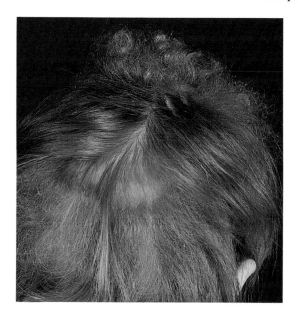

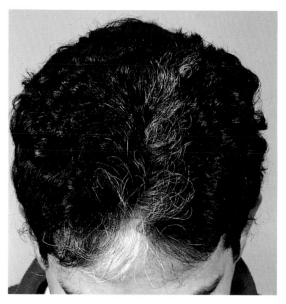

Fig. 16.11 *Woolly hair.* At birth the hair is tightly curled and does not grow to any great length. It may be a local or generalized defect (courtesy of the Institute of Dermatology).

Fig. 16.12 *Poliosis.* A forelock of completely depigmented hair occurs. It is inherited as an isolated finding or as part of piebaldism or Waardenburg's syndrome.

16.11) and rarely grows to any great length. The abnormality may be localized (woolly hair naevus) or involve all the scalp hair. The body hair is normal. Associated ophthalmic abnormalities have been described in some pedigrees.

MANAGEMENT

There is no treatment for the hair.

Poliosis

DEFINITION

A localized absence of pigmentation in the hair.

AETIOLOGY

It is hereditary. There is an absence or deficiency of melanin in the hair follicles. Poliosis may occur as an isolated finding or in association with generalized abnormalities such as piebaldism (see p. 154) or Waardenburg's syndrome.

CLINICAL FEATURES

A forelock of completely depigmented hair (Fig. 16.12) is present from birth and persists through life.

DIFFERENTIAL DIAGNOSES

1 Vitiligo: affected scalp hairs may become depigmented in vitiligo as an acquired phenomenon.
2 Alopecia areata: regrowth of hair in a localized area of alopecia areata may initially be depigmented, but the history should clearly differentiate the two conditions.
3 Waardenburg's syndrome: the poliosis is associated with deafness. There are associated facial anomalies including lateral displacement of the medial canthi and hypertrophy of the nasal root.
4 Vogt–Koyanagi–Harada syndrome: a rare disorder in which vitiligo, poliosis and uveitis follow a meningo-encephalitic illness.
5 Scalp hairs growing over a naevus or neurofibroma may occasionally be depigmented.

MANAGEMENT

1 Exclude any associated abnormalities.
2 Treatment is rarely requested, but the hair can be coloured in older individuals if desired for cosmetic reasons.

Conditions of increased hair growth

A clear distinction should be drawn between *hypertrichosis* (Fig. 16.13) and *hirsutism* (Fig. 16.14). Hypertrichosis is an excessive growth of normally vellous body hair which may subsequently differentiate into the terminal state. It can occur in a localized manner such as in a naevus or in a generalized way in such disorders as anorexia nervosa or porphyria or after certain drugs such as corticosteroids. Hirsutism is an increase in androgen–dependent hair growth and may be part of a more general disorder known as virilism. However, there is marked racial variation in the density of normal body hair which must be taken into account in assessing whether or not the hair growth is pathological.

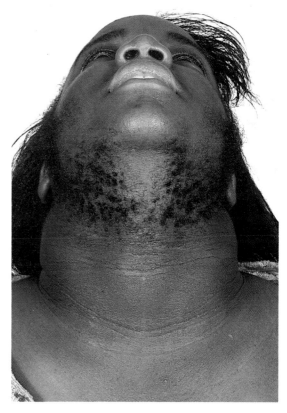

Fig. 16.14 *Hirsutism.* This is the growth of coarse terminal hairs in the female in a pattern simulating that of the sexually developed male, as in this girl with type A insulin resistance – acanthosis nigricans, hyperinsulinaemia and androgen excess without morbid obesity.

Hypertrichosis lanuginosa

DEFINITION

An extremely rare syndrome in which fetal lanugo hair persists throughout life.

AETIOLOGY

The condition is inherited as an autosomal-dominant trait.

CLINICAL FEATURES

The child is covered in a profusion of soft lanugo

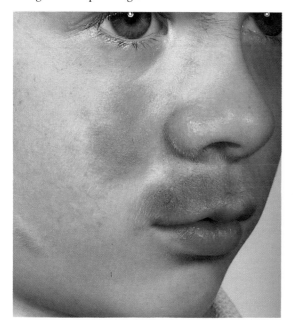

Fig. 16.13 *Hypertrichosis.* This term means the growth of terminal hairs in an area which is not normally hairy. It may be localized to a congenital naevus such as this, known as a Tierfel naevus because of its resemblance to animal fur.

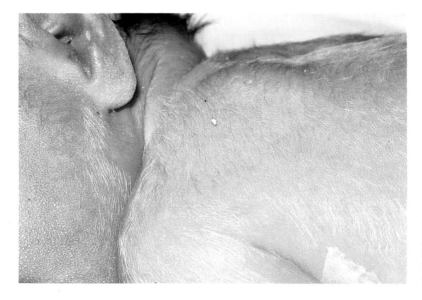

Fig. 16.15 *Lanugo hairs in the premature.* It is normal for the fetus to be covered by fine, downy hair *in utero.* This is usually shed before birth but is still evident in very premature babies.

hair over most of the body surface, with the exception of the palms and soles. The hair may grow to a considerable length, and may be especially long and dense around the ears and nostrils. The lanugo persists throughout life.

DIFFERENTIAL DIAGNOSES

1 It is normal for the fetus to be covered by fine, downy lanugo hair *in utero*, but this is usually shed before birth. However, it may still be evident in premature babies (Fig. 16.15), although it will be lost during the neonatal period.
2 Fetal-alcohol syndrome: hypertrichosis may be an obvious part of the syndrome, but is rarely as extensive as in hypertrichosis lanuginosa and is associated with other congenital defects, such as mental retardation.

MANAGEMENT

1 Regular shaving helps to improve the appearance. Body hair may only need shaving every few months, although conspicuous areas such as the face may need to be shaved several times a week. There is no other more specific treatment.
2 The initial whole-body shave in a neonate requires a general anaesthetic.

Circumscribed naevoid hypertrichosis (faun-tail naevus)

DEFINITION

A tuft of long hairs in the lumbosacral region, which may be associated with a spinal defect.

AETIOLOGY

This localized hypertrichosis is a developmental abnormality.

CLINICAL FEATURES

Long, coarse, darkly pigmented terminal hairs are present in the centre of the lower back (Fig. 16.16). The descriptive term 'faun-tail naevus' highlights its resemblance to an animal's tail. The abnormality is important as it draws attention to the possibility of underlying spinal dysraphism.

MANAGEMENT

1 The naevus may also occur in isolation.
2 The lumbosacral spine should be X-rayed to exclude a congenital skeletal abnormality, and if such a problem is identified, specialist advice should

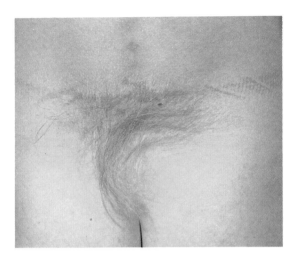

Fig. 16.16 *Faun-tail naevus.* Long, coarse, darkly pigmented terminal hairs are present in the centre of the lower back. It may be associated with spinal dysraphism.

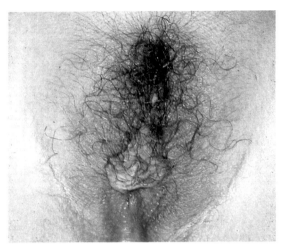

Fig. 16.17 *Congenital adrenal hyperplasia.* This 2-year-old girl has undergone precocious puberty secondary to her congenital adrenal disease (courtesy of Dr. C. Buchannan).

be sought from a neurosurgeon and orthopaedic surgeon.

Congenital adrenal hyperplasia (CAH)

DEFINITION

An inherited deficiency of one of the enzymes in the biosynthetic pathway of cortisol synthesis, resulting in increased synthesis of androgenic steroids and marked virilization.

AETIOLOGY

The defect is most commonly a C21-hydroxylase deficiency. The block in the synthetic pathway results in low cortisol levels and a loss of negative feedback on the pituitary with consequent increased production of adrenocorticotrophic hormone and therefore stimulation of other metabolites, especially androgens.

CLINICAL FEATURES

Depending on the severity of the enzyme deficiency, the individual may be affected either in early childhood (precocious puberty, Fig. 16.17) or in adolescence (with hirsutism and mild virilization).

Female babies with CAH have ambiguous genitalia at birth with pseudohermaphrodism. Thirty per cent of infants with CAH have an associated impairment of aldosterone synthesis, which results in marked electrolyte disturbances.

DIFFERENTIAL DIAGNOSES

1 Cushing's syndrome: excess cortisol production of either adrenal or pituitary origin may produce hypertrichosis and some degree of virilization, but this can be clearly distinguished from CAH on biochemical grounds, by the finding of a raised midnight cortisol.
2 Virilizing ovarian tumours: these may mimic CAH, but are rare in the young.

MANAGEMENT

1 Any infant with ambiguous genitalia should be investigated to exclude CAH.
2 The finding of a raised serum 17-hydroxyprogesterone is confirmatory.
3 Rapid diagnosis may be achieved by random urine analysis for the 11-oxygenation index (the ratio of steroids without a hydroxyl group at the 11-position to those with such a moiety). The index is raised in CAH.

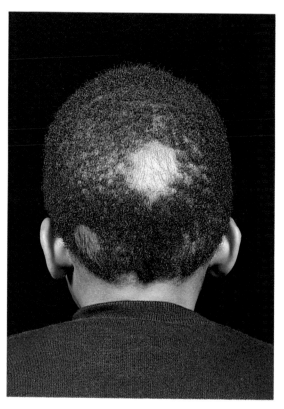

Fig. 16.18 *Alopecia areata.* Well-circumscribed discoid areas of hair loss without inflammation appear suddenly. In black children, the hair may initially grow back as fine, straight hairs.

Acquired hair disorders

Alopecia areata

DEFINITION

Patchy hair loss occurring on a normal scalp in a well patient.

AETIOLOGY

The sudden hair loss is due to premature telogen in the affected area. In the majority of individuals it is idiopathic, but various factors have been described which are important in the pathogenesis of alopecia areata. The condition may be familial and there is an association with HLA-DR3, HLA-DR4 and HLA-DR5. It may be associated with auto-immune disease (e.g. thyroid disease and diabetes), and can also occur in association with the development of hypertension. In children there is a link (33%) with atopy. Alopecia areata is found with an increased prevalence in Down's syndrome.

CLINICAL FEATURES

Well-cirumscribed, discoid areas of hair loss appear suddenly. They may be solitary (Fig. 16.18) or, if

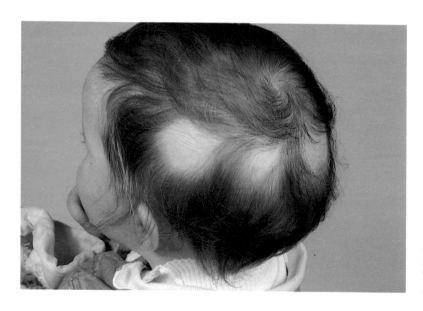

Fig. 16.19 *Alopecia areata.* Alopecia in childhood does not ultimately carry a good prognosis. Although recovery may occur, there is a tendency to relapse. The skin of the scalp is quite normal in appearance.

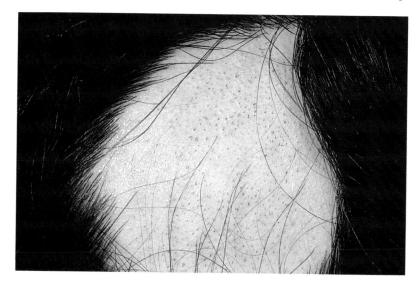

Fig. 16.20 *Alopecia areata.* Short broken off hairs rather like exclamation marks are present in the active phase of hair loss.

the condition is progressive, multiple areas may be involved (Fig. 16.19). Lesions vary in size from less than 1 cm to many centimetres in diameter (Fig. 16.20). Sometimes the hair loss is more diffuse (Fig. 16.21), in which case the diagnosis may prove more difficult. The scalp itself appears healthy and in particular there is no scarring and the follicles are preserved. At the borders of the affected areas, short, broken (exclamation mark) hairs (Fig. 16.20) are diagnostic. The areas of alopecia may gradually enlarge and coalesce to produce large areas of hair loss.

The eyelashes and eyebrows may be affected. Involvement of the whole scalp is known as alopecia totalis (Fig. 16.22). If the whole body is affected, the condition is called alopecia universalis. It is estimated that 1% of patients with alopecia areata progress to either alopecia totalis or universalis. Alopecia totalis is more common in children than in adults.

In the majority of patients with alopecia areata the hair eventually regrows, although the outlook is quite variable. The chance of recovery is estimated at >90% in cases of a solitary patch of alopecia, and 60% of children experience spontaneous regrowth within 1 year. However, involvement of the occipital region (ophthiasis) is associated with a lower rate of remission. Extensive alopecia of early onset also carries a poor prognosis, and regrowth is unlikely in a child who develops alopecia totalis before puberty.

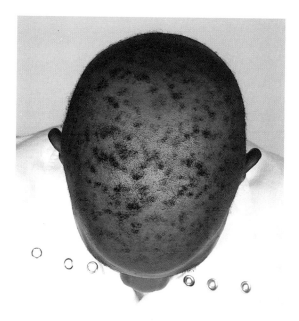

Fig. 16.21 *Alopecia areata.* Occasionally the hair loss may be diffuse with multiple islands of healthy hair in between.

When regrowth occurs, the hair may initially be depigmented. In black children, the first hairs after recovery are often straight rather than curly (Fig. 16.18).

A pitted nail dystrophy may be found in associa-

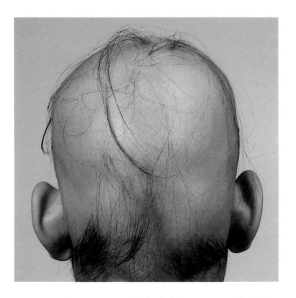

Fig. 16.22 *Alopecia areata.* This boy's hair regrew completely, but has fallen out again subsequently. The prognosis of such alopecia areata is not usually good.

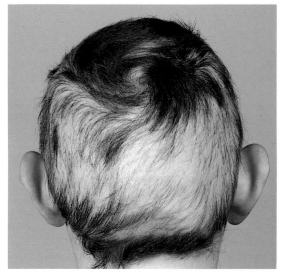

Fig. 16.23 *Trichotillomania.* This is a self-induced loss of hair due to unhappiness. It is usually temporary in childhood. The hair loss is partial, localized and often asymmetrical.

tion with alopecia areata, most frequently in patients with extensive hair loss.

DIFFERENTIAL DIAGNOSES

1 Tinea capitis (see p. 102): in contrast to alopecia areata, the residual hairs are broken and the scalp is scaly and may be inflamed. The definitive difference is the positive mycological investigations.
2 Trichotillomania (see p. 266 and Fig. 21.3): the pattern of short, broken hairs (Fig. 16.23) is usually characteristic, with peripheral sparing. However, confusion may occasionally arise in cases of diffuse alopecia areata.
3 Traction alopecia (see p. 206): the hair loss occurs in association with tight hairstyles which exert undue force on the hair roots.
4 Telogen effluvium: a large number of follicles may synchronously and prematurely enter telogen following systemic illness, high fever or psychological stress, culminating in sudden hair loss 2–3 months after the precipitating event.
5 Diffuse hair loss of systemic disease: nutritional deficiencies and a variety of endocrinopathies (e.g.

thyroid disease) may be associated with diffuse hair loss.
6 Cicatricial alopecia: several inflammatory dermatoses (e.g. lichen planus or lupus erythematosus) severe infection, (especially kerion) and trauma may damage hair follicles sufficiently severely to produce scarring and areas of permanent hair loss (Fig. 16.24). However, cicatricial alopecia is rare.

MANAGEMENT

1 The psychological impact of hair loss on children and their families should not be underestimated.
2 In very limited cases, simple observation may be most appropriate as the chances of spontaneous recovery are high.
3 The mainstay of treatment is the application of superpotent topical or intralesional steroids. Most benefit is achieved if treatment is used early in the disorder. Established disease is much more resistant to therapeutic intervention. Systemic steroids rarely produce a sustained benefit, and their use in children cannot often be justified.
4 Inducing a reactive dermatitis (either allergic

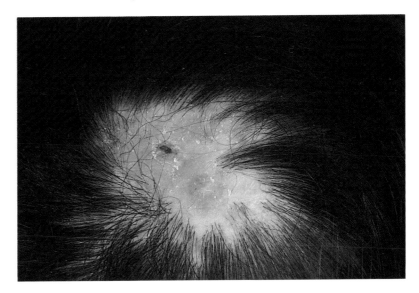

Fig. 16.24 *Scarring alopecia.* Permanent alopecia due to scarring is uncommon in childhood, but may be due to lupus erythematosus, lichen planus or kerion.

by using dinitrochlorobenzene or diphencyprone, or irritant by using dithranol) has been found to be beneficial in a proportion of patients.

5 Limited success has been reported from ultraviolet (UV) light therapy, both UVB and psoralens and UVA (PUVA), presumably as a result of inducing local immunosuppression.

Occipital hair loss in infants

DEFINITION

A band of localized alopecia over the back of the head during the first year of life.

AETIOLOGY

Occipital hair loss beginning at the age of 2–3 months may be due to a localized delayed first telogen, but later, friction from rubbing the head in the cot is contributory.

CLINICAL FEATURES

A transient band of hair loss commonly develops over the back of the head (Fig. 16.25) in babies from the age of 2 months. If rubbing is playing a part, the scalp may appear slightly red.

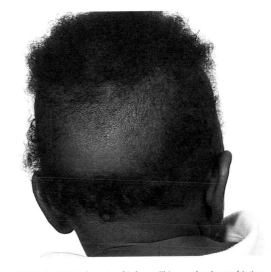

Fig. 16.25 *Occipital alopecia of infancy.* This may be due to friction or may be a localized form of delayed first telogen. The hair loss may be quite marked occipitally, but always recovers.

MANAGEMENT

No treatment is warranted and reassurance that the hair will regrow normally over the next few months is all that is required.

Traction alopecia

DEFINITION

Localized hair loss resulting from mechanical trauma.

AETIOLOGY

The condition arises from prolonged traction on the hair root as a result of certain hairstyles (Fig. 16.26). Mild forms may arise as a result of pulling

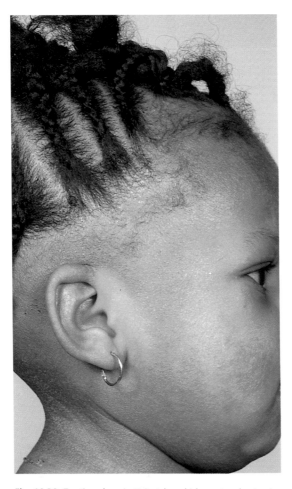

Fig. 16.26 *Traction alopecia.* Hair styles which exert undue tension and traction on the hair follicle may cause hair loss. It is common in Afro-Caribbeans and may be permanent.

the hair back in a ponytail over long periods, but more commonly it is associated with the tight, twisted ethnic hairstyles popular in some races.

CLINICAL FEATURES

Gradual hair loss develops at sites of maximum tension on the hair. Typically this is around tight partings and in the bitemporal region.

MANAGEMENT

1 It may be very difficult to persuade the parents of a younger child that the hairstyle is responsible, and fashion-conscious teenagers may be reluctant to change their hairstyle.
2 The hair should not be tied back for long periods. Styles should be changed every so often to vary the points of tension, and the hair released at night.
3 If the above advice is not heeded, the alopecia may become permanent.

Pityriasis amiantacea

DEFINITION

Localized, firmly adherent, heaped-up hyper-keratotic plaques common on the scalp in children.

AETIOLOGY

The cause is not known. The condition may occur in isolation or in conjunction with an inflammatory dermatosis, particularly psoriasis. Nineteen per cent of patients with pityriasis amiantacea have a family history of psoriasis and 6% of children with it are atopic.

CLINICAL FEATURES

Pityriasis amiantacea is more common in girls, and is more prevalent in children than adults, often starting around the age of 6 years. Thick, tightly adherent white scales develop on the scalp. They may be seen attached to the hair shaft (Fig. 16.27) as the hair grows out. In florid cases there may be some

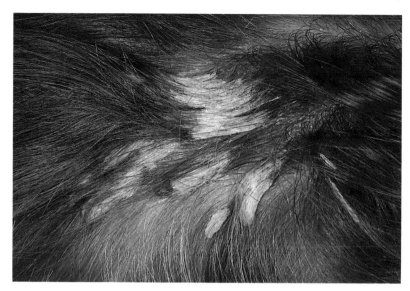

Fig. 16.27 *Pityriasis amiantacea.* Thick tightly adherent white scales develop on the scalp and attach to the hair shaft, rather like tiles overlapping on a roof.

hair loss due to the mechanical effect of the scale. It may be a solitary finding, but up to 15% of children have been observed to develop psoriasis later.

DIFFERENTIAL DIAGNOSES

1 Tinea capitis (see p. 102): this may be considered a possibility in cases of pityriasis amiantacea associated with alopecia, but in the latter mycology is negative.
2 Pediculosis capitis (see p. 115): the adherent flakes of scale attached to the hair shaft have often been mistaken for nits by the unwary.
3 Cradle cap (see p. 49): this consists of large, thick, heaped-up, greasy, yellow scales which may become matted with the hair. It is seen in young babies, often in association with seborrhoeic dermatitis, whereas pityriasis amiantacea most often affects older children.

MANAGEMENT

1 Salicylic acid 5–10% in emulsifying ointment, applied to the affected scalp, left on overnight and shampooed out in the morning, will reduce scale.
2 Unguentum cocois compound applied overnight under a shower cap and shampooed out is also effective, but slightly messier to use.

Trichostasis spinulosa

DEFINITION

A disorder of hair follicle metabolism resulting in the production of multiple unmedullated vellous hairs from a single hair follicle.

AETIOLOGY

The cause is unknown.

CLINICAL FEATURES

The condition particularly affects the seborrhoeic regions including the front (Fig. 16.28) and back of the torso, shoulders and upper outer arms. There are black dots which may be mistaken for comedones, but on closer inspection are revealed as projecting tufts of multiple fine hairs (Fig. 16.29). It is not uncommon in adolescence.

MANAGEMENT

Wax depilatories have been used successfully and retinoic acid applied topically may be effective.

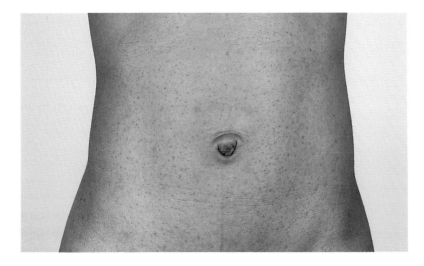

Fig. 16.28 *Trichostasis spinulosa.* There are a myriad of black dots to be seen which rather resemble blackheads. The torso is a common site.

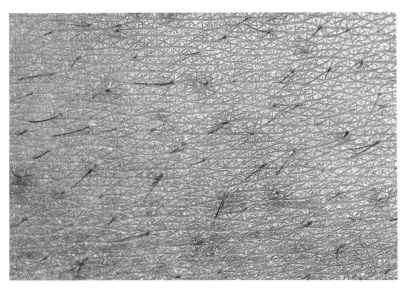

Fig. 16.29 *Trichostasis spinulosa.* On close inspection of the lesions in Fig. 16.27, multiple vellous hairs are seen emanating from each pore.

Chapter 17
Nail Disorders

Introduction

The nail consists of layers of keratin. It develops from an invagination of the epidermis which covers the dorsum of the distal phalanx. Nails begin to form in the embryo at the age of 9 weeks, cover a significant portion of the finger tip by 22 weeks, and are full length at birth. Nail growth is thus a facet of age, and nails are incomplete in premature babies. Toe-nail development lags behind that of the finger-nails. Nail disorders are not uncommon in children and may be due to physiological, congenital or acquired factors.

Physiological disorders

Linear melanonychia

DEFINITION

Longitudinal streaks of pigmentation may occur as a common normal variant in black individuals (Fig. 17.1).

AETIOLOGY

The pigmentation is due to the presence of melanin granules within the nail plate, produced by the melanocytes in the nail matrix.

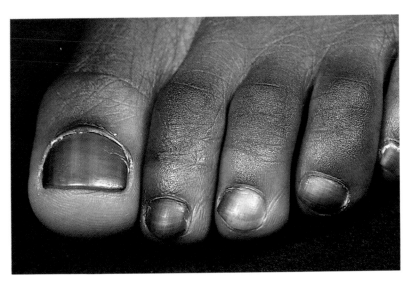

Fig. 17.1 *Linear melanonychia.* Longitudinal streaks occur as a normal variant in Afro-Caribbeans. There may also be diffuse pigmentation.

CLINICAL FEATURES

Linear bands of black or brown pigmentation occur along the length of the nail. Their frequency increases with age, and they are found in 25% of black children aged between 3 and 10 years. Several nails are usually affected.

DIFFERENTIAL DIAGNOSES

1 Subungual haematoma: there is usually a history of trauma. The black discoloration is diffuse and rather speckled at the edges, and the russet tinge of haemorrhage is usually visible.
2 Subungual melanoma: this is exceedingly rare in childhood. Unlike in linear melanonychia, the pigmentation is non-linear, extends onto the proximal nail fold and affects only one nail.

MANAGEMENT

If the bands of pigmentation are causing concern, simple reassurance that these are a common normal variant with no pathological significance is all that is required.

Congenital and inherited dystrophies

The nails may be affected in a variety of rare congenital syndromes as part of a generalized disorder (such as anhidrotic ectodermal dysplasia, epidermolysis bullosa and mucocutaneous candidiasis) and are described elsewhere. Absence of nails, or hyponychia, may occur as a result of fetal exposure to drugs (e.g. anticonvulsants or alcohol) during pregnancy. The more common disorders are discussed here.

Nail–patella syndrome

DEFINITION

A genetically inherited disorder characterized by a nail dystrophy occurring in association with skeletal abnormalities.

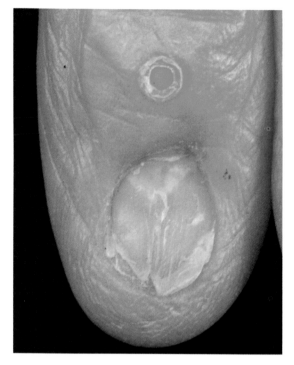

Fig. 17.2 *Nail–patella syndrome.* The thumb-nails in particular are either totally or partially absent, as are the patellae (Fig. 17.3). The lunula is triangular.

AETIOLOGY

The condition is inherited as an autosomal-dominant trait, and affects tissues derived from both the ectoderm and the mesoderm. The gene responsible for the disorder is carried on chromosome 9 and there is close linkage between the inheritance of the nail–patella syndrome and the ABO blood groups.

CLINICAL FEATURES

The nails are partially or completely absent. In milder cases the nails may simply be ridged and split easily. The thumb-nail (Fig. 17.2) is most severely affected and the toe-nails may be spared. A triangular lunula is characteristic, but only present in about half the cases. The most consistent skeletal abnormality is an absent or hypoplastic patella (Fig. 17.3), but involvement of other bones (e.g. iliac spurs) and renal abnormalities have also been described.

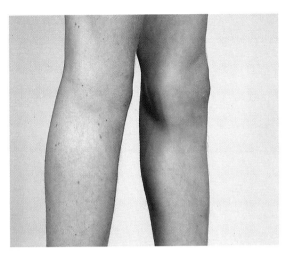

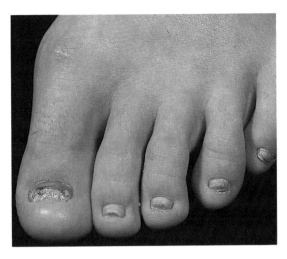

Fig. 17.3 *Nail–patella syndrome.* The patellae are either absent or hypoplasic.

Fig. 17.4 *Pachyonychia congenita.* There is marked subungual hyperkeratosis and a wedge-shaped appearance to the nails associated with hyperkeratosis of the palms and soles.

DIFFERENTIAL DIAGNOSIS

The skeletal abnormalities and lack of paronychia distinguish the nail–patella syndrome from pachyonychia congenita (p. 211).

MANAGEMENT

1 Diagnosis is confirmed by an X-ray of the knees.
2 Other associated abnormalities should be excluded.
3 There is no means of correcting the nail deformity.

Pachyonychia congenita

DEFINITION

An inherited ectodermal dysplasia with prominent nail dystrophy, palmoplantar keratoderma and hyperhidrosis occurring in association with mucocutaneous and ocular abnormalities.

AETIOLOGY

The inheritance is autosomal dominant, but the extent of the syndrome may be quite variable. Several subtypes have been described.

CLINICAL FEATURES

The nails may appear quite normal at birth, but by the age of 6 months they have developed a brown discoloration. The nails become progressively thickened, hard and curved. There is marked subungual hyperkeratosis and the distal portion of the nail lifts off the nail bed (Fig. 17.4). Recurrent infection (paronychia) can result in shedding of the nail. All the nails may be affected, but the thumbnail is the most severely dystrophic, and the abnormality characteristically diminishes towards the fifth digit.

Associated features include follicular hyperkeratoses, palmoplantar keratoses, pigmentation of the elbows and knees, oral changes, partial alopecia, cataract, and, in rare cases, short stature and mental retardation.

MANAGEMENT

1 The nails are very difficult to manicure and pose a considerable cosmetic problem. Occasionally, surgical removal of a severely affected nail may be justified.
2 There is some evidence that oral retinoids are helpful, but their use in children is limited by side effects.

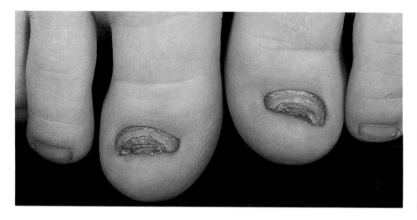

Fig. 17.5 *Congenital malalignment of the nails.* The great toe-nails are affected at birth and deviate laterally, often embedding into the nail fold. The nails are thickened, ridged and discoloured.

Congenital malalignment of the great toe-nails

DEFINITION

A congenital condition in which the nail plate of the first toes is distorted and grows laterally in an angulated fashion, with resultant nail dystrophy.

AETIOLOGY

It has been postulated in the past that the abnormality arose as a result of poor fetal positioning, but evidence now suggests that it is a familial entity with autosomal-dominant inheritance.

CLINICAL FEATURES

The great toe-nails are deviated laterally at birth (Fig. 17.5). As they grow, they embed in the lateral nail fold, resulting in an ingrown nail. Minor trauma results in ridging, thickening, onycholysis and brown discoloration of the nail due to subungual haemorrhage.

DIFFERENTIAL DIAGNOSES

1 Fungal infection of the toenails: this can be excluded by mycology, but is usually asymmetrical, whereas in congenital malalignment, the toe-nails are affected symmetrically.
2 Ingrown toe-nail: this is usually solitary rather than bilateral and acquired through wearing tight footwear or poor nail clipping.

MANAGEMENT

1 If the condition is diagnosed before the age of 2 years, surgical realignment of the nail is possible and results in cure.
2 Spontaneous correction of the disorder has been reported.

Acquired disease

The nails may become dystrophic in any inflammatory disease affecting the distal digits. Psoriasis (Fig. 17.6), eczema (Fig. 17.7) and lichen planus

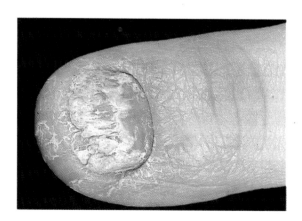

Fig. 17.6 *Psoriasis.* Irregular pitting of the nail plate may be accompanied by separation of the distal nail from its bed (onycholysis).

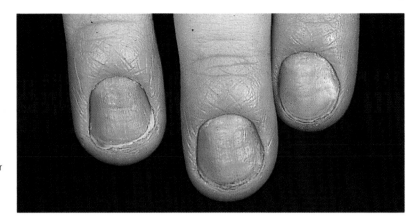

Fig. 17.7 *Eczema of the nails.* Previous eczema overlying the posterior nail folds disturbs growth in the underlying nail matrix and results in horizontal ridging of the nails.

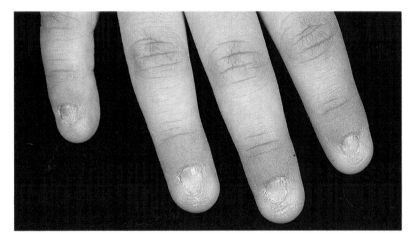

Fig. 17.8 *Lichen planus.* This is a destructive nail dystrophy. The lymphocytic infiltration of the basal cell layer of the epidermis may result in an adhesion between the skin of the posterior nail fold and the nail plate. This is known as a pterygium.

(Fig. 17.8) are all described elsewhere, but their nail changes are illustrated here for comparison with other nail disorders.

Koilonychia

DEFINITION

A concave curvature in the nail plate.

AETIOLOGY

At birth the nails are thin and soft and easily traumatized. Upward curvature of the great toe-nails is very common in babies and is transient.

In older individuals, koilonychia may arise from iron-deficiency anaemia, but in children it may occur as a familial (autosomal-dominant) condition. It may also be seen in association with other congenital abnormalities, e.g. monilethrix (see p. 193).

CLINICAL FEATURES

The edges of the nail are curved upwards to produce a central depression, resulting in a 'spoon-shaped' nail (Fig. 17.9). The changes are most severe on the index finger.

MANAGEMENT

A remedial cause (e.g. iron deficiency) should be sought and treated.

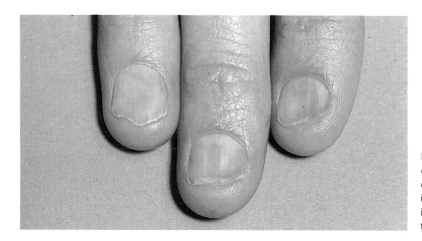

Fig. 17.9 *Koilonychia.* The nail is concave rather than convex, being curved at its edges. When present since infancy it is congenital. In young babies it may be a transient phenomenon due to immaturity of the nails.

Beau's lines

DEFINITION

A single horizontal ridge occurring across all the nails, representing a temporary arrest of nail growth, secondary to an intercurrent systemic illness.

AETIOLOGY

Nail formation may be interrupted by any major disease (e.g. zinc deficiency in acrodermatitis enteropathica), infection (e.g. measles) or following chemotherapy for cancer, but will sometimes be noticed after a relatively minor febrile illness.

Beau's lines are also reasonably common in babies before the age of 3 months as a transient idiopathic finding.

CLINICAL FEATURES

A deep transverse depression is seen in the nail plate (Fig. 17.10). Normally all the nails are affected simultaneously, most obviously across the fingernails but also across the toe-nails. The changes become visible several weeks after the causal illness.

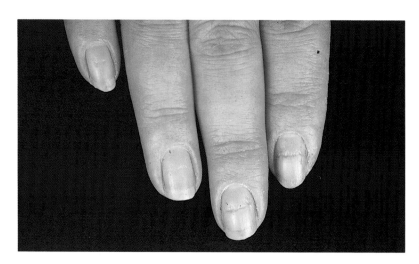

Fig. 17.10 *Beau's lines.* A transverse depression occurs across all the nails. It becomes visible a few weeks after an illness and subsequently grows out.

The band is first apparent proximally but it progresses distally with subsequent nail growth.

MANAGEMENT

No treatment is required.

Habit tic deformity

DEFINITION

A median nail dystrophy resulting from repeated trauma either to the nail plate or the cuticle itself.

AETIOLOGY

The nail matrix may be damaged by repetitive trauma from a subconscious nervous habit of picking at the cuticle or scratching the thumb-nail with the ipsilateral forefinger.

CLINICAL FEATURES

Multiple small, horizontal grooves are seen in a linear fashion down the median aspect of the nail (Fig. 17.11). Habit tics are most common on the thumb-nail of the non-dominant hand.

MANAGEMENT

Many children find such subconscious repetitive actions gratifying. If they grow out of the habit, the nail deformity will correct, but it often persists into adolescence and adult life. The principle is the same as in the case of nail biting (onychophagia, Figs 17.12 and 21.2) and it is often difficult to persuade the child to give it up. However, it is totally harmless and therefore is best ignored as usually, in the fullness of time, the habit is abandoned, and the nail recovers.

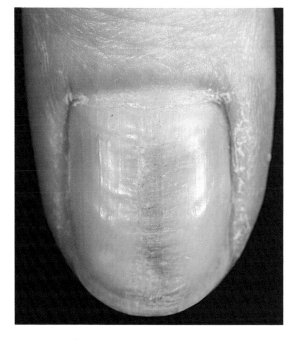

Fig. 17.11 *Habit tic deformity.* A linear depression consisting of many small horizontal grooves occurs along the length of the thumb nail. It may persist into adult life.

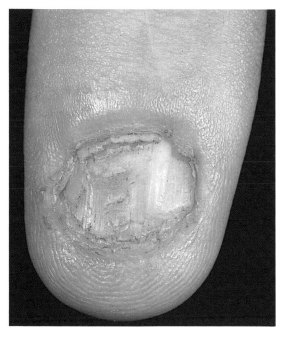

Fig. 17.12 *Onychophagia.* Nail biting is a common and often temporary habit tic in childhood and adolescence. The nail is short and the edges are irregularly fractured.

Parakeratosis pustulosa

DEFINITION

A self-limiting inflammatory condition of unknown aetiology, affecting the distal finger-tip and nail, usually in a solitary manner.

AETIOLOGY

The condition has been considered as a variant of both eczema and psoriasis, but probably has more in common with the latter. A small percentage of children certainly develop psoriasis vulgaris elsewhere later on.

CLINICAL FEATURES

Parakeratosis pustulosa is not uncommon, usually beginning before the child reaches the age of 5 years. Like childhood psoriasis, it more often affects girls. The condition is usually confined to one digit (Fig. 17.13) and is more common on the fingers than the toes. Erythema and scale develop around the terminal phalanx, and there may be a few pustules initially. As the disease continues, subungual hyperkeratosis becomes prominent and the nail becomes onycholytic and progressively dystrophic with pitting.

MANAGEMENT

1 The condition may persist for several years but it eventually resolves spontaneously.
2 Treatment is unsatisfactory, but a moderately potent topical steroid can limit the cutaneous changes.

Nail dystrophy of alopecia areata

DEFINITION

A pitted nail dystrophy seen in association with alopecia areata.

AETIOLOGY

Alopecia areata is an auto-immune disease.

CLINICAL FEATURES

The nail changes of alopecia areata may develop before the onset of hair loss and persist after re-growth of the hair. It has been estimated that 66% of patients with alopecia areata have nail changes, but in our own experience nail involvement is much less frequent. The most common nail change is fine pitting, with the pits arranged in transverse rows (Fig. 17.14). In more severe cases, multiple fine,

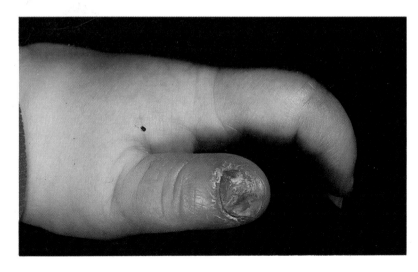

Fig. 17.13 *Parakeratosis pustulosa.* Erythema and scaling occur around the skin of the terminal phalanx and there is distal subungual hyperkeratosis. It ultimately resolves spontaneously.

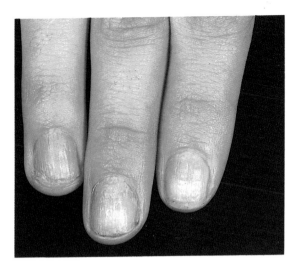

Fig. 17.14 *Alopecia areata.* Pitting occurs often in a regular manner, along either the longitudinal or the horizontal axis of the nail and sometimes both, as in this 14-year-old.

longitudinal ridges may produce 'sandpaper' nails. The nail dystrophy may not affect all of the nails.

DIFFERENTIAL DIAGNOSES

1 Psoriasis (see Fig. 17.6): the pitting is irregular, coarser and associated with onycholysis.
2 Twenty-nail dystrophy (see below): the nail changes occur in isolation, with no evidence of associated hair loss.

MANAGEMENT

Eventually, the nail changes resolve spontaneously.

Twenty-nail dystrophy

DEFINITION

A symmetrical dystrophy of all the nails, occurring in children in the absence of any other overt skin disease.

AETIOLOGY

It is not clear whether twenty-nail dystrophy represents a distinct entity or is merely an inflammatory dermatosis confined to the nail matrix. It has been suggested that if a nail biopsy were performed, most cases of twenty-nail dystrophy might be reclassified as lichen planus or alopecia areata.

CLINICAL FEATURES

The nails are opalescent and longitudinally ridged. All the nails are affected (Fig. 17.15), but the magnitude of the changes may be variable.

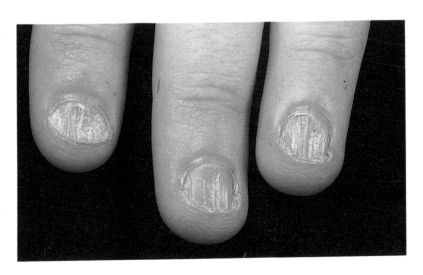

Fig. 17.15 *Twenty-nail dystrophy.* All twenty nails are affected by excess ridging and an opalescent discoloration. It is self-limiting.

MANAGEMENT

1 A longitudinal nail biopsy can be useful to look for an underlying cause (e.g. lichen planus), but it is not often justified in children.
2 No specific treatment is effective.
3 The condition may resolve spontaneously.

Subungual exostosis

DEFINITION

A painful osseous nodule beneath the nail.

AETIOLOGY

The lesion develops as an outgrowth of normal bone and is not a true exostosis. There is some evidence that the lesions may result from trauma.

CLINICAL FEATURES

The lesions are most common on the first toes, but can affect any digit. A hard, vascular nodule develops beneath the nail, lifting up the distal nail plate (Fig.

17.16). The lesion is exquisitely tender and pain often precludes the wearing of shoes.

MANAGEMENT

1 The diagnosis is confirmed on X-ray of the digit (Fig. 17.17).
2 Surgical excision is necessary to remove the lesion.

Infections

Paronychia

DEFINITION

A painful pustular infection of the nail fold, which may be acute or chronic.

AETIOLOGY

Any deformity of the nail will predispose towards infection of the nail fold (e.g. congenital malalignment of the great toe-nail: see p. 212), but the most common factor in the development of paronychia in childhood is the habit of thumb-sucking. Habitual

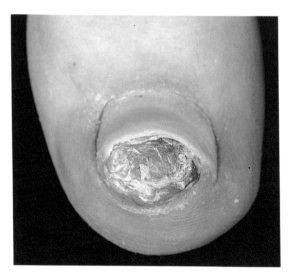

Fig. 17.16 *Subungual exostosis.* A hard, tender nodule develops under the distal nail plate, particularly of the great toe.

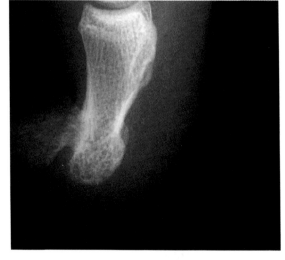

Fig. 17.17 *Subungual exostosis.* The exostosis may be confirmed radiographically as an opacity.

sucking of the digits results in maceration of the tissues, providing a ready portal of entry for infection. Acute paronychia is usually caused by staphylococci, but occasionally Gram-negative enterococci may be responsible. Chronic infections are almost always due to *Candida*, as a result of immersion of the hands in water. Chronic paronychia is not common in children but may occur in late adolescence as a result of an occupation, e.g. catering or hairdressing.

CLINICAL FEATURES

Acute paronychia

The nail fold is erythematous, tender and swollen. A bead of pus may be expressed from the side of the nail by gentle pressure (Fig. 17.18).

Chronic paronychia

In chronic cases the posterior nail fold is swollen, the surface of the nail plate becomes ridged and discoloured and the cuticle is lost (Fig. 17.19). In cases of severe candidal nail infection affecting several nails, the possibility of an inherited abnormality of immune function, chronic mucocutaneous candidiasis (see p. 109), should be considered.

DIFFERENTIAL DIAGNOSIS

Blistering distal dactylitis is a localized superficial lake of pus which forms on the finger pulp, due to infection by *Streptococcus A*. Although on the finger tip, it does not involve the nail fold, and is less tender than a paronychia. It responds to a course of antibiotics.

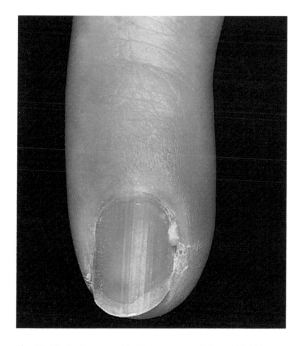

Fig. 17.18 *Acute paronychia.* The area around the nail fold is acutely painful, red and swollen, and pus is visible (courtesy of Mr C. Chandler).

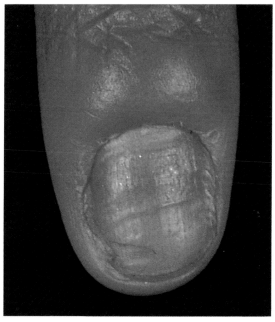

Fig. 17.19 *Chronic paronychia.* The cuticle is destroyed by constant immersion in water. *Candida* enters under the nail folds, which become swollen. The nail plate is subsequently deformed by a series of horizontal ridges.

MANAGEMENT

Acute paronychia

1 The nail fold should be swabbed for microbiological culture.
2 Appropriate antibiotics should be given orally.
3 Acute surgical drainage may occasionally be required to release the pus.

Chronic paronychia

1 In all instances, but especially in the case of chronic candidal infections, resolution depends upon keeping the area dry, but this may be difficult in the case of thumb-suckers.
2 The topical application of an antiseptic (e.g. sulphacetamide 15% in spirit t.d.s) can be helpful.

Periungual warts

DEFINITION

A viral infection affecting the nail fold and producing hyperkeratotic changes.

AETIOLOGY

The infection is caused by one of the common human papillomaviruses responsible for hand warts in children. Nail-biting both predisposes to and spreads the infection.

CLINICAL FEATURES

Periungual warts are asymptomatic, hyperkeratotic papules, which may spread along the nail fold and coalesce (Fig. 17.20). If the surface becomes fissured, the wart may then become painful. A secondary nail dystrophy, in which a groove appears in the adjacent nail, may develop in chronic cases.

MANAGEMENT

Warts are eventually self-limiting but periungual warts are particularly recalcitrant. Conservative measures (see p. 93), such as salicylic acid paints, are

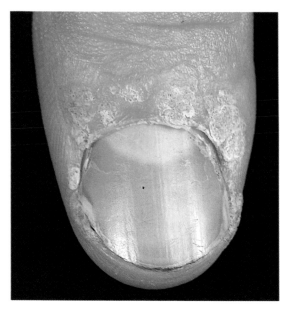

Fig. 17.20 *Periungual warts.* Well-defined hyperkerototic papules occur along the nail folds. They are common in nail-biters.

to be preferred, as cryotherapy is uncomfortable and poorly tolerated in children.

Onychomycosis

DEFINITION

A dermatophyte fungal infection of the nail.

AETIOLOGY

Infection is due to invasion of the nail by dermatophyte fungi. Conditions which promote maceration of the digits (e.g. prolonged immersion in water) predispose to fungal infections. Onychomycosis in children is nearly always the result of cross-infection from an adult member of the household with tinea pedis.

CLINICAL FEATURES

Tinea of the nail is not common in immunocompetent children, but since it is treatable, the diagnosis should not be missed. The infection commences at

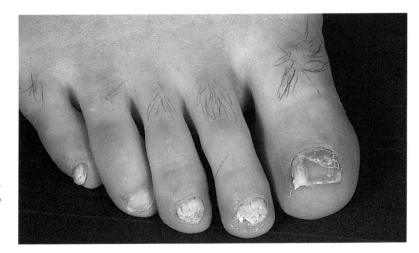

Fig. 17.21 *Onychomycosis.* Tinea of the nails is uncommon in childhood, although it may commence in the toe-nails in adolescence. In this case there is white discoloration and hyperkeratosis to a varying degree, with sparing of the fourth toe.

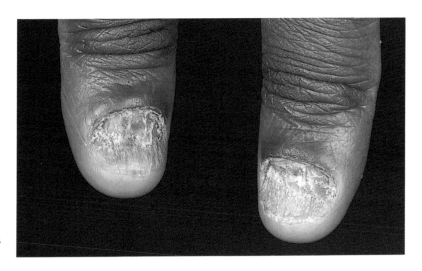

Fig. 17.22 *Onychomycosis.* The nails of this African boy are pigmented, hyperkeratotic and dystrophic. Cultures grew *Trichophyton soudanense.*

the side of the nail plate with discoloration (Fig. 17.21) and subsequently with onycholysis and subungual hyperkeratosis (Fig. 17.22) develop. Nails may be affected partially or completely, but the infection is usually asymmetrical.

MANAGEMENT

1 The diagnosis should be confirmed by microscopy and culture of nail clippings.
2 Oral griseofulvin is the only treatment currently licensed for use in children. However, the more potent fungicidal agent terbinafine will become

available soon and is the treatment of choice in adolescence.

Herpetic whitlow

DEFINITION

A localized, painful primary herpetic infection of the nail fold.

AETIOLOGY

Herpes simplex virus may be inoculated into the

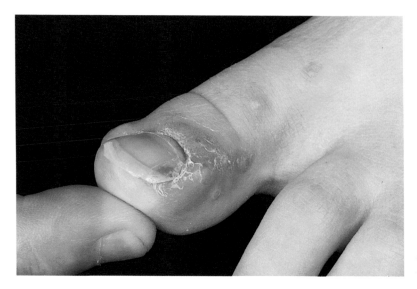

Fig. 17.23 *Herpes simplex.* Clusters of tense vesicles with oedema occur along the nail fold.

finger tip at any site of minor trauma such as through nail-biting.

CLINICAL FEATURES

Localized tenderness and pain precede the eruption of clusters of tense vesicles along the nail fold (Fig. 17.23), which take up to 2 weeks to resolve. Following the initial infection, recurrent episodes are common.

MANAGEMENT

1 Topical acyclovir 5% cream applied five times daily for 5 days may reduce the intensity of an attack. Systemic acyclovir may be required during the primary attack.
2 The vesicles contain active virus and care should be taken to prevent cross-infection.
3 The diagnosis may be confirmed by culture or virus or visualizing it electronmicroscopy of the virus.

Chapter 18
Disorders of Sebaceous and Sweat Glands

Introduction

This chapter discusses inflammatory disorders and developmental cysts affecting the adnexal glands of the skin. Syringomas are described in Chapter 11.

Acne

Acne is a common disorder. While most cases will be straightforward acne vulgaris, other variants of acne need to be taken into account in assessing the patient (Table 18.1).

Acne vulgaris

DEFINITION

An inflammatory disorder of the pilosebaceous apparatus, common on the face and upper trunk in adolescence.

Table 18.1 Classification of acne

Acne vulgaris
Acne conglobata
Acne fulminans
Infantile acne
Drug-induced acne
Pomade acne
Hormonal acne due to an endocrinopathy
Acne excoriee des jeunes filles*

* See Chapter 21.

AETIOLOGY

Acne develops as a result of increased sebum excretion and altered follicular keratinization, conditions which allow follicular bacteria to flourish.

The primary abnormality in acne vulgaris is increased sebum production. Patients have oily skin and often complain of greasy hair. Sebum secretion is androgen dependent. It may be high at birth, as a result of maternal androgens, but rapidly declines in infancy. It begins to increase again from the age of 6 years onwards, until the sebaceous glands are fully mature in the teenage years. The follicles of the head and chest are colonized by lipophilic bacteria, especially the anaerobic diptheroid, *Propionibacterium acnes*. The levels of this bacteria are higher in acne sufferers, and *P. acnes* is responsible for most of the inflammatory changes in acne. Hereditary factors also play a part and teenagers with severe acne often have a positive family history.

Very occasionally, persistent acne may be a marker for an endocrinopathy such as the adrenogenital syndrome or polycystic ovaries. Certain drugs may induce or exacerbate acne, e.g. systemic steroids and isoniazid. Substances which occlude the follicular orifice (e.g. oily moisturizers and some cosmetics) are said to be comedogenic and will exacerbate acne. Acne confined to the forehead may be entirely due to hair oil running down onto the skin and producing follicular occlusion: *pomade acne*.

CLINICAL FEATURES

Acne has traditionally been considered to be a teenage

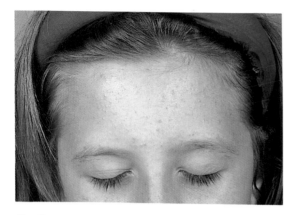

Fig. 18.1 *Acne vulgaris.* Acne is an early physical sign of impending puberty as in this 9-year-old. It usually begins earlier in girls than boys.

disorder, but there is evidence that the trend now is for individuals to develop acne later and for the condition to persist into the third decade. However, over 70% of the population will develop physiological acne during their teenage years. Acne is an early sign of impending puberty, and a significant number of children will develop some degree of acne before the age of 10 years. In 15% of the population the acne is of sufficient severity to warrant medical advice. Acne usually begins earlier in girls (Fig. 18.1), but tends to be more severe in boys. Acne most commonly begins on the face (cheeks, forehead or chin), but frequently also involves the upper back (Fig. 18.2) and chest, especially in boys.

Acne is a polymorphic condition with comedones, papules, pustules (Fig. 18.3), nodules, cysts and

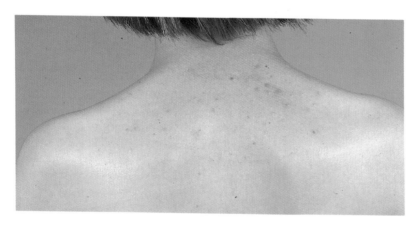

Fig. 18.2 *Acne vulgaris.* The disorder frequently involves the torso in addition to the face.

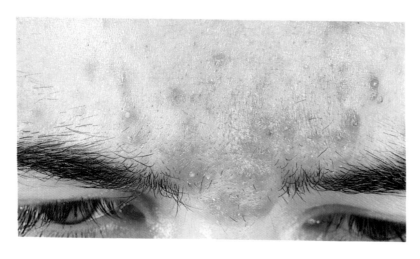

Fig. 18.3 *Acne vulgaris.* Acne is a polymorphic condition of comedones, papules and pustules associated with greasy skin.

scars making up the spectrum of clinical signs in association with greasiness of the skin. The hallmark of acne is the comedone. Closed comedones (whiteheads) are small white papules, composed of keratin cysts containing sebaceous material, which may be confused with milia. If the follicular orifice becomes dilated, the contents are visible as a dark plug (Fig. 18.4), the open comedo (or blackhead). Comedones are often more prominent in boys. Rupture of a closed comedo results in the inflammatory component of acne, the papules, pustules and in more severe cases nodules and cysts (acne conglobata; Fig. 18.5). Large inflammatory nodules and cysts may communicate through deep connecting sinuses (Fig. 18.6). Individual lesions resolve within 2–4 weeks but the overall condition is chronic. The face (Fig. 18.7), chest and back are involved either individually or all together. Scarring may result, which is usually in the form of small pits but may be hypertrophic. In black patients, pigmentation around the scars may be very disfiguring.

COMPLICATIONS

Acne fulminans: A rare systemic reaction to severe nodulocystic acne, with fever, arthralgia and lytic lesions developing within joints. It requires in-patient treatment with oral steroids, in addition to conventional acne treatment to suppress the reaction. The steroids need to be tapered slowly to prevent relapse.

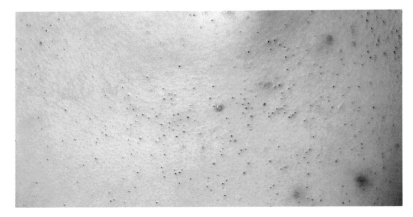

Fig. 18.4 *Acne vulgaris.* Comedones are the hallmark of acne. If the follicular orifice is dilated with a black plug, it is known as an open comedo or blackhead.

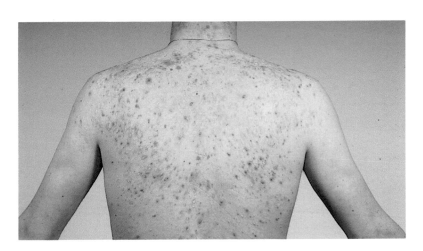

Fig. 18.5 *Acne conglobata.* In more severe cases, nodules, cysts and scarring are added to the physical signs of acne vulgaris. This form of acne requires treatment with isotretinoin.

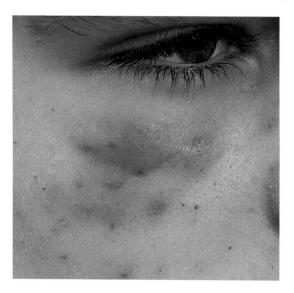

Fig. 18.6 *Acne conglobata.* Large inflammatory nodules and cysts may communicate via deep connecting sinuses.

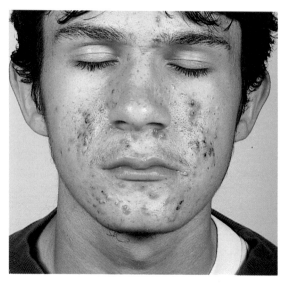

Fig. 18.7 *Acne conglobata.* This is a disastrous condition psychologically, as well as being destructive because of the scarring. This adolescent should be treated with isotretinoin, rather than antibiotics.

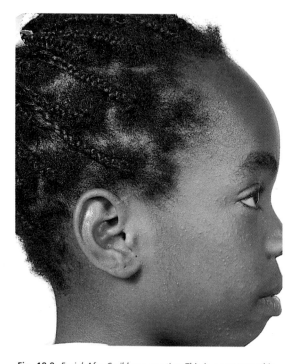

Fig. 18.8 *Facial Afro-Caribbean eruption.* This is a monomorphic papular eruption of unknown cause lasting 1–2 years in young black children.

DIFFERENTIAL DIAGNOSES

1 Facial Afro-Caribbean childhood eruption (FACE) is a distinctive monomorphic papular eruption (Fig. 18.8), most marked around the periorbital region. It is seen in young black children, and tends to begin rather earlier than acne, at around the age of 8 years. There are no pustules, and the condition is self-limiting, resolving spontaneously within 1–2 years without scarring.

2 Perioral (or periorbital) dermatitis: this is a disorder resulting from the inappropriate use of topical glucocorticosteriods on the skin, and may even occur with the weakest, hydrocortisone. Papules and pustules, which are often itchy, occur either around the mouth (Figs 18.9 and 18.10) or eyes. Although they appear to subside when treated with the steroid, they recur a few days later. The process continues inexorably until the steroid is stopped and the acne is treated with oral antibiotics.

3 Comedo naevus: this is a developmental abnormality of the hair follicle. It appears in childhood or adolescence and is permanent. It consists of numerous blackheads, often in a linear distribution (Fig.

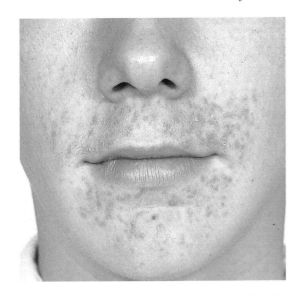

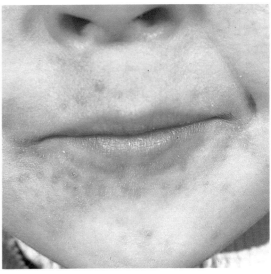

Fig. 18.9 *Perioral dermatitis.* Topical steroids are contraindicated in acne and result in a perioral eruption of scaly red papules which respond to stopping the steroid and instituting oral antibiotics.

Fig. 18.10 *Perioral dermatitis.* If topical steroids are used inappropriately on the face, an acneiform eruption will occur, particularly around the mouth.

18.11). The lesions may become inflamed and resemble acne but are unilateral.

4 Pomade acne: this is acne occuring on the forehead (Fig. 18.12) and is secondary to blockage of the pilosebaceous follicles by grease or oil used on the hair. It is common in Afro-Caribbeans.

MANAGEMENT

The psychological effect of acne on a teenager during a vulnerable period in their social development should not be underestimated and is not necessarily directly related to the severity of their disease. Many patients require considerable reassurance during their therapy, particularly as the treatment takes several months and results may be slow initially.

Topical therapy

This is useful in the treatment of mild to moderate acne, especially if systemic treatment is contraindicated.

1 Benzoyl peroxide is an antibacterial and keratolytic agent most usually used in combination with topical

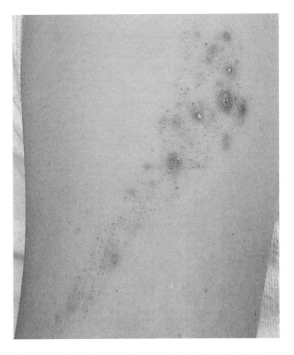

Fig. 18.11 *Comedo naevus.* These are keratin-filled pits that look like blackheads. They may become inflamed and resemble acne, but occur in a linear unilateral distribution.

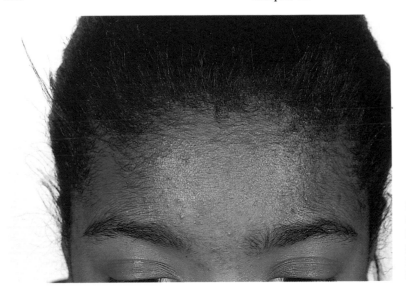

Fig. 18.12 *Pomade acne.* Afro-Caribbeans tend to grease their scalp hair to make it more manageable. If the grease is permitted to cover the forehead, the pilosebaceous orifices become blocked and acne results.

antibiotics. The lotion is applied once or twice daily, but its use may be limited by its irritant properties. Treatment usually begins at a strength of 2.5% and is built up to 10% according to the patient's tolerancce.

2 Retinoic acid reduces the follicular hyperkeratosis, preventing further comedo formation. It is very irritant and produces considerable erythema and scale with initial use. Treatment should begin with the mildest 0.025% preparations and the strength titrated according to the results and side effects.

3 Topical antibiotics: clindamycin, tetracycline and erythromycin lotions are available to treat mild to moderate acne. They should be applied to the whole area, not just the individual spots, are well tolerated and resistance is rare. Preparations of topical erythromycin in combination with zinc are particularly effective. Topical tetracycline may be less cosmetically acceptable because it produces a yellow discoloration on the skin.

Systemic antibiotics

Tetracyclines are the standard oral treatment for acne (usually as oxytetracycline or minocycline), but should not be used in younger patients, because of the risk of staining the teeth. Vibramycin and demeclocycline hydrochloride are also potent photo-sensitizers. Erythromycin or trimethoprim are the preferred alternatives. Antibiotics should always be given for a prolonged period (3–6 months, and sometimes longer) to achieve the best results. It is often useful to combine oral antibiotics with topical therapy.

Anti-androgens

A combination preparation of cyproterone acetate and ethinyloestradiol is a useful alternative in older teenage girls, who want the benefit of an oral contraceptive.

Oral retinoids

Isotretinoin has revolutionized the management of severe acne over the last decade. It is given in a dose of 1 mg/kg/day for 4 months. However, it is expensive and highly teratogenic, so that its use needs to be carefully monitored and restricted to appropriate cases of severe or treatment-resistant acne vulgaris. It is the treatment of choice in nodulocystic acne, but sexually active girls need adequate contraception. The retinoids act by reducing sebum secretion, but have the side effect of producing drying/cracking of the lips and nasal mucosa (with occasional epistaxis) and drying of the cornea.

However, the benefits are so great that most patients tolerate these side effects without difficulty. Muscle pains are not uncommon in adolescents during treatment and vigorous physical exercise should be reduced. The drug can cause premature closure of the epiphyses and therefore should not readily be given to children who are still actively growing.

Infantile acne

DEFINITION

Acneiform papules and pustules occurring on the face in young children.

AETIOLOGY

Transient facial pustules are not uncommon in the immediate neonatal period (Fig. 18.13), due to the increased activity of the sebaceous glands as an effect of maternal androgens. However, acne may persist beyond the neonatal period, or arise *de novo* in a young child, but the mechanisms for this process are not clear. Children who have suffered from infantile acne are more likely to have severe acne during the teenage years. Rarely, acne in infancy may be associated with a virilizing endocrinopathy such as congenital adrenal hyperplasia.

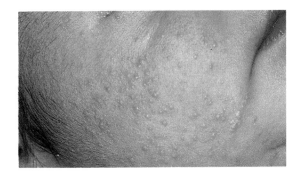

Fig. 18.13 *Sebaceous gland hyperplasia.* Transient facial pustules are common in the neonatal period, secondary to the effect of maternal hormones (courtesy of Dr M. Clement).

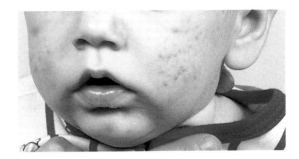

Fig. 18.14 *Infantile acne.* It is more common in boys and is usually confined to the face, particularly the cheeks

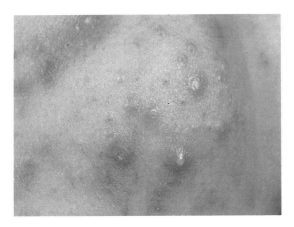

Fig. 18.15 *Infantile acne.* The lesions consist of comedones, papules and pustules as in this close-up picture of the 4-month-old baby in Fig. 18.13.

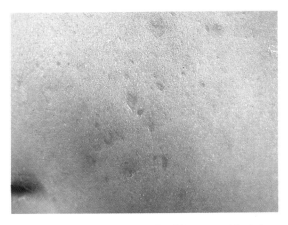

Fig. 18.16 *Infantile acne.* Occasionally, if there are nodular lesions, scarring results as in this child, now aged 4 years, whose lesions are shown in Figs 18.13 and 18.14 in infancy.

CLINICAL FEATURES

Infantile acne is more commonly found in boys. Involvement is usually confined to the face, and often localized to the cheeks alone (Fig. 18.14). The lesions are primarily comedones with small inflammatory papules and pustules (Fig. 18.15). Nodular lesions which cause scarring are rare (Fig. 18.16).

MANAGEMENT

1 Topical antibiotics either alone or in combination with weak keratolytic agents constitute first-line treatment.
2 A prolonged course of oral erythromycin may be required. Tetracyclines are contraindicated.
3 Oral retinoids (0.3–0.6 mg/kg) have been reported to be effective in particularly severe cases, but the theoretical risk of bony complications should limit use to treatment-resistant cases.

Hyperhidrosis

DEFINITION

Excessive sweating, especially of the palms, soles or axillae.

AETIOLOGY

Primary hyperhidrosis may be familial and occur in association with palmoplantar keratoderma or the nail–patella syndrome. Rarely, unilateral hyperhidrosis may be secondary to neurological disease involving the sympathetic pathway. However, the majority of cases of hyperhidrosis are idiopathic.

CLINICAL FEATURES

Excessive sweating usually begins in later childhood around puberty and may persist into adult life. It may be continuous or phasic. The axillae, palms (Fig. 18.17) and soles may be involved together or in isolation. The affected area is clinically moist and cold to the touch. In severe cases, sweat may be seen to drip from the palms. The disorder is not only of cosmetic embarrassment to the sufferer, but may also interfere with schoolwork and their later professional life.

DIFFERENTIAL DIAGNOSIS

Endocrine diseases: Thyrotoxicosis should be excluded, though it is usually associated with warm, moist hands rather than cool peripheries as in hyperhidrosis.

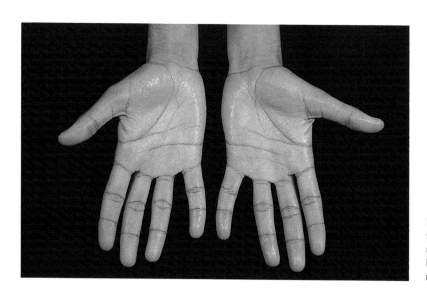

Fig. 18.17 *Hyperhidrosis.* Excess sweating of the palms interferes with manual dexterity. Iontophoresis or laparoscopic sympathectomy may be necessary.

MANAGEMENT

1 Proprietary antiperspirants are of little use, but 20% aluminium chloride hexahydrate solution may be effective.

2 Iontophoresis is the introduction of an ionized substance into the skin by the passage of a direct current. It may be carried out with either tap water or anticholinergic agents. The latter, however, produce anticholinergic side effects. It can be very helpful, but needs to be repeated every few weeks, although remissions do occur.

3 In cases of localized axillary hyperhidrosis, surgical excision of the skin of the axillary vault is effective, provided it is practical.

4 Laparoscopic sympathectomy via the axilla provides a simple permanent surgical cure for palmar sweating, but is only available in a few referral centres. Although the operation has a high success rate, it may be complicated by compensatory sweating of the trunk and lower limbs.

Hidradenitis suppurativa

DEFINITION

A chronic, deep inflammatory process affecting the apocrine sweat glands, resulting in suppuration, sinus formation and severe fibrotic scarring.

AETIOLOGY

The exact aetiology is unknown. However, it is more common in females and hormonal factors appear to be important, especially relatively low oestrogen states. The condition is exacerbated by the presence of progesterones. Most cases develop in isolation, but the condition may occur in association with acne conglobata and dissecting cellulitis of the scalp (the *follicular occlusion triad*). It is sometimes familial.

CLINICAL FEATURES

The condition usually begins in postpubertal teenagers, but tends to persist into adulthood. Multiple, erythematous papules develop, which discharge

purulent material and heal with cord-like fibrotic scarring. It affects the axillae (Fig. 18.18) and groin and occasionally lesions develop around the areola in females. The condition usually follows a chronic course and can be very debilitating and embarrassing for the patient.

MANAGEMENT

1 Long-term antibiotic therapy with erythromycin may limit the extent of the disease, but is rarely curative.

2 Hormonal therapy with a combined contraceptive pill incorporating an oestrogen and cyproterone acetate has been reported to be helpful.

3 Limited disease, particularly in the axilla, may be successfully treated by surgical excision of the involved area with grafting if necessary.

4 Some patients have responded to treatment with oral retinoids.

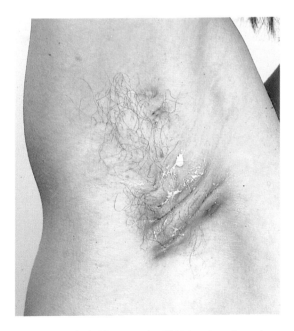

Fig. 18.18 *Hidradenitis suppurativa.* Multiple red papules and nodules develop which discharge purulent material and result in scarring. The axillae and groin are predominantly affected.

Steatocystoma multiplex

DEFINITION

Multiple, small, firm, white cysts containing sebum, most common on the anterior chest wall.

AETIOLOGY

The condition is inherited as an autosomal-dominant trait. However, cysts rarely appear before adolescence.

CLINICAL FEATURES

Small, firm, domed cysts of a whitish-yellow colour (Fig. 18.19) develop within the dermis from the time of puberty. There is no visible punctum (Fig. 18.20). The cysts are most numerous over the sternum (Fig. 18.19), but may also occur on the back and upper limbs. Individual lesions frequently become inflamed by secondary infection and may rupture.

DIFFERENTIAL DIAGNOSES

1 Syringomata: these lesions are derived from sweat rather than sebaceous glands. They are smaller, more uniform in size and flesh-coloured, rather than waxy-white.
2 Epidermoid cysts: these are rarely so numerous and they tend to be larger and have a distinct punctum.

MANAGEMENT

1 Surgical excision of so many lesions is usually impractical.
2 The contents of the cysts may be successfully expressed through a small incision with good cosmetic results.

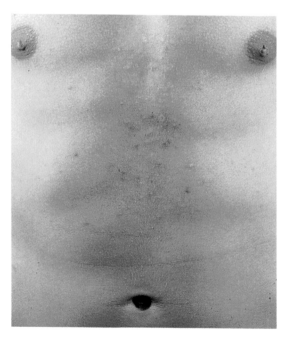

Fig. 18.19 *Steatocystoma multiplex.* This disorder is inherited as an autosomal dominant and is composed of sebaceous cysts. It presents in adolescence as the sebaceous glands mature under the influence of androgens.

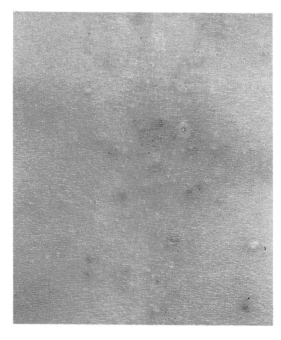

Fig. 18.20 *Steatocystoma multiplex.* This close-up view of the teenager's chest in Fig. 18.19 shows multiple flesh-coloured smooth-surfaced cysts.

Fordyce spots

DEFINITION

A prominence of the sebaceous glands in the oral cavity, which is a variant of normal.

AETIOLOGY

The lesions are made up of normal sebaceous glands, but unlike those of the skin, they occur in isolation and are not associated with hair follicles.

CLINICAL FEATURES

Multiple, small, discrete, yellow papules occur on the buccal mucosa, lips (Fig. 18.21) and elsewhere in the mouth. They are common, and become more prominent after puberty. Their presence sometimes gives rise to anxiety, but they are entirely benign.

MANAGEMENT

Reassurance is all that is required.

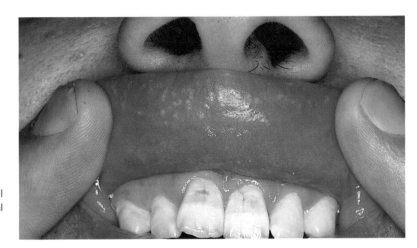

Fig. 18.21 *Fordyce spots.* These small yellow papules on the lips are a normal variant and represent sebaceous glands.

Chapter 19
Orogenital Disease

Introduction

Many of the disorders which affect mucous membranes in children are part of a more generalized disease process, such as lichen planus (see Fig. 6.18) and Stevens–Johnson syndrome (see Fig. 15.11), which are discussed elsewhere. The more specific disorders are dealt with here.

Lichen sclerosus et atrophicus

DEFINITION

A pruritic condition characterized by atrophic white patches, most commonly in the genital area.

AETIOLOGY

The cause of the condition is unknown. It may occur in conjunction with morphoea (see p. 250) and has therefore been classified as a connective tissue disease but there is some evidence that genetic, endocrine and auto-immune factors may each play a part in the pathogenesis. Immunoglobulin and complement deposition may be demonstrated along the dermo-epidermal junction in lesional skin. Trauma (e.g. from elastic in underwear) may exacerbate the condition as an isomorphic (Koebner) phenomenon.

CLINICAL FEATURES

Although the condition is most common in adults, it

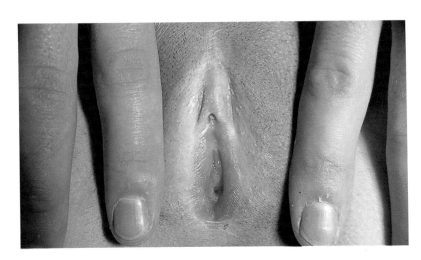

Fig. 19.1 *Lichen sclerosus et atrophicus.* Well-circumscribed, white sclerotic plaques occur around the vulva. The skin may become atropic and minor haemorrhages result.

is well recognized in children, but may be under-reported. The onset in childhood is most often between the ages of 2 and 5 years and it appears to be much more common in girls. Well-circumscribed, white sclerotic (Fig. 19.1) and subsequently atrophic plaques develop at affected sites. The epidermal surface is puckered and easily wrinkled. Erosions, purpura and haemorrhagic blisters may complicate more severe disease.

In boys, lichen sclerosus may cause a scarring phimosis and is responsible for a significant number of elective (non-ritual) prepubertal circumcisions. In girls, the condition usually begins around the vulva, but may extend to involve the perianal region in a figure-of-eight pattern (Fig. 19.2). Pruritus and dis-comfort are the main symptoms. The condition may be associated with significant dysuria or pain on defaecation leading to enuresis and constipation, respectively. As a result the child may present to other medical disciplines less familiar with lichen sclerosus than dermatologists, with consequent diag-nostic delay. Ignorance of the condition has resulted in some cases being misdiagnosed as sexual abuse.

Extragenital disease, involving sites such as the wrists and shoulders, has similar physical signs and occurs in about 20% of girls, but is not reported in boys.

MANAGEMENT

1 Reassurance that the condition is benign and not related to any form of abuse is essential.
2 The condition tends to be chronic, but childhood cases have a better prognosis than adults with the disease. There is a tendency for spontaneous impro-vement and 50% of cases remit at puberty. Extra-genital disease appears to carry the best prognosis.
3 Bland emollients provide some symptomatic relief.
4 In severe cases, short courses of potent topical steroids (e.g. 0.05% clobetasol propionate ointment) once daily is the best treatment.
5 Topical 1% progesterone applied twice daily for 3 months is suggested to be effective in the treatment of girls.
6 Laxatives to soften the stool are required in cases associated with pain on defaecation and constipation.

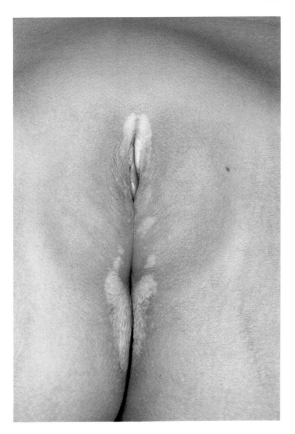

Fig. 19.2 *Lichen sclerosus et atrophicus.* The sclerotic change often extends to form a figure-of-eight pattern around the vulva and anus. Potent topical steroids reduce pruritus and discomfort.

Aphthous ulceration

DEFINITION

A common disorder of recurrent, localized, short-lived and painful ulceration in the mouth.

AETIOLOGY

The cause of the problem is unknown but genetic, immunological and infective factors have been implicated.

CLINICAL FEATURES

The disorder is especially common between the ages

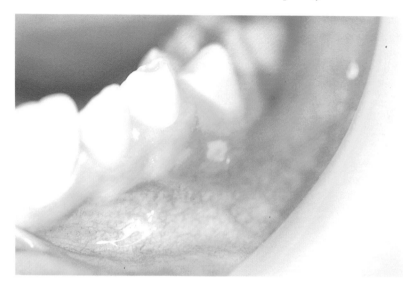

Fig. 19.3 *Aphthous ulcer.* Minor aphthae are small, irregular-shaped ulcers which are painful, but heal within a week (courtesy of Miss K. Barnard).

of 5 and 10 years, particularly in girls. The lesions may be classified as minor or major aphthae depending on size, depth and hence severity. Minor aphthae (Fig. 19.3) are small, irregular, shallow ulcers with a grey-white slough at the base occurring on the oral mucosa and tongue, which heal without scarring. The ulcer may be preceded by a burning sensation and is often very tender. Lesions are usually single, lasting between 7 and 10 days, but they may recur anywhere within the mouth. In contrast, major

aphthae (Sutton's ulcers) are rare, larger, more severe and may heal with scarring. The genitalia may be involved in these patients and in females a premenstrual flare may occur. Attacks may be virtually continuous and present a difficult therapeutic challenge.

DIFFERENTIAL DIAGNOSES (see Table 19.1)

1 Herpes simplex infection: primary attacks often involve the mouth (herpes stomatitis). Recurrent episodes usually affect the lips (Fig. 19.4) and tend to recur at the same site. Clusters of vesicles are the hallmark of the condition. Swabs for viral culture will confirm the correct diagnosis.
2 Hand, foot and mouth disease (see p. 95): the presence of vesicles at acral sites (Fig. 19.5) helps to distinguish this infective disorder.
3 Herpangina: this may be caused by a variety of different group A Coxsackie viruses. Early white papulovesicular lesions develop on the soft palate and fauces, which progress to ulceration.
4 Crohn's disease: oral ulceration may occur in patients with inflammatory bowel disease. Thickening of the mucosae produces a folded or 'cobblestone' appearance and the lips may be swollen and split (Fig. 19.6) due to chronic granulomatous inflammation.

Table 19.1 Classification of mouth ulcers

Infective	Herpes simplex
	Herpangina
	Hand, foot and mouth disease
Immunological	Stevens–Johnson syndrome
	Chronic bullous disease of childhood
	Pemphigus
Systemic	Behçet's disease
	Crohn's disease
Drug-induced	Chemotherapy
	Fixed drug eruption
Idiopathic	Aphthous ulcers
	minor
	major

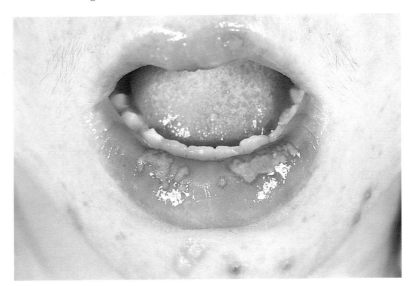

Fig. 19.4 *Herpes simplex.* The initial lesions are vesicular and erosion and ulceration follow subsequently. Primary attacks often involve the mouth.

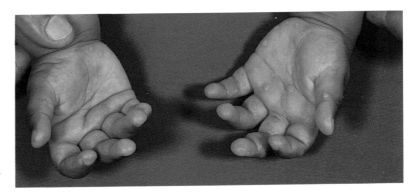

Fig. 19.5 *Hand, foot and mouth disease.* The presence of vesicles at acral sites such as the palms and soles help to make the diagnosis.

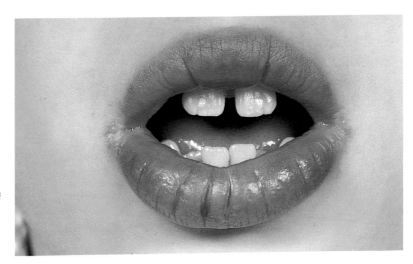

Fig. 19.6 *Crohn's disease.* There may be swelling, thickening and splitting of the lips. Biopsy shows non-caseating granulomas but investigation of the gastrointestinal tract is necessary to establish the diagnosis.

5 Stevens–Johnson syndrome: crusted labial erosions and oral ulceration are associated with erythema multiforme (see p. 98).

6 Behçets disease: this is a multisystem disorder in which recurrent aphthous (Fig. 19.7) and genital ulceration occur in association with pathergy and ophthalmic, articular and neurological involvement. It is rare before the age of 20 years, but cases in the young are reported and may be under-recognized.

The primary presenting feature in paediatric cases is recurrent aphthous-type ulceration which may precede other evidence of systemic disease by many years.

7 Leucopenia: patients who become neutropenic on chemotherapy regimes frequently develop painful mouth ulcers.

8 Fixed drug eruption: red oedematous swellings occur in the same sites each time the drug (usually

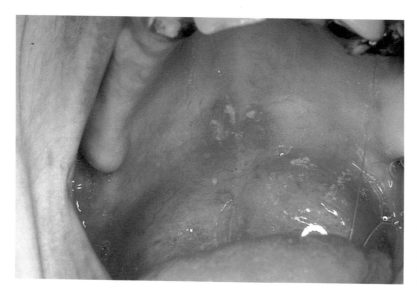

Fig. 19.7 *Behçet's disease.* This is very rare before the third decade but recurrent aphthous ulceration is the initial presentation in most patients, followed by painful genital ulcers.

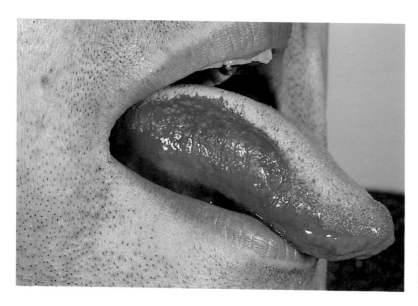

Fig. 19.8 *Fixed drug eruption.* This 18-year-old had taken a sulphonamide and developed ulceration on his tongue and penis (Fig. 19.9) and a red swelling on the back of his hand.

phenolphthalein, a sulphonamide or a tetracycline) is ingested. When the mucosae are affected, ulceration may occur in the mouth (Fig. 19.8) or on the genitalia (Fig. 19.9). It is rare in childhood, but may occur in adolescence.

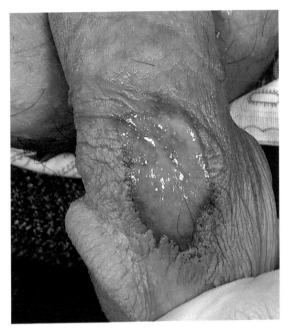

Fig. 19.9 *Fixed drug eruption.* The condition recurs in the same site each time the allergen is ingested.

MANAGEMENT

1 Minor aphthae are treated with simple antiseptic mouth washes. If pain is a problem, local topical steroids (e.g. hydrocortisone pellets or triamcinolone in orabase) may be helpful.

2 Major aphthae are much more resistant to treatment. Oral steroids, levamisole and thalidomide have all been used with some success, but such therapy should be carefully monitored because of possible side effects.

Granulomatous cheilitis (Miescher's cheilitis)

DEFINITION

A chronic swelling due to granulomatous inflammation of the lip.

AETIOLOGY

The cause of the condition is unknown but a small percentage may be associated with inflammatory bowel disease. There is no evidence to implicate an infective agent in the aetiology, but genetic factors may be important. Histology reveals granulomatous inflammation within the dermis.

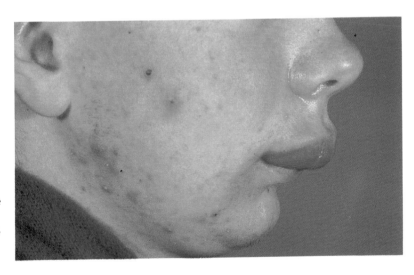

Fig. 19.10 *Granulomatous cheilitis.* The swelling is sudden in onset, diffuse and most commonly affects the upper lip. If there is concomitant facial palsy, it is known as the Melkersson–Rosenthal syndrome.

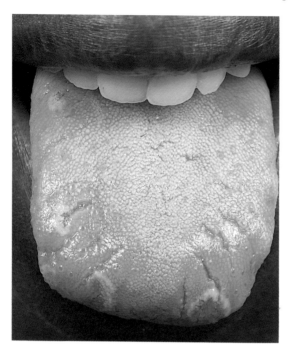

Fig. 19.11 *Scrotal tongue.* A scrotal or fissured tongue may occur on its own and is of no clinical significance, but may also be associated with the Melkersson–Rosenthal syndrome. The configuration of the lesions constantly changes.

CLINICAL FEATURES

The condition usually begins in later childhood or adolescence. The swelling is acute and most frequently involves the upper lip (Fig. 19.10), the lower lip, or even the cheeks which may become grossly enlarged. The lip feels firm and deep fissures may develop within the vermillion border. An associated fissuring of the tongue (scrotal tongue) occurs in 20% of patients (Fig. 19.11).

DIFFERENTIAL DIAGNOSES

1 Melkersson–Rosenthal syndrome: granulomatous cheilitis and scrotal tongue occur in association with facial palsy.
2 Angioedema: type I hypersensitivity reactions are acute and may be associated with periorbital oedema. Pruritus is prominent but the attacks are of short duration.
3 Sarcoid: although the histology reveals granulomas, discrete papules and nodules are usually apparent on the lips clinically and there is often systemic evidence of sarcoid.
4 Exfoliative cheilitis (factitial cheilitis): the ver-

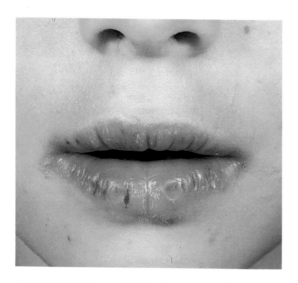

Fig. 19.12 *Exfoliative cheilitis.* The lips are persistently scaly and cracked due to chronic biting of the lips and occurs in the emotionally labile. It eventually recovers.

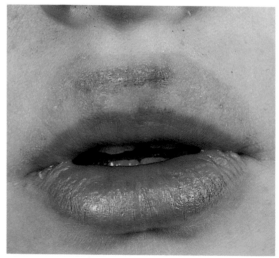

Fig. 19.13 *Lip-licking.* This is a habit tic due to constant licking of the lips and occurs around the lips. The condition is resistant to therapy, but ultimately disappears.

million borders of the lips are persistently scaly (Fig. 19.12). It starts in the centre of the lower lip and spreads to both lips and is probably due to interference. It may spread around the lips (Fig. 19.13) due to lip-licking and be quite persistent but it eventually disappears. Many of the patients have emotional problems.

5 Contact dermatitis, e.g. to flavourings or tooth paste.

MANAGEMENT

1 Surgical reduction is rather unsatisfactory.

2 Local infiltration with triamcinolone under local anaesthetic cover may be effective in reducing the swelling.

3 Oral clofazimine may also be helpful.

Chapter 20
The Skin in Systemic Disease

Introduction

The skin may be involved in a variety of multisystem diseases. The cutaneous signs are important as they are readily visible and may point to the correct diagnosis at an early stage. In addition, generalized pruritus in the absence of any cutaneous signs other than excoriation (Figs 20.1 and 20.2) may be the presenting feature of a spectrum of internal diseases (Table 20.1).

Table 20.1 Systemic causes of generalized pruritus

Metabolic	Hepatic dysfunction
	Obstructive jaundice
	Renal failure
Endocrine	Thyroid disease
Haematological	Iron-deficiency anaemia
	Myeloproliferative disorders
	Lymphoma
Psychological	Psychogenic pruritus

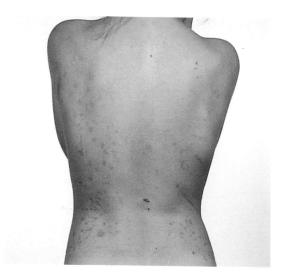

Fig. 20.1 *Generalized pruritus.* This girl had generalized itching and excoriations secondary to the Crigler–Najjar syndrome of unconjungated hyperbilirubinaemia.

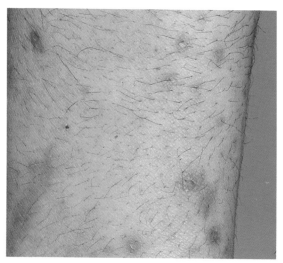

Fig. 20.2 *Generalized pruritus.* Linear and punctate areas of excoriation and hyperpigmentation secondary to scratching are evident in this teenager with iron-deficiency anaemia.

Nutritional and metabolic disorders

Acrodermatitis enteropathica

DEFINITION

An erosive dermatitis of the perioral and genital area occurring in infancy as a result of zinc deficiency.

AETIOLOGY

The condition is a manifestation of zinc deficiency. The majority of cases occur in infants who either have hereditary zinc deficiency or who are receiving milk from zinc-deficient mothers. The condition is most accentuated in premature babies. However, breast milk is a better source of zinc than cow's milk, so that some cases develop at the time of weaning. Rarely, the disease is acquired later in life as a result of malabsorption syndromes, dietary insufficiency or malignancy.

CLINICAL FEATURES

The disease is most prevalent in infants and usually becomes manifest shortly after birth. An erosive dermatitis develops around the mouth and anus (Fig. 20.3) and on the acral regions of the hands

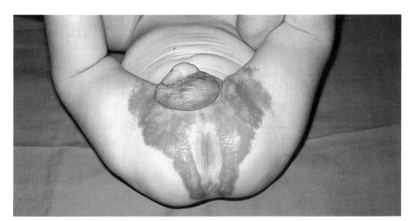

Fig. 20.3 *Acrodermatitis enteropathica.* An erythematous, glazed, somewhat eroded eruption occurs around orifical openings such as the anus, usually in association with diarrhoea and failure to thrive (courtesy of Dr M. Clement).

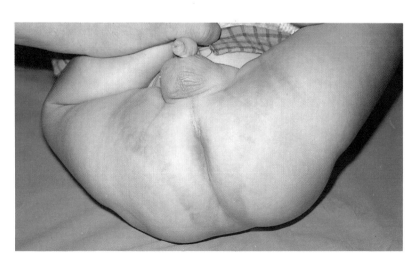

Fig. 20.4 *Acodermatitis enteropathica.* The condition responds dramatically to treatment with zinc (courtesy of Dr M. Clement).

and feet. The skin of the affected areas is red, glazed and may be vesicular. A florid paronychia may be present. Secondary infection with *Candida* is common. Diarrhoea is a frequent but not consistent finding, but is usually preceded by the cutaneous signs. The child may exhibit failure to thrive, and in untreated cases, progressive alopecia and photophobia develop.

MANAGEMENT

1 The clinical picture is usually highly suggestive of zinc deficiency.
2 The diagnosis is confirmed by detection of low serum zinc levels.
3 Dietary zinc supplements produce rapid resolution of the disease (Fig. 20.4).

Xanthomatosis

DEFINITION

A disorder of lipid metabolism resulting in its deposition in the skin.

AETIOLOGY

In childhood and adolescence, the most common causes are either hyperlipoproteinaemia or secondary to biliary obstruction, especially primary biliary hypoplasia (Alagille's syndrome).

CLINICAL FEATURES

Lipid may be deposited as yellow material around the eyes (xanthelasma), in the palmar creases, as nodules (often eruptive) on the trunk, elbows and knees (Fig. 20.5) and in the tendons. Tendon xanthomas may occasionally be seen in adolescents with familial hypercholesterolaemia, but the other types of deposits are not seen although they may occur in adult life.

MANAGEMENT

The cause must be established and the underlying disorder treated.

Collagen vascular disorders

Lupus erythematosus (LE) in childhood

Lupus erythematosus in the young may be classified according to the age of onset of the disease as either neonatal LE, in which the primary pathology is maternal, or childhood LE, which may take any

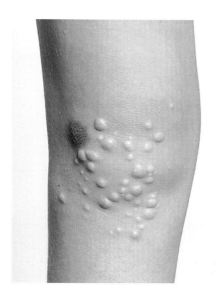
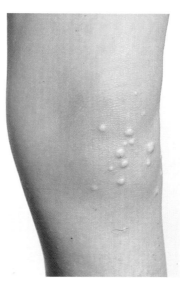

Fig. 20.5 *Xanthomatosis.* Yellow nodules and papules are present on the knees of this child with primary biliary hypoplasia. They disappeared after liver transplantation.

of the forms recognized in adult disease, namely systemic, discoid and subacute LE or lupus profundus.

Neonatal lupus erythematosus

DEFINITION

A rare syndrome in which transient cutaneous lesions and sometimes heart block occur in babies born to mothers with circulating LE antibodies.

AETIOLOGY

The condition develops because of the transplacental transfer of maternal antibodies, particularly Ro (or occasionally La).

CLINICAL FEATURES

Annular erythematous lesions with central atrophy and fine scaling are seen most notably on the forehead, cheeks and around the eyes (Fig. 20.6). They may develop anytime during the first 2 months of life, but are normally present at birth in affected infants. Hypopigmentation is common. Congenital heart block is a serious associated finding, but its incidence varies in different racial groups, being relatively rare in the Japanese compared with Europeans. Some babies may also develop a mild anaemia, hepatosplenomegaly or lymphadenopathy. The diagnosis is confirmed by the presence of the appropriate serum antibodies in the mother and child.

MANAGEMENT

1 The most important aspect of management is to exclude a cardiac conduction defect. A pacemaker may be necessary for neonates with congenital heart block.
2 No specific treatment is required for the cutaneous lesions, but the parents should be advised about sun protection.
3 It is important that parents are advised that neonatal cardiac problems may complicate subsequent pregnancies.

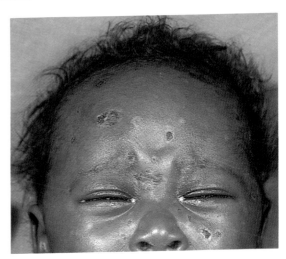

Fig. 20.6 *Neonatal lupus erythematosus.* Annular erythematosus lesions with central atrophy on the forehead and cheeks develop as a result of transplacental transfer of maternal antibodies, particularly Ro and La.

Systemic lupus erythematosus (SLE)

DEFINITION

An auto-immune multisystem connective tissue disorder involving the skin, joints and renal system.

AETIOLOGY

Systemic lupus erythematosus is an auto-immune disorder, the hallmark of which is the presence of circulating antibodies to antinuclear factor and double-stranded DNA. Genetic and hormonal factors are important in the development of the disease, which is much more common in females. Rarely, it may be associated with complement deficiency (especially C2 and C4). Occasionally, SLE may be drug-induced (e.g. by isoniazid or anticonvulsant therapy).

CLINICAL FEATURES

SLE is primarily a female disease and is rare before puberty. However, 90% of children who develop LE 90% have cutaneous involvement and the

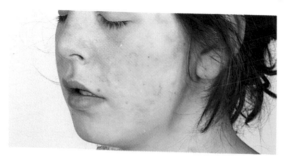

Fig. 20.7 *Systemic lupus erythematosus.* A patchy, maculopapular, mauve erythema occurs on the cheeks.

skin signs are the usual presenting feature of the syndrome.

Classically, SLE is associated with a maculo-papular erythema (Fig. 20.7) or discoid plaques (Fig. 20.8) in a photosensitive distribution (Fig. 20.9). When both cheeks and the nose are affected the distribution is said to be butterfly-like in appearance. Other features include a prominent livedo reticularis, oral ulceration, periungual telangiectasia, Raynaud's phenomenon and digital infarcts (Fig. 20.10). Histologically in the skin, there is hyper-keratosis with follicular plugging and a peri-appendageal lymphocytic infiltrate resulting in liquefaction degeneration of the basal layer of the epidermis and subsequent atrophy. There may be granular deposits of IgG at the dermo-epidermal junction on direct immunofluorescence.

SLE is a multisystem disorder in which joint

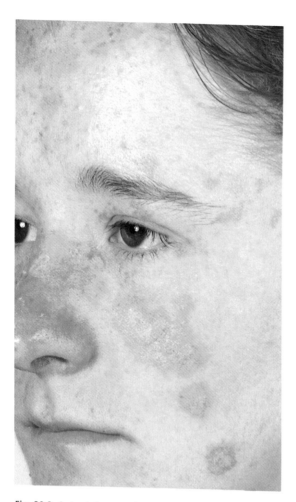

Fig. 20.8 *Systemic lupus erythematosus.* Well-defined, red scaly discoid plaques occur over the nose and cheeks.

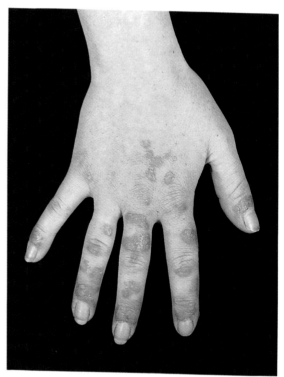

Fig. 20.9 *Systemic lupus erythematosus.* Similar lesions occur on other light-exposed areas such as the backs of the hands in the same teenager as in Fig. 20.8.

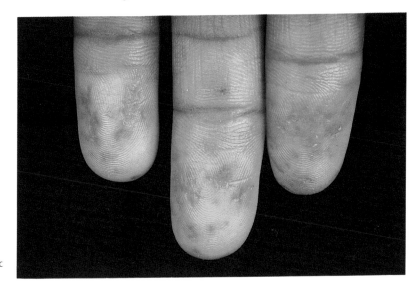

Fig. 20.10 *Systemic lupus erythematosus.* Mauve, chilblain-like, uncomfortable lesions develop on the finger tips in both discoid and systemic lupus erythematosus.

involvement is common. It may affect the heart, lungs and central nervous system, but it is the renal involvement which is life-threatening. Over 50% of children with SLE will develop renal disease.

Rarely, LE may affect the skin in other ways (see below). While these may be quite common in adult disease, they are more unusual in children.

Other variants of lupus erythematosus

1 Discoid LE: annular or discoid erythematosus plaques (Fig. 20.11) with prominent scaling, follicular plugging and sometimes hyperpigmented margins especially on the face (Fig. 20.12) and scalp. These heal with scarring and atrophy. In adults,

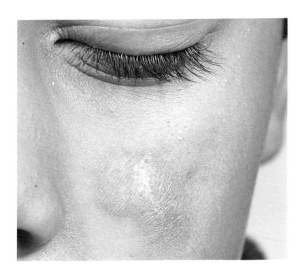

Fig. 20.11 *Discoid lupus erythematosus.* A well-defined, discoid, red plaque is present on the cheek with a tenacious scale.

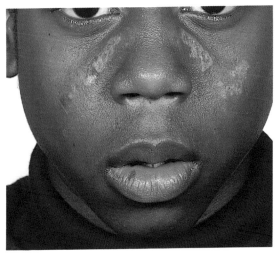

Fig. 20.12 *Discoid lupus erythematosus.* In older lesions the margin may be hyperpigmented, especially in Afro-Caribbeans, and the central area is atrophic and scarred.

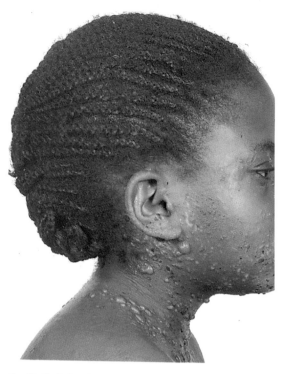

such lesions are normally associated with disease limited to the skin with no internal involvement. However, isolated cutaneous LE is rare in younger patients, and discoid lesions are usually a manifestation of systemic disease.

2 Subacute LE: this has only occasionally been reported in the teenage years, but is not dissimilar to the eruptions described in neonatal LE. Extensive, urticated maculopapular erythematous lesions are associated with marked photosensitivity and arthralgia. Renal involvement is less common and a high percentage of patients have positive anti-Ro/La antibodies.

3 Bullous LE: this photosensitive eruption may present as a widespread bullous dermatosis (Figs 20.13 and 20.14). It is extremely rare and may initially be confused with childhood pemphigoid. Skin biopsy, immunofluorescence and auto-antibody profiles reveal the true diagnosis, which is usually relentless in its progression.

4 Lupus profundus: a deep, panlobar panniculitis may occur in SLE, usually in association with arthralgia and fever. Firmly indurated, deep inflammatory nodules develop on the face, upper limbs and buttocks, which are very slow to resolve. They eventually heal to leave disfiguring atrophy at the sites of involvement.

Fig. 20.13 *Bullous lupus erythematosus.* Blistering is rare in lupus but occurs in a photosensitive distribution. This girl had systemic disease with renal involvement.

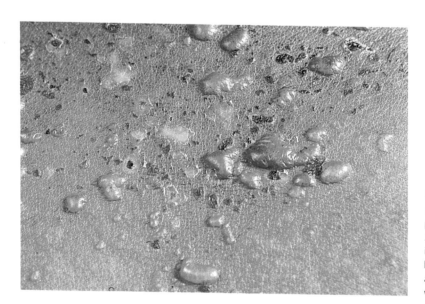

Fig. 20.14 *Bullous lupus erythematosus.* Tense blisters were present on the child shown in Fig. 20.13. Skin biopsy and immunofluorescence distinguish the blisters from childhood pemphigoid, and in this case the antinuclear factor was strongly positive.

MANAGEMENT

1 The diagnosis should be confirmed by means of auto-antibodies and skin biopsy for histology and immunofluorescence.

2 Each patient requires careful assessment of the extent of systemic involvement, especially renal function.

3 Local cutaneous disease can be treated with potent topical steroids. However, the response to systemic steroids in more severe disease is often very disappointing. Extensive, disfiguring cutaneous disease may require treatment with antimalarials, but these agents are very toxic in young children and the dose should not exceed 4 mg/kg/day.

4 Sun protection advice is imperative.

Juvenile dermatomyositis

DEFINITION

An auto-immune disorder with severe inflammatory changes in skin, blood vessels and muscles.

AETIOLOGY

The precise aetiology of this connective tissue disease remains unknown, but it is thought to be auto-immune in origin and mediated through immune complexes. A significant percentage of adult disease is associated with malignancy, but there are only sporadic reports of such associations in juvenile disease. Circulating auto-antibodies demonstrated in juvenile dermatomyositis include anti-Jo-1, which is linked to the HLA-DR3 phenotype. There is also a higher incidence of HLA-B8 in childhood dermatomyositis. There is some evidence for a viral aetiology, especially Coxsackie B infections, with an increased incidence in the spring.

CLINICAL FEATURES

Childhood dermatomyositis occurs in all racial groups, is more prevalent in girls, and is more severe than the adult disease. Juvenile dermatomyositis begins before the age of 10 years in the majority of cases. The cutaneous signs usually precede or coincide with the onset of muscular disease. Violaceous macules and papules develop over bony prominences, especially the knuckles (Gottron's papules). A macular, violaceous erythema (heliotrope in colour), which may be accompanied by oedema, develops in the periorbital region, especially over the upper eyelids (Fig. 20.15). Some patients

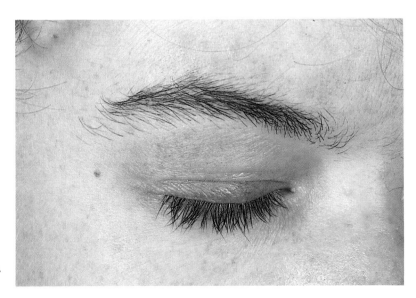

Fig. 20.15 *Juvenile dermatomyositis.* A mauve colour around the eyes, sometimes associated with swelling, is very characteristic.

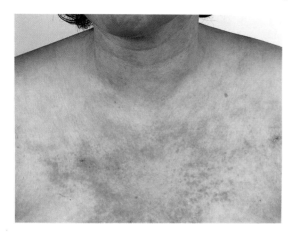

Fig. 20.16 *Juvenile dermatomyositis.* A mauve blotchy erythema may also occur in a photosensitive distribution on the front of the chest as in this 16-year-old.

develop a more widespread blotchy erythema in a photosensitive distribution (Fig. 20.16). The nail fold capillaries are dilated, producing a blush at the proximal border of the nail, and there may be splinter haemorrhages from thromboses within these vessels. The cuticle often appears ragged. Rarely panniculitis and cutaneous ulceration may occur.

The inflammatory myopathy is the most disabling feature of the syndrome, primarily affecting the proximal muscles and producing difficulty in such movements as climbing stairs, rising from a chair or brushing the hair. In young children, it is often the parents who first notice their decreased mobility. There may be some degree of myalgia, but the weakness is constant and progressive. Subcutaneous calcification, which may be very extensive, develops in over half of childhood cases. Other features which may occur include a florid vasculitis, myocarditis and progressive dyspnoea secondary to pulmonary fibrosis.

DIFFERENTIAL DIAGNOSES

1 SLE: this may be very similar in cases where the cutaneous signs predominate.
2 Infectious myositis (e.g. poliomyositis): pain is a more prominent feature of the muscle weakness and skin changes are absent.

MANAGEMENT

1 The diagnosis is made on the basis of a raised serum creatine phosphokinase (CPK), abnormal electromyogram (EMG) and muscle biopsy, together with the auto-antibody profile. The cutaneous histology is often non-specific.
2 Each individual should be assessed for cardiac and pulmonary disease with electrocardiogram (ECG), chest X-ray and pulmonary function tests.
3 Prednisolone 1 mg/kg/day is the primary treatment, and should be tapered slowly according to the clinical response. Monitoring the CPK is most useful in this respect, and low-dose maintenance steroids may be required for a considerable time.
4 Bed rest is essential in the acute phase, but physiotherapy is important in preventing contractures.

Morphoea

DEFINITION

A localized sclerotic change in the skin, producing thickened white plaques.

AETIOLOGY

Morphoea is thought to represent a localized form of systemic sclerosis and to share a similar immunological basis. There is a higher incidence of auto-immune disease in the families of patients with morphoea. Infections have been implicated in the aetiology, especially measles and Lyme disease, but the current evidence is inconclusive. Some lesions have been reported to follow bacille Calmette–Guérin (BCG) vaccination.

CLINICAL FEATURES

Morphoea is more common in adults, but linear morphoea (Fig. 20.17) occurs more often in childhood. The lesions develop spontaneously and consist of thickened, ivory-coloured plaques (Fig. 20.18) which may develop anywhere on the skin. Active lesions frequently have a mauve border which later fades to brown. The surface of the skin is usually smooth, but may appear atrophic, and lichen sclero-

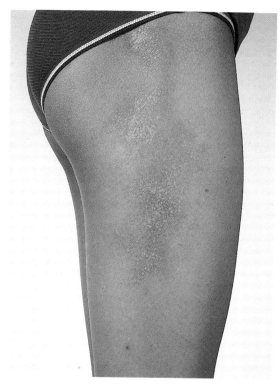

Fig. 20.17 *Linear morphoea.* White sclerotic plaques are surrounded by a hyperpigmented border. A linear appearance is more common in children.

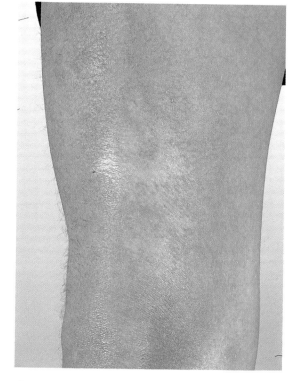

Fig. 20.18 *Morphoea.* This is a localized form of scleroderma. The sclerotic plaques are shiny, tethered and have a mauve outline.

sus et atrophicus (Fig. 20.19) and morphoea may coexist. The skin appendages are destroyed in morphoea, so that hairs are usually absent and sweating ceases.

Histologically, there may be a mild non-specific lymphocytic infiltrate in the early lesions. Established lesions show an atrophic epidermis with an expanded featureless dermis, in which the collagen appears eosinophilic and homogenous.

Morphoea may also occur in a linear manner with marked contraction/scarring of the subcutaneous tissues. It most frequently involves the lower limbs, but may also occur on the forehead and be associated with facial hemiatrophy (en coup de sabre).

MANAGEMENT

1 Most cases of morphoea are self-limiting and require no specific treatment.

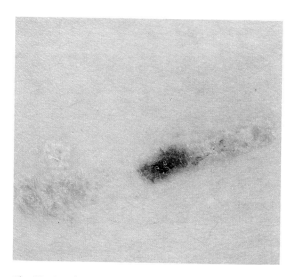

Fig. 20.19 *Lichen sclerosus et atrophicus.* The plaques are made up of white sclerotic papules which become atrophic and often, as shown here, haemorrhagic (see also Chapter 19).

2 If there is significant atrophy of the deep tissues, which might lead to developmental complications (e.g. of a limb), therapy with either prednisolone or penicillamine may be justified, but needs to be carefully monitored.

Haematological disorders

Langerhans cell histiocytosis (LCH) (histiocytosis-X, Letterer–Siwe disease)

DEFINITION

A rare multisystem reactive proliferation of histiocytes which accumulate in various organs.

AETIOLOGY

The cause of LCH is unknown, but the proliferative process is now considered to be reactive rather than malignant. The lesional cell has now been identified as the Langerhans cell, supporting the hypothesis of an immunological aetiology in the disorder. Rod-shaped structures within the Langerhans cell (Birbeck granules) are detected on electron microscopy and are pathognomonic of the disorder. It has been suggested that these represent viral inclusion bodies and most recent attention has focused on the possible implications of human herpes virus type 6, which causes roseola.

CLINICAL FEATURES

Historically, the term histiocytosis-X covered a broad spectrum of diseases which were given a variety of eponymous names depending on the main organ involved (e.g. Letterer–Siwe disease, Hand–Schüller–Christian syndrome and eosinophilic granuloma). The skin may be affected alone or as part of a more severe multisystem disease, usually affecting bone, liver and the reticulo-endothelial system.

Cutaneous involvement most frequently occurs on the scalp, with small crusted, greasy scales (Fig. 20.20) arising on an erythematous base, which may be mistaken for seborrhoeic dermatitis (Fig. 20.21). However, the lesions become quite haemorrhagic and ooze especially when they involve the external ear. Small, ovoid brownish-yellow papules (Fig. 20.22) develop on the body. They may be quite sparse (Fig. 20.23) or coalesce into large plaques. The lesions may become scaly and purpuric, and frequently become eroded especially at flexural sites. They occur anywhere on the skin, including the palms and soles, but especially on the trunk. Bony involvement may lead to purulent otitis media and

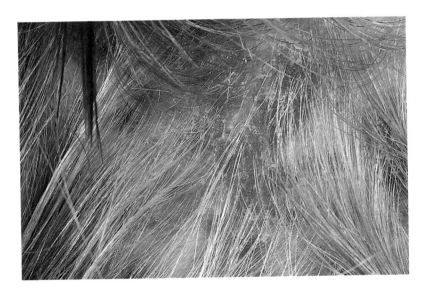

Fig. 20.20 *Langerhans cell histiocytosis.* The yellow-brown papules are discreet and well defined in this 1-year-old, who is also depicted in Figs 20.22 and 20.23.

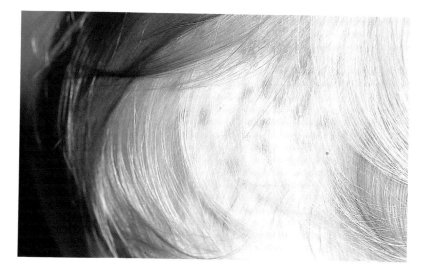

Fig. 20.21 *Langerhans cell histiocytosis.* In infants, the scalp is most frequently involved with small crusted papules with a haemorrhagic base, which are easily mistaken for seborrhoeic dermatitis.

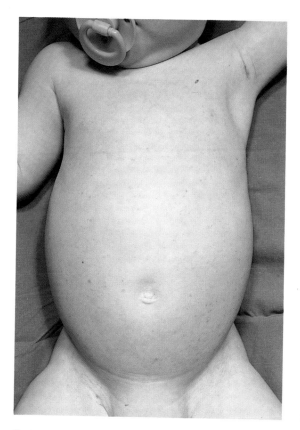

Fig. 20.22 *Langerhans cell histiocytosis.* Small, brown-yellow, ovoid papules are present. The diagnosis can be confirmed quite simply by a skin biopsy and histopathology.

Fig. 20.23 *Langerhans cell histiocytosis.* The trunk is particularly affected, but also the napkin area. The lesions may be quite sparsely distributed and the diagnosis subtle.

involvement of the alveolar margin with loss of teeth. Other possible features of the syndrome include hepatomegaly, splenomegaly, diabetes insipidus, lymphadenopathy and bone-marrow involvement.

DIFFERENTIAL DIAGNOSES

1 Seborrhoeic dermatitis: involvement of the scalp may appear quite similar, but is rarely as oozy and there is no purpura.
2 Disseminated juvenile xanthogranuloma: these are usually larger and more yellow (Fig. 20.24) than the papules of LCH, but the definitive diagnosis may be established histologically.
3 Benign cephalic histiocytosis: although the clinical lesions are quite similar, the infiltrate is S100-negative immunohistochemically, unlike skin biopsies from LCH which are S100-positive.
4 Xanthoma disseminatum: a rare disorder, more prevalent in boys, in which there is a proliferation of foamy histiocytes with secondary lipid deposition affecting the skin, eyes, upper respiratory tract and meninges.

MANAGEMENT

1 Confirmation of the diagnosis requires skin biopsy for routine histopathology, immunohistochemistry (Langerhans cells are S100-positive) and for the identification of Birbeck granules by electron microscopy.
2 A full and detailed assessment of the extent of involvement should include a full blood count, liver function tests, urinary osmolarity, chest X-ray and skeletal survey.
3 Treatment depends on the severity and extent of the disease. In contrast with the previous practice of aggressive chemotherapy, it has now been shown that many patients with single-system disease require no specific treatment. If treatment is required, the cutaneous lesions respond to topical nitrogen mustard or the combination of psoralens and ultraviolet A (PUVA) therapy. Multisystem disease is usually treated initially with oral prednisolone, but more aggressive treatment with chemotherapy (e.g. etopiside) may occasionally be required.

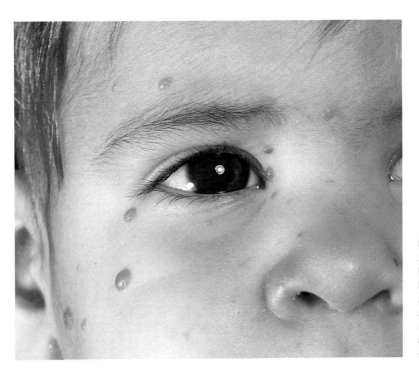

Fig. 20.24 *Disseminated juvenile xanthogranuloma.* The papules are larger and more yellow than those of histiocytosis. The histology shows an admixture of lymphocytes, xanthoma and giant cells, as opposed to the more uniform infiltration of histiocytes with eosinophilic cytoplasms and irregular vesicular nuclei seen in histiocytosis.

Mastocytosis

DEFINITION

A proliferation of mast cells most often confined to the skin, in which disseminated pigmented cutaneous macules and papules occur, which urticate on rubbing.

AETIOLOGY

The disorder is believed to be a reactive proliferation of mast cells mediated through cytokines, but the exact aetiology is unknown. A small percentage of cases of mastocytosis are malignant and follow an aggressive course.

CLINICAL FEATURES

Urticaria pigmentosa is the most common variant of mastocytosis. Over half the cases begin before the age of 2 years and in 90% involvement is confined to the skin. Small discrete, monomorphic pigmented

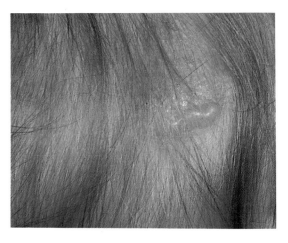

Fig. 20.26 *Urticaria pigmentosa.* The lesions may blister with trauma.

papules occur in a widely disseminated fashion on the body (Fig. 20.25). Rubbing a lesion produces piloerection, erythema and urtication (Darier's sign) due to local histamine release (Fig. 20.25). The lesions are usually intensely pruritic and may even

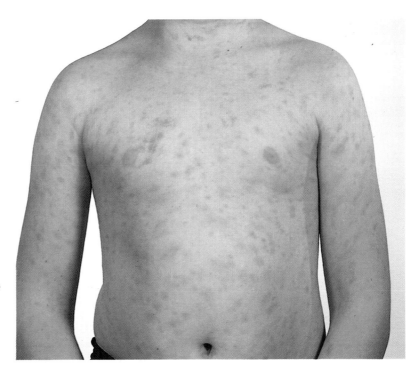

Fig. 20.25 *Urticaria pigmentosa.* Discrete monomorphic red-brown papules are widely distributed over the body. Urtication is visible over this boy's right breast. The condition usually presents before the age of 2 years, and most cases are confined to the skin.

become bullous on rubbing (Fig. 20.26). The pruritus may subside with time and blistering usually disappears spontaneously after a few years.

Variants of mastocytosis

1 Telangiectasia macularis eruptiva perstans: numerous telangiectatic macules occur with little pigmentation and no whealing. It is more usually seen in adults.
2 Diffuse cutaneous mastocytosis: widespread yellowish plaques produce a diffuse, leathery thickening of the skin (Figs 20.27 and 20.28). It is

rare, but is associated with intense pruritus and blistering. There is a higher incidence of systemic involvement, especially hepatosplenomegaly in this type of mastocytosis.
3 Solitary mastocytoma (see p. 140): a localized naevoid collection of mast cells, which urticates when rubbed (Fig. 20.29).
4 Systemic mastocytosis accounts for 10% of all cases of mastocytosis, but not all patients will have evidence of skin involvement. Instead, hepatic, bony and haematological involvement are most common. A small number of patients may subsequently develop a malignant proliferation of mast cells.

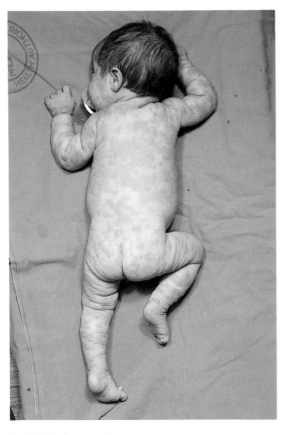

Fig. 20.27 *Disseminated cutaneous mastocytosis.* Extensive reddish-brown nodules were evident at birth. They urticate with minimal trauma and the child is restless due to the itch.

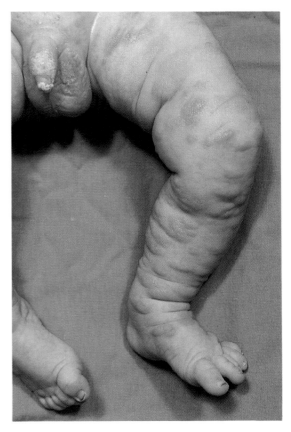

Fig. 20.28 *Disseminated cutaneous mastocytosis.* The affected skin is thickened and pigmented.

MANAGEMENT

1 The diagnosis is usually clinical, but confirmed by demonstrating increasing numbers of mast cells in a skin biopsy, stained with toluidine blue.

2 Localized disease usually requires no treatment.

3 Antihistamines may provide some symptomatic relief.

4 Superpotent topical steroids applied in a rotational manner to different areas of involvement can provide fairly long-lasting relief.

5 Extensive disease often responds very well to PUVA, but this needs to be used cautiously in younger patients, because of the long-term risk of carcinogenesis.

6 If there is any question of systemic involvement, assessment by a paediatric haematologist should be arranged.

7 Childhood urticaria pigmentosa usually regresses spontaneously after a few years.

Mycosis fungoides

DEFINITION

A disorder of T-helper lymphocytes which infiltrate

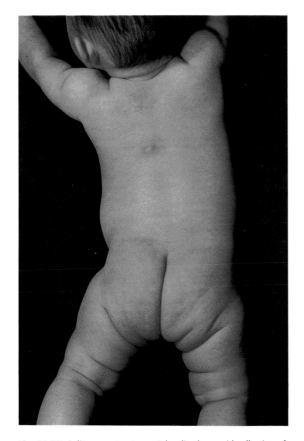

Fig. 20.29 *Solitary mastocytoma.* A localized naevoid collection of mast cells which resolves spontaneously. It presents as a single, or occasionally multiple, plaque or nodule which urticates when rubbed.

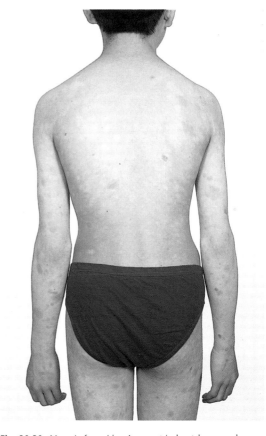

Fig. 20.30 *Mycosis fungoides.* Asymmetrical patches, papules and plaques of varying red, some with odd angulated shapes, are scattered over the skin. Some areas are hypopigmented.

the skin and occasionally lymph nodes and other viscera.

There is disagreement as to whether this is a primary T-cell malignancy or more likely, given the very slow progression of the disorder, a reactive process possibly due to chronic stimulation of an as yet unidentified allergen leading very occasionally to malignant transformation.

CLINICAL FEATURES

The condition quite frequently begins in childhood or adolescence as asymmetrical macules or patches on the trunk (especially buttocks) and limbs (Fig. 20.30). It is usually misdiagnosed as eczema for many years, but a well-defined, often angulated outline to some of the lesions with central atrophy may help make the distinction. If the condition progresses, the patches thicken becoming palpable plaques. Tumours and lymphadenopathy are extremely rare before adult life.

MANAGEMENT

A biopsy is required to establish the diagnosis. The cutaneous changes can be controlled by photochemotherapy (PUVA) or tropical nitrogen mustard.

Endocrine disorders

Cushing's disease and syndrome

DEFINITION

An endocrine disorder with multisystem involvement due to excessive production (or intake) of glucocorticoids.

AETIOLOGY

Cushing originally described the disease in association with a pituitary adenoma. If the disease is adrenal, ectopic or exogenous in origin it is known as Cushing's syndrome.

CLINICAL FEATURES

The patient appears obese with markedly round and plethoric facies. Purplish striae are prominent and extensive (Fig. 20.31). Hirsuitism is common and acne may develop. In pituitary-dependent disease, there may be widespread pigmentation due to the associated overproduction of melanocyte-stimulating hormone. Associated features include hypertension, glucose intolerance, gastric ulceration, immunosuppression and osteoporosis.

DIFFERENTIAL DIAGNOSES

1 Growth striae: horizontal striae are a common finding across the lower back (Fig. 20.32) in adolescent boys following a growth spurt. They are physiological and their localization points to the

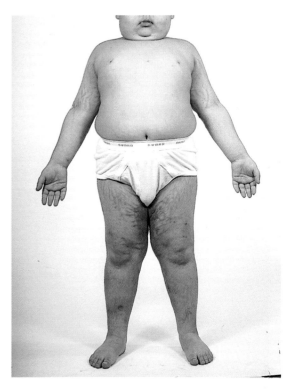

Fig. 20.31 *Cushing's syndrome.* This 7-year-old is small and obese, has a round plethoric facies and gross purple striae due to overtreatment with systemic glucocorticosteriods.

correct diagnosis. Milder striae may be seen on the upper, inner arms and thighs in obese adolescents, particularly black females.

2 Iatrogenic striae: excessive use of potent topical steroids may result in local atrophy and damage to the collagen with striae formation (Fig. 20.33), without evidence of systemic involvement as in Cushing's syndrome.

MANAGEMENT

1 The diagnosis is confirmed by the finding of a raised serum cortisol and loss of the normal diurnal fluctuation in cortisol production. The dexamethasone suppression test will determine whether the disease is pituitary or adrenal in origin, but the patient should be referred to an endocrinologist for further detailed assessment and appropriate treatment.

2 If exogenous steroids are the suspected cause, there will be evidence of adrenal suppression. The steroids should be stopped, but may need to be weaned down slowly to prevent an adrenal crisis developing.

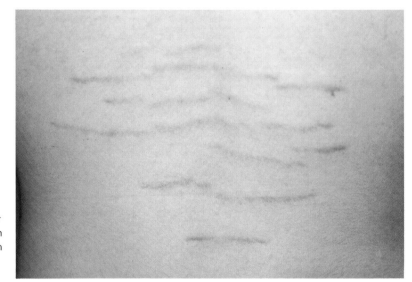

Fig. 20.32 *Physiological striae.* Linear purple stretch marks are quite common across the lower back in adolescence in association with a marked growth spurt.

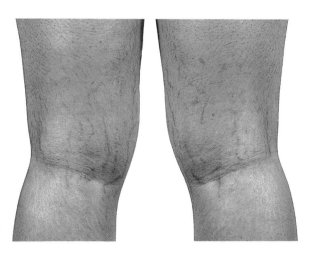

Fig. 20.33 *Topical steroid-induced striae.* Misuse of topical steroids for the wrong condition or overuse for the right one results in atrophy and striae of the skin.

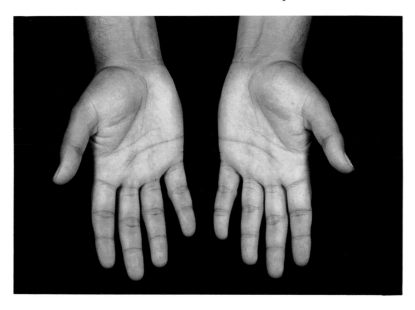

Fig. 20.34 *Addison's disease.* Increasing pigmentation slowly occurs all over the skin, shown here at the wrists with specific involvement of the palmar creases (courtesy of Professor A. McGregor).

Addison's disease

DEFINITION

Adrenal insufficiency with low circulating levels of cortisol and mineralocorticoids.

AETIOLOGY

The disease is usually auto-immune in the young, but it may follow any destructive disease of the adrenals (e.g. tuberculosis) or be secondary to pituitary dysfunction. Iatrogenic hypocorticism occurs as a result of abrupt withdrawal of corticosteroid therapy.

CLINICAL FEATURES

The cutaneous hallmarks of the primary syndrome are those of a gradual darkening of the skin visible as a diffuse generalized hyperpigmentation with particular involvement of the buccal mucosa and palmar creases (Fig. 20.34). Scars may become hyperpigmented and the hair may darken. The patient complains of dizziness and fatigue, loses weight, is weak and hypotensive. There is often severe electrolyte imbalance.

DIFFERENTIAL DIAGNOSIS

The presence of pigmentation differentiates primary adrenal disease (in which the loss of negative feedback results in increased melanocyte-stimulating hormone production) from pituitary disease, hypopituitarism, in which pallor is common.

MANAGEMENT

1 The diagnosis is confirmed by the demonstration of a low serum cortisol. The results of a synacthen stimulation test will establish if the disease is adrenal or pituitary in origin.
2 Intravenous fluid replacement and careful attention to fluid balance are imperative acutely.
3 Steroid replacement therapy may be required long term, but should be supervised by an endocrinologist.

Diabetes mellitus

Generalized pruritus, and superficial cutaneous infections such as candidosis and very rarely furunculosis may accompany diabetes mellitus. However, the most common abnormality positively associated with the disorder is necrobiosis lipoidica. The association with granuloma annulare is more tenuous.

Necrobiosis lipoidica diabeticorum

DEFINITION

A condition associated with diabetes mellitus in which collagen degeneration results in waxy plaques, usually on the shins.

AETIOLOGY

The majority of patients with necrobiosis lipoidica have diabetes mellitus, but skin disease may precede the glucose intolerance. In a small number of patients, the skin changes seem to occur in isolation, without any subsequent evidence of diabetes. It is thought that the vascular insufficiency as a result of micro-angiopathy in diabetics is responsible for the collagen degeneration.

CLINICAL FEATURES

Waxy, yellow, atrophic and telangiectatic plaques develop on the lower legs (Fig. 20.35). Any site may be affected, but the disorder is most common in the pretibial region. The plaques usually have a characteristic erythematous border. The disease is most frequently seen in teenagers and young adults, with the majority of cases occurring in females. Ulceration may complicate the lesions and is very slow to heal.

MANAGEMENT

1 Glucose intolerance should be excluded in patients without an established diagnosis of diabetes.
2 Topical or intralesional steroids may produce some improvement, but atrophy usually persists. The disorder is unsightly, but may well be best left alone.

Granuloma annulare

DEFINITION

A localized inflammatory process of unknown aetiology producing focal destruction of dermal collagen.

AETIOLOGY

The cause of the disorder is unknown, but there is considerable overlap with necrobiosis lipoidica (see above). About 5% of patients with granuloma annulare have glucose intolerance.

CLINICAL FEATURES

The disease may occur at any age, but predominantly affects children and adolescents and is more common in girls than boys.

Most cases are localized and consist of a ring of flesh-coloured or red, firm dermal papules producing a

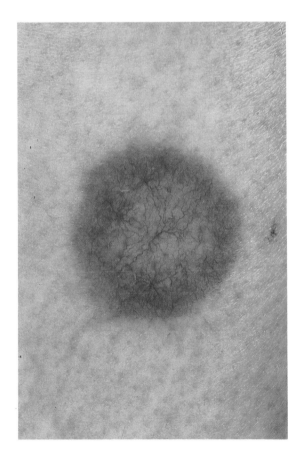

Fig. 20.35 *Necrobiosis lipoidica.* The lesion is a yellow waxy plaque with overlying telangiectasia occurring particularly over the front of the shins.

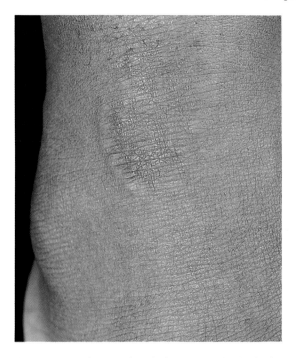

Fig. 20.36 *Granuloma annulare.* The lesion is round with a border which consists of flat-topped papules producing a beaded appearance. The ankle is a common site.

plaque a few centimetres in diameter with a beaded border (Fig. 20.36). The plaque may be slightly erythematous and slowly extends outwards in an annular fashion. Lesions may be single or multiple and are most frequent over the dorsal aspects of the hands (Fig. 20.37) and feet. Rarely, granuloma annulare may become disseminated. The lesions are usually self-limiting and eventually resolve spontaneously within a few months. However, recurrence is common in up to 40% of patients.

MANAGEMENT

1 The diagnosis is usually clinical, but may be confirmed by characteristic histology on biopsy. Sometimes the stimulus of surgical incison may induce remission.
2 Superpotent topical steroids or intralesional triamcinolone may accelerate resolution.
3 Often no treatment is required as spontaneous resolution is the norm.

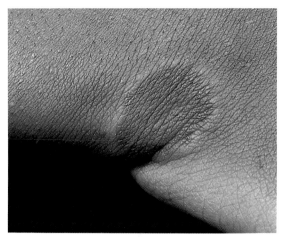

Fig. 20.37 *Granuloma annulare.* The raised margin of flesh-coloured papules is clear, surrounding an area of hyperpigmented skin in this Asian child. The wrist is often involved.

Acanthosis nigricans

DEFINITION

An epidermal disorder resulting in hyperkeratosis and pigmentation of the skin in flexural areas associated with insulin resistance.

AETIOLOGY

There are five types of acanthosis nigricans. The malignant type is very rare and usually occurs in adult life. The commonest (pseudo-acanthosis nigricans) is associated with obesity which probably causes insulin resistance. It is seen in dark-coloured skins and is reversible. There is a hereditary dominant type not associated with endocrinopathy and a drug-induced variety (e.g. due to stilboestrol, oral contraceptives and nicotinic acid). Benign acanthosis nigricans occurs in association with many endocrine disorders, including hyperandrogenism in females.

CLINICAL FEATURES

There is a velvety thickening and pigmentation in the flexural areas (Fig. 20.38), a drug-induced variety (e.g. due to stilboestrol, especially the axillae, neck and groin.

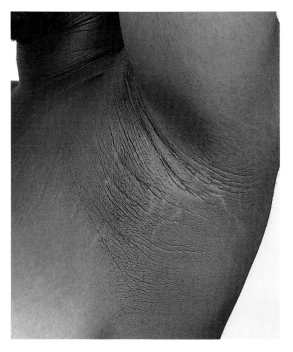

Fig. 20.38 *Acanthosis nigricans.* The skin is pigmented, thickened and velvety to touch in flexural areas, such as the axillae. This 14-year-old also had hirsutism and hyperandrogenism.

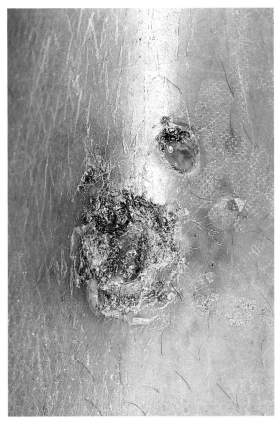

Fig. 20.39 *Pyoderma gangrenosum.* The lesions begin as red pustules or nodules which break down to produce necrotic ulcers, often with overhanging violaceous edges. The lower legs are common sites.

MANAGEMENT

Most cases are confined to the skin, but endocrine causes should be looked for and malignant cases may have mucous membrane involvement.

Miscellaneous

Pyoderma gangrenosum

DEFINITION

A rapidly progressive, non-infective, necrotizing ulceration of the skin.

AETIOLOGY

The disease is reactive in origin and may be precipitated by trauma. There is some evidence for it representing an abnormal immune response. In young patients the majority of cases are associated with inflammatory bowel disease, but it may also rarely complicate a haematological malignancy or immune defect, e.g. congenital hypogammaglobulinaemia. A severe bullous form of the disorder may occur in patients with haematological malignancies.

CLINICAL FEATURES

The lesion usually begins as a small red nodule which becomes pustular and then rapidly breaks down to produce a large necrotic ulcer with a violaceous, often overhanging, edge. Any area may be involved, including the face, but the lesions are most commonly seen on the lower leg (Fig. 20.39). There is no accompanying lymphadenopathy, but the patient may be febrile with arthralgia during the acute stages. The histopathological features are often non-specific.

DIFFERENTIAL DIAGNOSES

1 Infections causing localized gangrene, such as *Cryptococcus* and blastomycosis should be considered, but can be excluded by skin biopsy for histopathology and appropriate culture.
2 Behçet's disease: this may appear quite similar and there is considerable clinical overlap between the two diseases.

MANAGEMENT

1 Once infection has been excluded by aerobic and anaerobic culture, treatment with high-dose steroids should be instituted and usually produces a rapid response, with settling of any systemic upset particularly fever within 24 hours. Dapsone may be more effective than prednisolone in childhood cases.
2 Cyclosporin has been found to be effective in steroid-resistant cases and low-dose minocycline may be useful in subacute cases in older individuals.
3 Investigations should be directed towards finding an underlying cause, particularly inflammatory bowel disease, which should be treated appropriately.

Chapter 21
Psychological Disorders

Introduction

There is considerable overlap between psychological disorders and the skin. They may be classified in any one of the following ways:

1 Reactive disorders: certain disfiguring skin diseases, such as birthmarks or acne, may understandably present a patient with psychological difficulties.

2 Inappropriate reactions: some patients may be convinced that they have a skin problem, despite the absence of objective physical signs; a state known as *dysmorphophobia*. Alternatively they may become obsessed with minor imperfections which may prevent their going out, socializing or leading a normal life. This preoccupation with the skin often complicates cases of acne, and in some instances the patient may continue to perceive that there is a problem with the skin, long after the physical condition has been treated. Somatization, (anxiety, neurosis or depression manifest as a physical complaint or symptom) may occur particularly with facial and genital conditions, and are usually due to anxiety, depression or anorexia nervosa.

3 Psychological disorders: in other cases patients may do something to the skin, hair or nails as a result of a psychological problem or having had something inflicted on them (non-accidental injury or sexual abuse) which results in a cutaneous evidence of the abuse.

This chapter will concentrate on the types of psychological problems outlined in 2 and 3 above.

Habit tics

DEFINITION

A repetitive subconscious action from which the patient derives comfort, but which results in localized damage to the skin or associated structures.

AETIOLOGY

Mild habit tics are common in children, particularly during the first decade, and rarely represent significant psychological disturbance. They usually resolve spontaneously after a period of months or years, but if they persist into adulthood may signify deeper emotional problems.

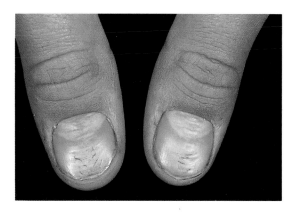

Fig. 21.1 *Habit tic.* Repeated running of the index finger-nail along the thumb-nail and damaging of the cuticle produces a linear groove along the affected nails.

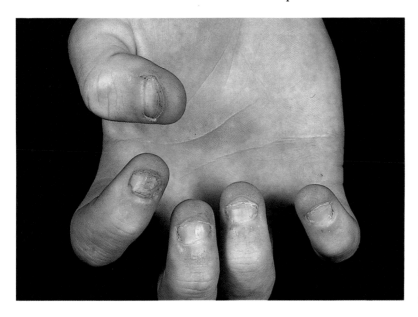

Fig. 21.2 *Onychophagia.* Nail-biting is a common form of habit tic representing a minor neurosis of no great significance.

CLINICAL FEATURES

Habit tics may take many forms from an area of lichen simplex, produced by repeated scratching, to a more persistent picker's nodule. Other common forms include localized hair pulling (e.g. of eyebrows or eyelashes), lip-licking, picking of the nails (Fig. 21.1) and nail-biting (Fig. 21.2).

MANAGEMENT

1 Reassurance to all concerned that this is usually only a stage and that the child is likely to grow out of the habit. Parents sometimes need some convincing to understand that the problem is produced by a habit tic and does not imply any serious underlying skin disease.
2 If necessary (and practical) the affected area can be occluded to allow healing.

Trichotillomania

DEFINITION

Localized areas of hair loss resulting from an irresistable urge to pull the hair, with consequent breakage of the hair shaft.

AETIOLOGY

Mild forms of the disorder are a not uncommon finding in younger children as a habit tic associated with boredom (e.g. eyelash pulling). Occasionally, trichotillomania may be preceded by true alopecia areata, which appears to draw attention to that area of the scalp in younger children, who then start pulling the remaining hair. More extensive disease is usually seen in adolescents as a sign of severe emotional disturbance, and there is a high incidence of subsequent eating disorders in these patients.

CLINICAL FEATURES

The condition may be seen at any age, but particularly during the early teenage years, when it is more common in girls. A large patch of hair loss becomes apparent. Multiple short, stubbly broken hairs are seen in affected areas. The pattern of involvement is often striking, with preservation of a border of normal hair, especially around the occiput (Fig. 21.3). Trichotillomania may coexist with evidence of other nervous habits, e.g. nail-biting, which distinguishes the condition from other causes of alopecia.

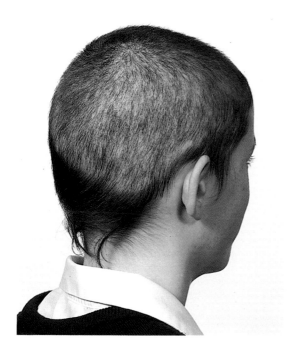

Fig. 21.3 *Trichotillomania.* Multiple, short, broken hairs occur in a well-delineated area on one side of the scalp due to the child's interference with it.

MANAGEMENT

1 This is a delicate problem, since there is often reluctance on the part of the family to accept that the condition is self-inflicted.
2 If the hair-pulling is mild and an isolated finding, resolution may be achieved by the application of bland emollients to 'treat and protect the hair', although it usually resolves on its own with time.
3 More significant disease usually requires some form of behavioural therapy. The cause of the emotional disturbance (unhappiness at school, domestic difficulties, parental divorce, child abuse) should be sought sensitively. The child's confidence needs to be built up gradually over several visits to allow the patient to open up. The assistance of a child psychologist can be most helpful in this respect.
4 Severely disturbed teenagers need specialist treatment from a child psychiatrist.

Acne excoriée des jeunes filles

DEFINITION

A condition seen in older girls which is often stress-related, in which widespread excoriations develop on the forehead and chin.

AETIOLOGY

Although there may be a history of mild acne, the primary abnormality is the patient's inability to leave the skin alone. Constant picking at the skin results in the clinical picture of superficial erosions. There are almost always significant emotional factors in the patient's life and the condition may be regarded as an abnormal stress response.

CLINICAL FEATURES

The condition is seen in females in their teenage years and twenties. Multiple, shallow erosions are evident on the cheeks, chin (Fig. 21.4) and to a lesser extent on the forehead. Usually the eruption is confined to the face, and although the patient constantly refers to 'acne', and may originally have had mild acne, there is often no clinical evidence of true acne.

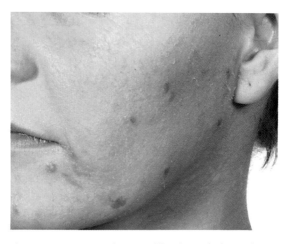

Fig. 21.4 *Acne excoriée des jeunes filles.* This results from picking at the skin of the face. There may be no actual acne to be seen.

MANAGEMENT

1 Getting to the root of the emotional problem is a difficult and delicate matter and may have to be explored over several visits to establish a rapport and build up the patient's confidence in the doctor.

2 The individual usually accepts that the lesions are induced/exacerbated by scratching and sometimes clears, but more often than not the condition is chronic.

3 Complex cleansing routines which necessitate long periods in front of a mirror should be discouraged as this tends to allow the patient to focus on their skin.

Dermatitis artefacta

DEFINITION

Self-inflicted, bizarre, chronic cutaneous lesions occurring as a result of severe psychological disturbance.

AETIOLOGY

The skin lesions are the manifestation of underlying emotional and psychological problems and will not improve until the primary problem is addressed.

CLINICAL FEATURES

The disorder is relatively uncommon, but is usually seen in adolescence, particularly in girls. Minor self-inflicted injuries are not uncommon in adolescence (Fig. 21.5) and are often only a transient problem. In contrast, older patients are often severely disturbed, with chronic disease and a poor prognosis. The clue to the diagnosis is the atypical nature of the skin lesions, which are often geometric in shape (Fig. 21.6), exoriated (Fig. 21.7) and do not fit into any recognized patterns of cutaneous disease (Fig. 21.8). Dermatitis artefacta may take many forms, but chronic ulceration is the commonest. The patient is usually extremely manipulative and very devious in managing to perpetuate the skin lesions in secret. Evidence of scarring from previous lesions is frequently seen.

MANAGEMENT

1 Occluding the area under bandaging (or in severe cases of unexplained ulceration of the limbs, a plaster-of-Paris cast) leads to rapid resolution.

2 The problem may be short lived in some teenagers if it is a simple attention-seeking response to some acute stress, e.g. examinations or a new sibling.

3 In more chronic cases, confronting the patient directly can precipitate a suicidal crisis. Management is aimed at slowly building up trust between the patient and the physician to enable gentle exploration of the full social and emotional circumstances. Specialist adolescent psychiatrists should gradually be introduced to enable a full psychiatric assessment and appropriate therapy.

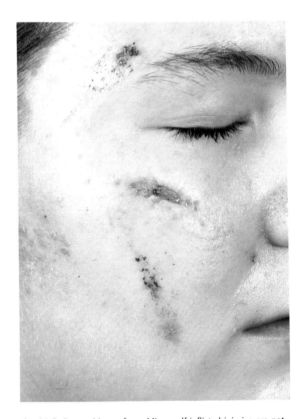

Fig. 21.5 *Dermatitis artefacta.* Minor self-inflicted injuries are not uncommon in adolescence and are often transient, as in this teenager who was having difficulties at school.

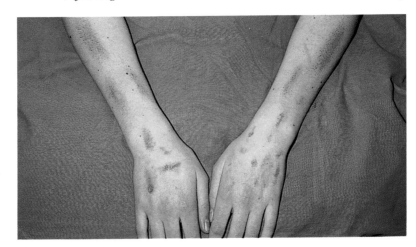

Fig. 21.6 *Dermatitis artefacta.* Linear or geometric shapes which do not conform to a known disease pattern may suggest the diagnosis.

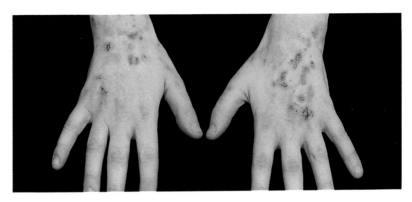

Fig. 21.7 *Dermatitis artefacta.* Excoriations predominate over the backs of the hands. They were also present on her face. They represent a *cri de coeur.*

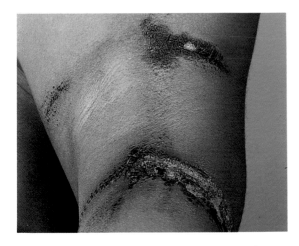

Fig. 21.8 *Dermatitis artefacta.* These bizarre linear areas of ulceration, pigmentation and scarring suggested the application of an external agent such as a ligature.

Non-accidental injury

DEFINITION

Deliberate harm inflicted upon a child by a third party.

AETIOLOGY

Non-accidental injury was first recognized over 20 years ago and has since been the subject of extensive research. It has been described in all social classes. Injury may be in the form of emotional deprivation or physical trauma such as shaking, blows (Fig. 21.11), burns (Fig. 21.12) or sexual abuse (Fig. 21.9). Although the perpetrator is usually a parent or step-parent, non-accidental injury may be inflicted by anyone in close contact with the child, including carers.

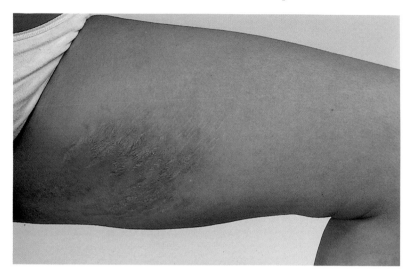

Fig. 21.9 *Sexual abuse.* This adolescent was abused by her grandfather. She complained to her doctor of genital irritation and was prescribed topical steroids. This resulted in striae, but there were no other signs. Finally a proper history revealed in the correct diagnosis.

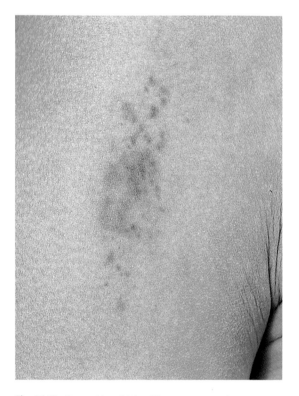

Fig. 21.10 *Non-accidental injury.* There was no satisfactory or plausible explanation for this area of purpura and bruising on the child's upper arm. An identical lesion was present on the other arm and the lesion almost certainly had resulted from undue pressure while shaking the child.

CLINICAL FEATURES

Children of any age may be subject to non-accidental injury, but infants are especially vulnerable. Suspicion that an injury may be non-accidental is aroused when the physical signs are either ignored or concealed or when there is a delay in presentation. The explanation given for the injury is often implausible, and fails adequately to account for the clinical findings. Non-accidental injury is usually a chronic process, so that there is often evidence of several old injuries (e.g. bruising, scars) as well as the current problem and X-rays may reveal evidence of old fractures. Non-accidental injury usually presents to the casualty department or paediatrics, but may be seen by dermatologists in the form of purpura, bruising (Fig. 21.10), cutaneous ulcers or unexplained scarring.

DIFFERENTIAL DIAGNOSES

1 *True accidents*: children frequently have genuine accidents, but multiple injuries in different stages of healing should always arouse suspicion.
2 *Mongolian blue spots*: these have been mistaken for bruising in neonates.
3 *Lichen sclerosus et atrophicus* of the genitalia (p. 234): in young girls this may be confused with sexual abuse by non-dermatologists.

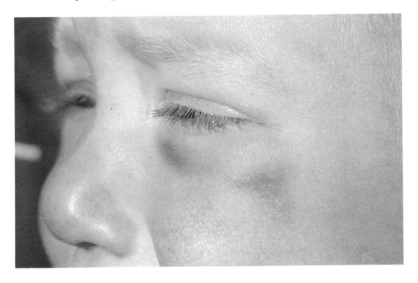

Fig. 21.11 *Non-accidental injury.* There is extensive bruising around the eyes (courtesy of Dr Black).

4 *Cupping*: cultural medicinal practices may leave bizarre pigmentary marks on the trunk.

5 *Munchausen's syndrome by proxy*: this is a more complicated form of psychological illness. Patients may mimic symptoms and signs of disease for personal gain (Munchausen's disease), often in a very convincing manner. In Munchausen's syndrome by proxy, the psychological problems of the parent are manifest by inducing/perpetuating signs of disease in their child. Unlike non-accidental injury, these parents seek early and repeated medical attention, and express great concern over the child's 'disease'.

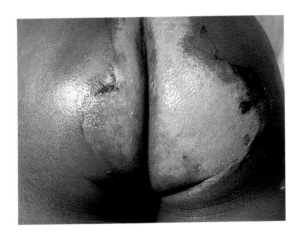

Fig. 21.12 *Non-accidental injury.* These burns arose as a result of dipping the child in a scalding bath.

MANAGEMENT

1 When a child is considered to be the subject of non-accidental injury, they should be placed on the at-risk register immediately.

2 The social services department should be informed and there should be close liaison between the social worker, family doctor, paediatrician and, if necessary, the police to monitor the family circumstances and child's welfare. If the child is considered to be in imminent danger, it may be necessary to remove the child into care.

Appendix
Guidelines for the
Use of Topical Steroids
in Children

It should always be remembered that young children, especially babies, have a relatively large surface area to volume ratio, and therefore absorb topical medicines more easily. Care should be taken in the administration of all forms of topical therapy in this age group, but especially in the use of topical steroids (Table A1). None the less, used judiciously and appropriately, they are invaluable agents in the treatment of inflammatory dermatoses. Table A2 shows the classification of topical steroids.

There is a discrepancy between the UK and the USA in the numbering of steroid classes. In the UK, there are four classes, where Class I is the most potent. In the USA there are seven classes where Class 1 is the most potent and Class 7 the weakest. In view of this, we have elected to categorize them as mild, moderate, potent and super-potent. Ointment formulations are usually preferred to creams because the latter contain preservatives which may act as contact sensitizers.

Table A1 Guidelines in prescribing requirements for BD application of a topical steroid for 2 weeks in children of different ages (weights shown in grams)*

Body site to be treated	6 months	1 year	4 years	8 years	12 years	16 years
Trunk (ant and post)	30	30	40	70	90	110
Arms and legs	40	50	70	100	130	170
Whole body	70	90	120	180	240	310

* Adapted from Maurice P.D.L. and Saihan E.M. *Br J Clin Prac* 1985;39:441–2.

Table A2 Classification of topical steroids

UK	Class	USA
IV	Mild	7
III	Moderate	4–6
II	Potent	2–3
I	Super-potent	1

Index

Page references in **bold** refer to figures, or where text and figures occur on the same page.